DYNAMICS of Fitness

fourth edition

A PRACTICAL APPROACH

George McGlynn
University of San Francisco

Brown & Benchmark
PUBLISHERS

Madison   Dubuque, IA   Guilford, CT   Chicago   Toronto   London
Caracas   Mexico City   Buenos Aires   Madrid   Bogota   Sydney

Book Team

Publisher *Bevan O'Callaghan*
Project Editor *Scott Spoolman*
Developmental Editor *Megan Rundel*
Production Editor *Terry Routley*
Proofreading Coordinator *Carrie Barker*
Art Editor *Miriam Hoffman*
Production Manager *Beth Kundert*
Production/Costing Manager *Sherry Padden*
Visuals/Design Freelance Specialist *Mary L. Christianson*
Marketing Manager *Pamela S. Cooper*
Copywriter *M. J. Kelly*

Basal Text *10/12 Times Roman*
Display Type *Times Roman*
Typesetting System *Aviion*
Paper Stock *50# Mirror Matte*

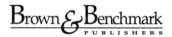

President and Chief Executive Officer *Thomas E. Doran*
Vice President of Production and Business Development *Vickie Putman*
Vice President of Sales and Marketing *Bob McLaughlin*
Director of Marketing *John Finn*

A Times Mirror Company

Cover design by Kay Fulton Design

Interior display designs by Kay Fulton Design

Cover image by © David Madison/Tony Stone Images

Copyedited by Anne Scroggin; Proofread by Barb Callahan

Library of Congress Catalog Card Number: 94–73463

ISBN 0–697–24651–5

Printed in the United States of America by Times Mirror Higher Education Group, Inc.,
2460 Kerper Boulevard, Dubuque, IA 52001

10   9   8   7   6   5   4   3   2   1

To my wife, Ingeborg, and my son, George

Contents

v

3

Chapter

Coronary Heart Disease and Exercise 25

4

Chapter

Fitness Evaluation 43

5

Chapter

Warm-Up and Flexibility 79

6

Chapter

Cardiorespiratory Endurance 99

7

Chapter

Starting Your Cardiorespiratory Endurance Program 121

8

Chapter

Muscle Strength and Endurance 135

9

Chapter

Nutrition 167

10
Chapter

Weight Control 207

11
Chapter

Drugs 227

12
Chapter

Exercise and Stress Reduction 241

13
Chapter

Other Risks to Health and Fitness 263

14

C h a p t e r

Special Considerations 277

Preface

Since the completion of the third edition, changes have continued to take place in the exercise and fitness habits of the American people. In addition, there have been a number of advances and refinements in the areas of exercise physiology, sports medicine, and nutrition. Physical health and nutrition have maintained a place of high priority in everyday living. Millions of individuals continue to be actively engaged in marathon running, jogging, tennis, weight programs, and a variety of other rigorous activities such as biathlons, triathlons, mountain biking, step aerobics, and water aerobics.

As in the earlier editions, the purpose of the present edition is to keep pace with these changes and provide a simple, logical, and individualized approach to developing and maintaining a high level of health and physical fitness. The text is intended as a practical guide for understanding and evaluating your wellness and exercise needs and developing a fitness program. The information presented here represents a consensus of presently available scientific evidence in the areas of exercise physiology and health. The text is intended primarily for college physical-fitness classes, such as aerobic conditioning, interval and circuit training, wellness and fitness, and weight reduction classes, but also it can be used for health-and-fitness-club exercise programs.

The previous edition emphasized the relationship between physical fitness and wellness in order to develop a greater awareness of one's maximum potential. In that context, wellness was presented as a comprehensive process related to your purpose in life and your responsibility to live life to its fullest. The third edition also expanded on the importance of nutritional assessment, behavior modification, eating disorders, diet guidelines, exercise during pregnancy, anabolic steroids, and stress.

The fourth edition has extended and refined many of these same areas. The chapter on heart disease has been expanded and updated including the American Heart Association's new Risk Assessment Questionnaire and risk factors. Also new information has been added on cholesterol levels. The chapter on evaluation has been revised to include new information on the Modified Sit-and-Reach Test, Girth Test, Head-and-Shoulder Raise Test, and a new table for the Walking Test. The chapter on warm-up and flexibility has been updated with information on excess flexibility, contraindicated exercises, new photos, and identification of appropriate muscles involved in stretching. The chapter on cardiorespiratory endurance now includes the revised rPAR-Q test for preexercise screening and additional information concerning those individuals who may be at risk during rigorous exercise. The chapter on starting your cardiorespiratory endurance program now includes information on water running, bench stepping, stationary bicycles, stair climbers, and treadmills. A diagram of skeletal muscles and of the individual muscle cell has been added to the chapter on muscle strength and endurance. The chapter on nutrition has received a major revision including new information on food labels, a diet evaluation quiz, beta carotenes, carbohydrate loading, antioxidants, and a new cholesterol table.

A great deal of knowledge is presently available concerning training and conditioning techniques, heart disease and exercise, and muscle physiology and nutrition. Unfortunately, it is very difficult for the layperson to sift through thousands of research papers and academic volumes on sports physiology, let alone the popular media, to find reliable answers to questions concerning fitness, exercise, and nutrition. My own experience as a researcher and professor of exercise physiology for over thirty-six years has supported my belief that it is important to provide information in a manner that is relevant, reliable, and understandable in order to rebut the misconceptions and confusion surrounding fitness and exercise. Ignorance about problems concerning exercise may not only result in wasted effort or temporary injury, but in some cases, it may lead to serious long-term health consequences. I am still appalled at the health-spa, diet-book mentality that dominates the popular media and contributes to ignorance in fitness and exercise.

A major concern of this text is to make you aware of your present level of fitness and how that can affect you the rest of your life. A sequence of simple tests enables you to analyze your present level of fitness and to compare it to established norms for your age and sex. After helping you to evaluate your present fitness, the text provides varying intensity levels of exercise that can be adapted to your individual needs, for short- or long-range fitness goals dealing with cardiorespiratory endurance, muscle strength and endurance, body composition, and flexibility. The text also provides record sheets and profiles for tracking your fitness-level changes.

Other chapters of the book deal with a variety of important factors associated with your health and fitness, including nutrition and weight control, common injuries, environmental exercise problems, drugs, maintaining fitness with age, females and exercise, heart disease, and stress reduction.

I hope the material in this text will increase your motivation to become actively involved in learning about fitness and in seeking a more productive and healthier life.

Acknowledgements

The following reviewers provided many valuable suggestions toward the development and preparation of this text:

Jack Benson, Eastern Washington University
Cindy J. Bross, Meredith College
Karla A. Kubitz, Kansas State University
Pamela MacFarlane, Northern Illinois University
Gary Oden, Sam Houston State University
Andrew L. Shim, Los Angeles Technical College
David J. Waters, University of Minnesota

1

chapter

Introduction

Chapter Concepts

After you have studied this chapter you should be able to

1. describe the relationship between wellness and physical fitness;
2. describe some of the common misconceptions concerning rigorous exercise;
3. describe the physiological benefits of physical exercise;
4. describe the psychological benefits of physical exercise;
5. describe the changes in fitness habits;
6. describe the changes in women's participation in physical activities;
7. define physical fitness;
8. describe health-related concepts of physical fitness;
9. describe cardiorespiratory endurance;
10. describe muscle strength and endurance;
11. describe body composition;
12. describe the difference between overweight and overfat;
13. describe flexibility; and
14. describe Healthy People 2000 Objectives.

Why This Book?

Wellness and Physical Fitness

We are all in a dynamic process of moving toward or away from behavior that is either destructive or beneficial to our health. It is therefore important for each individual to take responsibility for the direction in which he or she chooses to move. **Wellness** is a process of moving toward greater awareness of your human potential by developing a high level of physical fitness, good nutrition, positive relationships with others, and a concern about self-care and sensitivity to the environment. In this context, wellness is presented

1

as a style of living that requires self-responsibility to achieve your maximum potential. Acquiring a level of wellness requires change; it is related to your purpose in life and your determination to take control.

The emphasis on self-responsibility distinguishes wellness from the traditional medical model for health care and is the focal point of all health-related fitness programs. It is vital that the individual exert control over various factors or forces that determine where he or she is on the wellness continuum. The U. S. Department of Health and Human Services has issued specific health objectives for the nation. See table 1.1. These measurable objectives are based on an analysis of health problems in the United States and what should be done to reduce their magnitude by the year 2000. It is obvious from these objectives that there is a strong belief that proper exercise and nutrition throughout life is needed for optimum health.

The major purpose of this book is to provide a comprehensive guide to enable you to use your own innate abilities to improve all aspects of your physical and mental health so you can live life to its fullest. This book presents exercise as an integral part of your life. If you are already involved in a regular exercise program and know your way around the track and weight room, it will add to your interest by giving you new ideas and challenges. On the other hand, if you are sedentary, out of shape, self-conscious in your swimsuit, or turning into a piece of furniture in front of your television set, then this book is also for you. So, get ready for some exciting changes in your life.

It Doesn't Have to Hurt to Get in Shape

Unfortunately, many people associate physical exercise with pain, failure, and embarrassment. They view exercise as a Spartan ritual in which they must punish themselves physically to derive any benefit. Such a concept is probably a carryover from outdated high school athletic programs—in which the coach literally ran everybody into the ground in the name of ''getting in shape''—or from those grueling early morning boot camp calisthenics that all recruits endured. Also, the popular media reinforces this erroneous concept.

Certainly, when you leave the sedentary world and enter the realm of rigorous exercise, you will experience some discomforts—mild aches and pains, a slight breathing difficulty, and a feeling of fatigue. You also undoubtedly will be confronted with the morning-after symptoms of muscle soreness and fatigue. But these discomforts are usually minor and temporary and should not be of major concern. As you continue to exercise, these symptoms of beginning an exercise program will gradually disappear. Exercise should be enjoyable and relaxing, and its by-products should not be nausea and pain. In fact, if it does ''hurt'' when you exercise, this is a sign of overexercise and the need to moderate your activity.

Benefits of Regular Exercise

An increasing body of evidence suggests that physical activity and physical fitness contribute to good health. Studies[1] have shown that physical activity, be it occupational or recreational, is associated with decreased risks of coronary heart disease. Other studies[2] suggest that risks of colon cancer, stroke, and hypertension are reduced and that exercise can assist persons in managing diabetes, depression, and obesity.

The most compelling evidence to date comes from a comprehensive eight-year study of over thirteen thousand subjects.[3] This study has shown that even moderate physical fitness is associated with lower rates of cardiovascular disease and cancer mortality. Another landmark study of twelve thousand Harvard alumni showed that the death rate over eight years decreased by about 21 percent among men who had been sedentary but then became moderately active in various sports during middle age or later.

When those who regularly exercise are asked, "How have you benefited from exercise?" the answer inevitably is, "It makes me feel a lot better."

Feeling better reflects itself in a number of ways. First of all, exercise builds and maintains physical fitness. The basis for improved fitness is an increase in the work capacity of the heart and lungs, which enables the body to meet effectively those emergency conditions that require intense physical effort. This increased work capacity also provides a good physical foundation for the development of skills in a variety of sports.

It recently has been proposed that exercise may act to balance or stabilize the physiological consequences of emotional stress. Although the physiological mechanism is not yet known for certain, there is evidence of changes in hormones, neurotransmitters, and other body chemistry that may possibly help to prepare the body's response to stress situations.

1. Powell, K. E.; P. D. Thompson; C. J. Caspersen; and J. S. Kendrick. "Physical Activity and the Incidence of Coronary Heart Disease." *Ann. Rev. Public Health* (1987): 253–87.

2. Brownell, K. D.; G. A. Marlatt; E. Lichtenstein; and G. T. Wilson. "Understanding and Preventing Relapses." *Am. Psychol.* 41 (1986): 765–82.

Kohl, H. W.; R. E. LaPorte; and S. N. Blair. "Physical Activity and Cancer: An Epidemiological Perspective." *Sports Med.* 6 (1988): 222–37.

Paffernbarger, R. S.; and R. T. Hyde. "Exercise in the Prevention of Coronary Heart Disease." *Prev. Med.* 13 (1984): 3–22.

Siscovich, D. S.; R. E. LaPorte; and J. M. Newman. "The Disease-Specific Benefits and Risks of Physical Activity and Exercise." *Public Health Rep.* 100 (1985): 180–88.

Taylor, C. B.; J. F. Sallis; and R. Needle. "The Relation of Physical Activity and Exercise to Mental Health." *Public Health Rep.* 100 (1985): 195–201.

3. Blair, S. N.; H. W. Kohl, III; R. S. Paffernbarger, Jr.; D. G. Clark; K. H. Cooper; and L. W. Gibbons. "Physical Fitness and All-Cause Mortality: A Prospective Study of Healthy Men and Women." *JAMA* 262 (1989): 2395–401.

TABLE 1.1 Healthy People 2000 Objectives—Physical Activity and Fitness

Health status objectives

Objective 1.1. Reduce coronary heart disease deaths to no more than 100 per 100,000 people.

Objective 1.2. Reduce overweight to a prevalence of no more than 20 percent among people aged 20 and older and no more than 15 percent among adolescents aged 12 through 19.

Risk reduction objectives

Objective 1.3. Increase to at least 30 percent the proportion of people aged 6 and older who engage regularly, preferably daily, in light to moderate physical activity for at least 30 minutes per day.

Objective 1.4. Increase to at least 20 percent the proportion of people aged 18 and older and to at least 75 percent the proportion of children and adolescents aged 6 through 17 who engage in vigorous physical activity that promotes the development and maintenance of cardiorespiratory fitness 3 or more days per week for 20 or more minutes per occasion.

Objective 1.5. Reduce to no more than 15 percent the proportion of people aged 6 and older who engage in no leisure-time physical activity.

Objective 1.6. Increase to at least 40 percent the proportion of people aged 6 and older who regularly perform physical activities that enhance and maintain muscular strength, muscular endurance, and flexibility.

Objective 1.7. Increase to at least 50 percent the proportion of overweight people aged 12 and older who have adopted sound dietary practices combined with regular physical activity to attain an appropriate body weight.

Services and protection objectives

Objective 1.8. Increase to at least 50 percent the proportion of children and adolescents in 1st through 12th grade who participate in daily school physical education.

Objective 1.9. Increase to at least 50 percent the proportion of school physical education class time that students spend being physically active, preferably engaged in lifetime physical activities.

Objective 1.10. Increase the proportion of worksites offering employer-sponsored physical activity and fitness programs.

Objective 1.11. Increase community availability and accessibility of physical activity and fitness facilities.

Objective 1.12. Increase to at least 50 percent the proportion of primary care providers who routinely assess and counsel their patients regarding the frequency, duration, type, and intensity of each patient's physical activity practices.

Health status objectives

Objective 2.1. Reduce coronary heart disease deaths to no more than 100 per 100,000 people.

Objective 2.2. Reverse the rise in cancer deaths to achieve a rate of no more than 130 per 100,000 people.

Objective 2.3. Reduce overweight to a prevalence of no more than 20 percent among people aged 20 and older and no more than 15 percent among adolescents aged 12 through 19.

Objective 2.4. Reduce growth retardation among low-income children aged 5 and younger to less than 10 percent.

Risk reduction objectives

Objective 2.5. Reduce dietary fat intake to an average of 30 percent of calories or less and average saturated fat intake to less than 10 percent of calories among people aged 2 and older.

TABLE 1.1	Healthy People 2000 Objectives—Physical Activity and Fitness (Continued)

Objective 2.6. Increase complex carbohydrate and fiber-containing foods in the diets of adults to 5 or more daily servings for vegetables (including legumes) and fruits, and to 6 or more daily servings for grain products.

Objective 2.7. Increase to at least 50 percent the proportion of overweight people aged 12 and older who have adopted sound dietary practices combined with regular physical activity to attain an appropriate body weight.

Objective 2.8. Increase calcium intake so that at least 50 percent of youth aged 12 through 24 and 50 percent of pregnant and lactating women consume 3 or more servings daily of foods rich in calcium, and at least 50 percent of people aged 25 and older consume 2 or more servings daily.

Objective 2.9. Decrease salt and sodium intake so that at least 65 percent of home meal preparers prepare foods without adding salt, at least 80 percent of people avoid using salt at the table, and at least 40 percent of adults regularly purchase foods modified or lower in sodium.

Objective 2.10. Reduce iron deficiency to less than 3 percent among children aged 1 through 4 and among women of childbearing age.

Objective 2.11. Increase to at least 75 percent the proportion of mothers who breastfeed their babies in the early postpartum period and to at least 50 percent the proportion who continue breastfeeding until their babies are 5 to 6 months old.

Objective 2.12. Increase to at least 75 percent the proportion of parents and caregivers who use feeding practices that prevent baby bottle tooth decay.

Objective 2.13. Increase to at least 85 percent the proportion of people aged 18 and older who use food labels to make nutritious food selections.

Services and protection objectives

Objective 2.14. Achieve useful and informative nutrition labeling for virtually all processed foods and at least 40 percent of fresh meats, poultry, fish, fruits, vegetables, baked goods, and ready-to-eat carry-away foods.

Objective 2.15. Increase to at least 5,000 brand items the availability of processed food products that are reduced in fat and saturated fat.

Objective 2.16. Increase to at least 90 percent the proportion of restaurants and institutional food service operations that offer identifiable low-fat, low-calorie food choices, consistent with the *Dietary Guidelines for Americans*.

Objective 2.17. Increase to at least 90 percent the proportion of school lunch and breakfast services and child care food services with menus that are consistent with the nutrition principles in the *Dietary Guidelines for Americans*.

Objective 2.18. Increase to at least 80 percent the receipt of home food services by people aged 65 and older who have difficulty in preparing their own meals or are otherwise in need of home-delivered meals.

Objective 2.19. Increase to at least 75 percent the proportion of the Nation's schools that provide nutrition education from preschool through 12th grade, preferably as part of quality school health education.

Objective 2.20. Increase to at least 50 percent the proportion of worksites with 50 or more employees that offer nutrition education and/or weight management programs for employees.

Objective 2.21. Increase to at least 75 percent the proportion of primary care providers who provide nutrition assessment and counseling and/or referral to qualified nutritionists or dietitians.

Source: *Healthy People 2000: National Health Promotion and Disease Prevention Objectives.* U.S. Department of Health and Human Services, 1991.

For instance, increases in blood amines, glucose, androgens, lactic acid, and corticoid compounds resulting from exercise have been noted in research. Other evidence suggests that exercise causes the release of such chemicals as enkephalin, a euphoria-producing substance, and that physical conditioning programs facilitate the release from brain cells of beta-endorphin, a substance that produces relaxation. Some researchers attribute the beneficial effects of exercise on stress to reduced electrical activity in the muscles and an increased feeling of fitness. In combination, these factors may help to improve your self-concept, reduce your anxiety, insulate you from stress, and enhance your psychological functioning. (See chapter 12 for special stress-reduction exercises.)

Additional benefits of physical exercise include a possible delay in the aging process, protection from lower-back problems, the maintenance of body weight, and a possible reduction of the chances of getting coronary heart disease. Exercise also induces natural fatigue and relaxation and in some cases reduces a person's reliance on drugs that promote sleep. Finally, if you maintain good physical fitness levels, you will experience both the joy of participation in an intrinsically pleasing activity and the sense of well-being familiar to all who are involved in rigorous exercise. The most important benefit is that you not only feel good about your body, but you feel good about yourself.

To summarize, the benefits of regular exercise include:

1. Improved psychological functioning
2. Improved appearance
3. Increased efficiency of the heart and lungs
4. Increased muscle strength and endurance
5. Reduced stress response
6. Greater protection from lower-back problems
7. Possible delay in the aging process
8. Maintenance of proper body weight
9. Possible reduction of the risk of coronary heart disease
10. Naturally induced fatigue and relaxation

Changes in the Fitness Environment

A revolution has occurred on the exercise scene during the last fifteen years. Today, hundreds of thousands of individuals are engaged in fitness activities. An incredible transformation in sports participation has taken place! Almost half of all adults are now engaged in some type of fitness program. Close to forty million people are jogging today. In 1980, there were ten marathons in the United States and a few hundred dedicated runners. Today, there are about two hundred marathons and thousands of competitive runners. Other activities such as hiking, orienteering, rafting, climbing, cross-country skiing, and scuba diving have also attracted thousands.

The trend is toward a more flexible, all-inclusive fitness program that includes all sorts of beneficial exercises for people of all ages. Aerobic classes and jogging continue to attract exercisers. However, many people have shifted to activities such as fitness walking, low-impact aerobics, and dancing, as they have realized that even modest increases in lower-intensity activities, such as brisk walking thirty to sixty minutes a day, may add years to your life. Others are choosing more strenuous activities such as rock climbing, biathlons, triathlons, mountain biking, step aerobics, and water aerobics. Another new approach is **cross-training,** in which one combines a variety of complementary exercises to create a more challenging and efficient exercise program. Cross-training also prevents overuse of muscle groups and provides for a balance between muscle groups.

The social and physical environments today are much different than they were twenty years ago. The mass media—in particular, television—have had a major impact on our fitness habits by giving more coverage, not only to the more popular spectator sports, but also to such sports as marathon running, skiing, swimming, and cycling. In addition, there has been an astronomical rise in the general public's participation in tennis; racquetball; corporate fitness programs; aerobic dance programs; and health, running, and bicycling clubs. All of these factors have heightened most people's interest in health, nutrition, and physical fitness.

Women's participation in rigorous physical activities also has undergone marked changes in the last fifteen years. Traditionally, competitive sports and other physical activities were organized around male needs. Often, women were not welcome, and those who chose to participate were stigmatized by society. Because of society's rejection of this outmoded stereotype, changes in the perception of the female role, and mandated legislation, hundreds of thousands of young girls and women now are actively engaged in a wide variety of rigorous physical activities. In addition, the National Organization for Women and other support groups have given strong political and emotional support to women, encouraging them to feel good—not anxious—about being physically active and competitive. Title IX and gender equity have provided new opportunities in high school and college for sport participation.

The traditional view of exercise as physically exhausting and boring has been replaced by the contemporary view of it as enjoyable, healthful, and beneficial. Today, free of the demands of high-level skills or the fear of failure and ridicule,

7

almost anyone can identify himself or herself as an active individual by just putting on running shoes and shorts and heading for the jogging trail.

Participation has taken priority over spectating. You definitely gain a much more authentic experience from participating in physical activities than from watching others. More and more people are experiencing firsthand the joy, the satisfaction, the sense of accomplishment, and yes, even the pain and sometimes the failure of those who participate.

A more abstract, but nevertheless valuable, view of participation deals with the unique nature of the values accorded to this experience by those who participate. Existentialist philosopher Albert Camus once said that it is only the individual who gives value to life, that knowledge is a personal thing, and that the world is silent and irrational and yields no answer to us in our quest to know. According to Camus, whatever you experience depends upon your own individual perception. Thus, you are as old as you feel; the taste of vanilla ice cream is unique to each person; running, swimming, and hiking are experienced differently by each individual; and a song, a poem, a victory, or a defeat means whatever you think it does.

Our misconceptions about fitness are legends that persist despite recent change. Many people still find it surprising that professional athletes, such as baseball players and golfers, may have poor cardiorespiratory endurance. Some still expect that fitness automatically will be conferred upon them just because their work requires some physical exertion, such as lifting or moving. Others feel that bouncing, vibrating, and whirlpooling their muscles in a health spa are the shortest ways to fitness. These obvious misconceptions may stem partly from two varying definitions of fitness: performance-related fitness and health-related fitness.

Performance-Related Versus Health-Related Fitness

Performance-related fitness relates to many of the tests you may have taken, usually in school, that measured your levels of strength, skill, power, endurance, and agility in specific sports. These are performance-related tests and measure only limited aspects of fitness.

The main goal of this book is to develop the concept of **health-related fitness,** which concerns those aspects of our physical and psychological makeup that afford us some protection against coronary heart disease, problems associated with being overweight, a variety of muscle and joint ailments, and the physiological complications of our responses to stress.

The President's Council on Physical Fitness and Sports more comprehensively defines health-related fitness as the ability to carry out daily tasks with vigor, without undue fatigue, and with ample energy to enjoy leisure-time pursuits and to meet unforeseen injuries. This definition indicates that fitness is a relative term relating to your everyday activities. For example, some of us may have occupations that require higher levels of fitness than others (a construction worker compared to an office worker for instance), but all individuals must meet a minimum level of fitness to lead a healthy and productive life.

The four components of health-related fitness that are essential to leading a healthy life are cardiorespiratory endurance, muscle strength and endurance, body composition, and flexibility.

Cardiorespiratory Endurance

At the heart of physical fitness is **cardiorespiratory endurance,** which is the body's ability to deliver oxygen and nutrients to all of its vital organs in order to sustain prolonged, rhythmical exercise. How well the body provides oxygen is determined primarily by the efficiency of the heart and respiratory system. The cardiorespiratory system must be able to transport oxygen efficiently to provide energy to the heart, nervous system, and working muscles.

Aerobic fitness means in the presence of oxygen; as contrasted with anaerobic meaning in the absence of oxygen. **Aerobic fitness,** which is used interchangeably with cardiorespiratory fitness, is defined as the improvement with training of oxygen intake, transport, and use. Aerobic training mainly affects the skeletal muscles by increasing the level of enzymes necessary in the muscles' ability to produce energy. In addition, training increases the size and number of mitochondria, the cellular powerhouses that produce energy, and increases muscle ability to use fat as fuel. Aerobic fitness is attained when the metabolic rate and oxygen consumption of muscles are elevated long enough to overload the aerobic enzyme system; that is, push the system to its maximum level of production.

When insufficient oxygen is delivered to the muscles, their capacity to do work sharply declines. A heart in excellent condition and an efficient respiratory system are essential to a high level of physical fitness. Exercise increases the strength of the heart, which increases its ability to pump blood more efficiently throughout the body. One of the main benefits of this is the potential for increasing the supply of oxygen to the heart muscle. Exercise also results in the reduction of epinephrine production, heart rate, and blood pressure. When these three factors are reduced at rest, the amount of oxygen needed by the heart muscle is reduced.

In the past few years, there have been major advances in the research on heart disease and its relationship to exercise. Studies of the physiological adjustments and the demands made upon the heart during exercise have provided a basis for stress-testing programs. As a result, individualized exercise and re-habilitation programs have been adapted to the needs of those who are predis-posed to or who have coronary heart disease. In the past, when individuals suffered a heart attack, they were told to avoid exercise for fear of further injury to the heart. More recent research has now shown that aerobic exercise can be extremely beneficial to certain individuals who have suffered heart attacks. In fact, individually prescribed exercise programs may increase the efficiency of the heart to the point where it is possible to improve the circulation and reduce the risk of subsequent heart attacks.

The American Heart Association Committee on Exercise advocates physical activity as an adjunct to the control of blood pressure, blood lipid levels, and obesity. In recommending individualized exercise programs, the committee states that "exercise can enrich the quality of life and in combination with other mea-sures, such as low-fat diets and eliminating smoking, can help reduce coronary risk, and that exercise is the most significant factor contributing to the health of the individual."[4] The American Heart Association lists physical inactivity as a major risk factor for coronary heart disease.

Muscle Strength and Endurance

Muscle strength is the force produced when a muscle group is in the process of lifting, moving, or pushing a resistance. **Muscle endurance** is the ability of a muscle to maintain a continuous contraction or repeatedly contract over a period of time. Muscle endurance is to some degree dependent on muscle strength; however, it is possible to have a high level of muscle strength and a low level of muscle endurance. Strength is essential to a variety of everyday activities. Even though muscle strength is a relative factor related to the demand of the activity, a minimum level of strength is needed by all individuals. Those with lower levels of strength run a greater risk of injury when lifting or engaging in physical ac-tivities. Performance in recreational sports and athletics is enhanced by higher levels of strength. Power, the ability of the muscle to produce high levels of force in a short period of time, is also basic to a number of daily activities.

Strong abdominal muscles are an important component of body fitness. The abdominal muscles, for example, form a strong support for your internal organs. These organs exert considerable stress against the inner surface of the abdominal muscles. The more stretched the muscles become, as in the case of a protruding abdomen, the more heavily the internal organs press against the abdominal wall. Visceroptosis is a condition in which abdominal protrusion is so severe that the viscera (internal organs) drop down into new positions. The stomach, liver,

4. American Heart Association. "Subcommittee on Exercise and Cardiac Rehabilitation, Statement on Exercise." *Circulation* 64 (1981): 1302–4.

spleen, kidneys, and intestines all may be displaced, adversely affecting their functions. This forward displacement of the abdominal wall and the visceral contents is due to a lack of abdominal muscle strength. Adequate contraction of the abdominal muscles also prevents the muscles in the lower back from hyperextending the lumbar spine (that is, inward arching). Hyperextension can result in additional pressure on the spinal discs, which could cause pain and chronic injury.

As we grow older, we all incur losses in muscle strength. However, those who maintain a strength program can delay these losses. In addition, a strength program maintains greater maximum strength for dealing efficiently with everyday physical activities and sudden emergencies. Strength training may also play a role in increasing bone density, thus giving some protection against osteoporosis. Bone structure and density are maintained by the force of gravity and lateral forces acting on the bone from muscle contractions. Weight-bearing activities (walking and jogging) also aid in maintaining spine and hip mineral content. Better posture accompanied by a more aesthetic appearance are also benefits of strength maintenance.

Body Composition

Body composition refers to the proportion of body fat to lean body tissue. The relative balance of these two body components is a better gauge of an individual's fitness level than ordinary body weight. A recommended proportion of body fat for a man in his early twenties is approximately 12–17 percent; for a woman in the same age group about 19–24 percent is recommended. A male who is over 20 percent and a female who is over 30 percent body fat are considered to be obese. **Obesity,** therefore, is defined as being overfat. Overweight, a term often confused with obesity, is defined as exceeding the maximum weight listed for your height, sex, and frame size in a standardized table. It is possible to be classified as overweight on a standard height/weight table but have a normal percentage of body fat. Many athletes with large skeletal frames and large muscle mass may be erroneously classified as overweight but not obese. Other individuals who may be classified as having normal weight, on a standardized table, may in fact have more than a normal amount of body fat.

Obesity is one of the worst health problems confronting Americans today. Approximately 20 percent of the teenage population, 30 percent of all men, and 40 percent of all women weigh 15 to 20 percent more than they should. Obesity has important ramifications to health. Being overfat is one of the major risk factors associated with heart disease. Diabetes and high blood pressure also generally accompany being overfat. Exercise accompanied by weight loss can directly affect these two common problems. Obesity is also associated with gallbladder dysfunction, joint disease, and complications during surgery.

11

When you exercise, you inevitably burn up more calories than when you are sedentary; therefore, you start to lose fat, provided your food intake remains the same. An exercise program may result in an increase of muscle tissue with a decrease in stored fat. Because muscles weigh more than fat, you may actually gain a little weight even though you undergo a loss in body fat. Your body dimensions, however, will change, resulting in a slim waist, trim hips and thighs, and an improved overall appearance.

Obesity may also be defined in terms of waist to hip ratio. Waist to hip ratio can be calculated by dividing the number of inches around the waistline by the circumference of the hips. For example, a person who has a 27-inch waist and 38-inch hip would have a ratio of 0.71. A woman who has a ratio of 0.8 or higher and a man who is 0.95 or higher would be at high risk for weight-related health problems.

Flexibility

Flexibility is the movement of a joint through the full range of motion. Flexibility is important not only to learning athletic skills satisfactorily, but also to general health and fitness. Recent advances in physical medicine and rehabilitation indicate that flexibility is important to general health and physical fitness. Flexibility exercises are also valuable in reducing general neuromuscular tension and lower-back pain. A number of factors such as age, sex, weight, height, disease, and muscle definition affect flexibility. A decreased range of motion may limit proper movement and lead to inefficient movement, and to the possibility of injury to ligaments and tendons, poor posture, and lower-back problems. Decreases in flexibility are also associated with physical inactivity and aging.

How Long Before Results Show Up?

Now that you know what health-related fitness is all about, be patient. Fitness is not developed in a few days, so give yourself some time. However, after only a few weeks, you should begin to feel some physical changes, such as less breathlessness and fatigue. If you have been sedentary for a number of years, you should not expect to sense responses within a few weeks. Your body will take a number of months to adjust to the demands of exercise in order to gear up for increases in efficiency. Don't expect miracles to occur in a few weeks. Convince yourself that it will be necessary to invest a lot of time in training. Research indicates that people engaged in a rigorous physical exercise program start to experience increased efficiency in the cardiovascular system in approximately eight weeks, and progressive increases follow thereafter. There are also many individual differences that affect each person's responsiveness to training—age, sex, race, genetic disposition, obesity, exercise history, medical history, and motivation all play an important part. Remember, however, that gains are lost if exercise is not continued on at least a maintenance level.

If you follow the guidelines and the individualized exercises presented in this book, you will be following procedures based upon sound scientific principles, which will not only benefit your health, but also be a source of continued enjoyment to you.

Key Terms

Aerobic Fitness
Improvement with training of oxygen intake, transport, and use

Body Composition
The proportion of body fat to lean body tissue

Cardiorespiratory Endurance
The ability of the lungs and heart to take in and transport adequate amounts of oxygen to the muscles for activities that are performed over long periods of time

Cross-Training
A combination of complementary exercises to enhance strength, performance, and endurance

Flexibility
The extent and range of motion around a joint

Health-Related Fitness
Those aspects of our physical and psychological makeup that afford us some protection against coronary heart disease, problems associated with being overweight, muscle and joint ailments, and the physiological complications of responding to stress

Muscle Endurance
Ability to maintain continuous contraction or repeatedly contract over a period of time

Muscle Strength
The force produced by a muscle group

Obesity
Having above-normal body fat

Wellness
The process of moving toward greater awareness of your human potential by developing a high level of fitness

2

chapter

Motivation

After you have studied this chapter you should be able to

1. describe the importance of motivation in achieving fitness goals;
2. describe the chances of increasing overall physical fitness;
3. describe the value in achieving a high level of physical fitness;
4. describe present fitness and nutritional status;
5. describe ten psychological and social benefits of exercise;
6. describe guidelines that will help you in your fitness program;
7. describe important aspects of goal setting;
8. describe the importance of contracts; and
9. describe methods for changing behavior.

It's All Up to You

B   ehavior generally is motivated by a desire to attain goals that give value and meaning to our lives. **Motivation** is the energy that fuels the engines of behavior that drive toward these goals. Its presence explains why we strive, work, and persevere.

Research reveals that a considerable number of individuals who begin weight loss, drug rehabilitation, and similar programs drop out long before achieving much progress. Furthermore, as these programs progress, participants display decreased interest and reduce their efforts. The mainsprings of their actions appear to stop working, and they no longer are able to maintain their goal-directed activity. They apparently lack the capability of convincing themselves that they can complete a program. In other words, if you believe that you are capable of attaining a goal, you are more likely to achieve it. When people doubt their ability to achieve a goal, they often reduce their driving efforts or give up altogether when they run into obstacles.

Human motivation depends on a series of choices based on our perceptions. It is possible that the individuals who drop out of the previously mentioned improvement programs do value their goals but that the perceived relationships between program activity and goal achievement are uncertain, leading to reduced commitment. Generally, the force of effort maintained by individuals toward their goals is determined by two factors: their perceived chances of achieving the desired outcomes and the degree of value they place on the outcomes. In other words, each person internalizes his or her chances of success and also the value of that success to his or her well-being. ("What are my chances of losing those twenty-five pounds, and if I do lose them, of what value is that twenty-five-pound loss to me?")

Before starting an exercise program, it is important that you evaluate your present circumstances and satisfactorily answer two important questions:

1. What are my chances of increasing my overall physical fitness?
2. Will the changes brought about by exercise be of value to me?

The answer to the first question is relatively easy: Excellent. Research indicates that the low-fit or sedentary individual can look forward to substantial gains in cardiorespiratory and muscular fitness after only a few months of continuous, rigorous exercise.

You will have to answer the second question yourself. However, here are some thoughts to consider. If you are now sedentary, it is reasonable to assume that the physical and psychological changes discussed in chapter 1 that occur in your body as a result of exercise will be of some value to you. In addition, research indicates that we all have certain basic needs in common that must be fulfilled to lead a balanced life. For example, we all enjoy the satisfaction of achievement, whether it comes from a promotion at work or from jogging two miles without stopping. Also, knowing that we can achieve our goals is an important reinforcement of our need to experience some control over our environment. A sense of mastery, the completion of a task, or the learning of a valued skill that once seemed difficult to acquire can all lead to feelings of self-confidence and well-being. The desire to witness and control our environment, to enjoy it, to react to it, and to master it is the most significant factor in providing satisfaction. Furthermore, we gain satisfaction from meaningful activities and from opportunities to develop a sense of responsibility and self-direction. All of these needs can be met by a sound exercise program.

It's very easy to find excuses *not* to exercise. Too cold, too hot, too windy, too busy, too tired, will make it up next week—all are frequently heard. However, if you accept the goals of health-related fitness and are aware of how they relate to your self-concept, you soon will be looking for excuses *to* exercise.

Changing Behavior

It is difficult to change behavior without addressing the underlying causes, otherwise the same problems come back along with a new set of problems. Also many of our behaviors tend to be adaptive and not maladaptations to everyday events. That is, we tend to make adaptations that enable us to get through each day with a minimum amount of stress. Another difficulty is that when we make an attempt to change our behavior in a positive way, we tend to find ways to undermine it. Certain changes make us feel less free, and feeling free is often more important than concerns about our health. However, if we are presented with informed choices for behavioral change, reinforced by results that we can experience and measure, we tend to stay committed.

It is essential that fitness achieve a high priority in our lives. Efforts in increasing motivation must have that end in sight at all times. However, external rewards (**extrinsic motivation**) are viewed only as a temporary means in changing behavior. Behavior can only be continuously maintained by our own internal rewards (**intrinsic motivation**).

The following are some general steps that may aid you in changing behavior. Some of these steps can be eliminated or modified, or you can add others to the list, depending upon your needs.

Suggestions for Changing Behavior

1. Desire to change; it is your responsibility.
2. Analyze the history of your problem.
3. Record your current behavior.
4. Analyze your current status.
5. Set short- and long-term goals.
6. Sign a contract with a friend or your instructor.
7. List some possible strategies for change.
8. Select one or two strategies that may be useful.
9. Learn and adopt new coping skills (i.e., how to relax) and social skills.
10. Outline a maintenance program once your goal has been reached.

Goal Setting

It is important to establish goals so that your progress toward a healthier life can be observed and measured. In order to do this, it is vital to develop a greater awareness of yourself and your environment. Focus on your lifestyle and convince yourself that you are capable of self-assessment and of taking action in the process of moving toward your goals.

Many individuals attribute their failure to achieve goals to lack of ability. They tend not to try again or persist; they stop trying. Research tells us that the reasons for failure can directly affect the ability to carry on. The most common reasons are lack of effort, lack of ability, task difficulty, and bad luck. It is important to remember that motivation is changeable and under your control.

Some important aspects of goal setting:

1. Select a goal you can definitely attain if you exert sufficient effort.
2. Remember your level of success in achieving your goal is directly linked to the amount of effort you exert. Your willingness to undergo some discomfort is vital to achieving your goals.
3. If successful or unsuccessful in realizing your goals, determine why.
4. When you have achieved your goals, establish new ones.

Foremost in this procedure is the establishment of measurable short- and long-term goals. For example, short-term goals could be determining your target heart rate, degree of flexibility, range of motion, or the amount of resistance to use for weight training. Examples of long-term goals could be jogging a mile in ten minutes, reaching the recommended muscle strength for your age and sex, or reducing your body fat by 5 percent. It is also important to set new goals as the previous ones are reached.

Some Important Aspects of Goal Setting

1. Establish your own realistic goals.
2. Put them in writing.
3. Your goal must be attainable.
4. Your goal must be measurable.
5. Your goal should have target dates.
6. Your goal should allow for change.
7. Your goal should state the amount of effort as well as outcome.

An effective technique for conveying self-responsibility and continued awareness of change is a wellness inventory (see figure 2.1). The inventory will enable you to self-assess many aspects of your fitness, identify behaviors that are beneficial or detrimental, and target those areas that need change.

Suggested Lab Activity

Directions: Place a check in the appropriate box under your present status. Then place a check in the box for the goal you would like to achieve under future goals.

	Present status				Future goals			
	Always	Frequently	Occasionally	Sometimes	Never	Always	Frequently	Occasionally	Sometimes	Never

Physical fitness

1. I exercise vigorously at least three times a week for twenty minutes.

2. I warm up before exercising by stretching or jogging.

3. I am satisfied with my body weight.

4. My exercise includes a strength component.

5. I avoid sporadic exercise.

6. I avoid extremes of too much or too little exercise.

7. I am satisfied with my physical appearance.

8. I tire easily when exercising or doing strenuous work.

9. I cool down after rigorous exercise.

10. I get an adequate amount of sleep.

11. I have adequate physical strength for my age.

12. I need to improve my present physical fitness.

Figure 2.1 Self-scoring wellness assessment.

Chapter 1 focused more on the physical benefits of rigorous exercise. The following are some of the more psychological and social benefits:

1. **You Don't Have to Worry About Failing.** There are no complex skills to learn, no condescending instructors, no embarrassing situations, no last-place finishes, no critical peers, no intimidation.

	Present status					Future goals				
	Always	Frequently	Occasionally	Sometimes	Never	Always	Frequently	Occasionally	Sometimes	Never
Nutrition										
1. I avoid foods high in saturated fats such as beef, pork, cheese, and fried foods.										
2. I avoid fad diets.										
3. I eat high-fiber foods.										
4. I minimize salt intake.										
5. I eat fruits and uncooked vegetables daily.										
6. I select lean cuts of meat, poultry, and fish.										
7. I plan my diet so that I get sufficient vitamins and minerals.										
8. I avoid eating too much sugar, candy, sweets, and simple carbohydrates.										
9. I eat regularly.										
10. I drink sufficient water so my urine is light yellow.										
11. I eat a variety of foods.										
12. I am able to maintain proper body weight.										

Figure 2.1 *(Continued)*

2. **You See Results.** You are reshaping your body. Improving your cardiorespiratory endurance increases your feelings of health and energy. Moreover, weight-resistance training improves your sense of muscular strength and well-being.

3. **You Can Say Goodbye to Destructive Self-Criticism.** No racket throwing, no recriminations, no self-destructive thoughts. Certainly a progressive increase in exercise requires some adaptation of effort on your part, but what activity doesn't?

4. **You Compete Only with Yourself.** You can set your own goals and forget about peer pressure. There are no opponents to defeat, no times to overcome, no records to break.

5. **You Make All the Decisions.** You are truly master of your own fate. You can decide your own schedule and set your own rules and standards. You can exercise alone, exercise with a friend, or do your own thing.

6. **You Receive Social Approval.** Everyone admires people who exercise. You may find and make new friends. You are putting yourself in a no-lose social environment.

7. **You Experience an Improved Self-Image and Recognition.** Extra inches off the waistline, increased feelings of well-being and energy, a more aesthetic-looking body—these goals are all within your range of achievement.

8. **You Feel Satisfied.** Achieving goals that you personally have established, working toward more self-confidence, and getting a clear focus on your life all bring increased satisfaction.

9. **You Are Successful.** No one fails when they exercise, but don't expect a ''quick fix'' after only a few days. Be patient, and the outcome will be positive.

10. **You Have a Chance to Express Yourself.** Exercise provides one of the few opportunities for emotional release and free expression. You be the judge of what you want to do with your body. Tune in to its signals, and you'll be surprised at what you hear.

Guidelines to Keep You Exercising

Find a Convenient Location to Work Out. Choose a place to exercise that is close to where you work or live. Don't depend on others for transportation.

Vary Your Exercises. To avoid boredom, don't get locked into one routine, whether it's warm-up, jogging, swimming, or weights. Be creative. Select an activity you enjoy.

Stay Within Your Limits. Don't set goals that leave you exhausted. Set goals that are realistic and achievable.

Record Your Progress. If you keep track of what's happening to your body, heart rate, strength, and weight, you will be amazed at the changes. Such records also provide great feedback and reinforcement. Appendix B at the back of the book provides record sheets for most of the exercise regimens presented in this text.

Don't Be Obsessive About Exercise. Keep records, but don't keep score. You don't have to keep piling it on. Two miles a day is a lot safer and healthier than twenty miles, and besides, it's more enjoyable.

Work Out with a Friend or Your Family. Social support really helps.

Be Patient and Stay with It. The benefits do not come overnight. Generally, it takes a few months for physiological changes to become noticeable.

Set Your Own Time Schedule. It is important to organize a convenient schedule. Don't make it too rigid. Allow for some flexibility.

Comfort Zone. Interpret symptoms associated with exercise as positive signs of a good workout.

Keep It in Perspective. View your exercise program in the context of the total fitness goals expressed in chapter 1. Don't keep score or continually strive for that euphoric feeling. Be aware of why you are out there jogging or swimming, and set reasonable goals. Don't feel guilty because you have to miss a few days of exercise. Keep your own goals in mind as you listen to peers chatter about their experiences of ''runner's high'' during super long distances or if they ask condescending questions about your motivation and fitness if you are not training for the local marathon. Don't let others dictate your exercise program. If others want to set unreal, unnecessary standards for themselves—and possibly create emotional problems in the process—that's their problem. Don't let them make it yours.

Contracts

A contract can be an effective method in directing and maintaining behavior toward specific exercise goals. The contract is used to formalize a commitment to exercise. It is the written record of your entire exercise plan. Behavior to be changed is clearly and objectively defined within the contract so that one can determine when it occurs. The contract should specify short-term goals and focus on the positive consequences for the achievement of the goal. The contract allows you to play a role in directing your own behavior.

It is important to remember not to engage in unhealthy practices in order to achieve your objectives. For example, exercising three hours in one day to make up for three days of missed exercise is not a healthy practice. A commitment to a contract may be made between you and your instructor, a friend, or a family member. At the end of the contract, new goals can be renegotiated and renewed. See appendix B for examples of exercise contracts.

The ultimate purpose of most individuals is to be themselves and to achieve the realization of their personal self-concept. We all tend to be in perpetual pursuit of what we regard as our deserved role in life and want to be treated and rewarded in relationship to our ability. When our experience confirms this, we tend to stay committed and persevere toward our goals.

Exercise Planning Guidelines*

Begin Gradually and Progress Slowly. Results will show up in about two or three months; don't be in a rush.

Always Check Your Heart Rate During and Immediately After Exercise. Your heart rate response will tell you if you are doing too much, too soon, or too little.

Apply the Progressive Overload Principle. Gradually overloading a body system will lead to an increase in its capacity.

Exercise a Minimum of Three to Four Times Weekly for Thirty Minutes or More. Exercise duration below this will not substantially increase your capacity.

Alternate Light and Heavy Training. This will allow adequate recovery between work-outs and reduce the risk of injury.

Warm-Up Before Each Exercise Session. Warm-up will increase the work capacity of your muscles and heart and reduce the risk of injury.

Cool Down After Each Exercise Session. This will allow you to maintain the blood flow from the exercised muscles to the heart and decrease recovery time.

Use the Appropriate Training Programs Outlined in Each Chapter. The start of your exercise program should be based on the outcome of your fitness evaluation found in chapter 3.

Key Terms

Extrinsic Motivation
External rewards or motives

Intrinsic Motivation
Internal motives

Motivation
The basic reasons why we strive, work, and persevere toward our goals

*Each of these guidelines will be discussed in detail in the appropriate chapters.

23

3

c h a p t e r

Coronary Heart Disease and Exercise

Coronary Heart Disease

A major cause of premature death for men and women in the United States is **coronary heart disease,** a disease of the arteries that supply blood to the heart muscle. Coronary heart disease affects over five million people and accounts for over 1.5 million heart attacks each year. It is sometimes referred to as the "silent" disease because some individuals may have no symptoms that indicate its presence. Other individuals, however, may experience such manifestations of the disease as crushing pain in the chest, weakness, breathlessness, or sensations of burning or pressure.

25

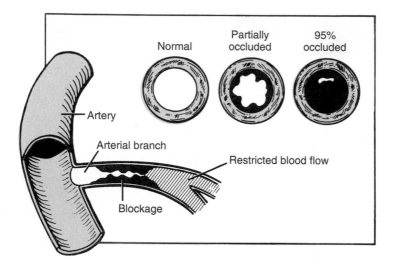

Figure 3.1 Atherosclerosis—the progressive narrowing of a coronary artery.
From Jack H. Wilmore and David L. Costill, Training for Sport and Activity, 3rd edition. Copyright © 1988 Times Mirror Higher Education Group Inc., Dubuque, Iowa. All rights reserved. Reprinted by permission.

The most common type of coronary heart disease is **atherosclerosis.** Atherosclerosis is caused by an accumulation of plaque on the inner walls of the arteries. **Plaque** forms from deposits of cholesterol, lipids, blood cells, calcium, and tissue debris. Because the coronary arteries are responsible for supplying the heart muscle with oxygen, any interruption in the flow of blood through these vessels can have serious consequences. Plaque can cause artery walls to lose their elasticity. Plaque also may narrow the lining of the artery walls, thus increasing pressure against the walls. If plaque narrows the lining enough, it may completely block the flow of blood. The result is death of tissue that depends on the artery to supply it with nutrients and oxygen.

The reasons for plaque formation are not completely understood. There seems to be agreement, however, that the smooth muscle cells lining artery walls are in some way injured, thus leaving a vulnerable spot for cholesterol and other substances that form plaque to collect. (See figure 3.1.)

The heart derives nutrition and oxygen not from the blood that fills its chambers, but from the arteries that lie on its surface. A heart attack, or **myocardial infarction (MI),** occurs when the circulation of blood to the heart muscle is cut off, resulting in the death of muscle cells in the heart. Atherosclerosis is the most common contributor to heart attacks, but they also can be caused by spasms of the coronary arteries, congenital defects, rheumatic heart disease, and a number of other factors. When the heart tissue dies as a result of arterial blockage, the damaged muscle cells secrete enzymes, which pass into the blood supply. The type and amount of enzymes are one means of diagnosing a heart attack.

Heart Attack Symptoms

When the fibrous plaque significantly narrows the coronary arteries, during exercise or stress, there will be a decreased blood supply to heart tissues, resulting in myocardial ischemia. The American Heart Association lists the following signs of a heart attack:*

1. Uncomfortable pressure, fullness, squeezing, or pain in the center of the chest lasting longer than two minutes.
2. Pain that spreads to the shoulders, arms, or neck.
3. Severe pain, dizziness, fainting, sweating, nausea, and shortness of breath.

Risk Factors of Coronary Heart Disease

According to the National Center for Health Statistics, the mortality from heart attacks in the United States has dropped by one-third since 1980. This success has been due not only to improved medical treatment of coronary heart disease, but also to preventive steps people have taken. Heart attacks are the leading killer of North American men and women however, accounting for about 500,000 deaths every year—about 20 percent in people under age sixty-five. Most of these deaths could be avoided, or at least postponed, if everyone paid attention to the risk factors for coronary heart disease and took preventive means to counter them.

There is considerable evidence that some individuals are at a greater risk of developing coronary heart disease than others. Table 3.1 represents the current thinking of the American Heart Association. The risk factors are divided into **primary** or major and **secondary** or contributing. A primary factor means that a factor alone increases the risk of coronary heart disease. A secondary factor means that a certain factor increases the risk of coronary heart disease only if one of the primary factors is already present or that its significance has not been previously determined.

Risk factors such as age, gender, and genetics obviously cannot be changed. However the majority of the others can be controlled and in some cases altered to reduce the risk of coronary heart disease. The American College of Sports

*Some individuals may have all or only a few of these symptoms.

27

TABLE 3.1	Coronary Heart Disease Risk Factors

Primary or major risk factors

Heredity*

Male sex*

Increasing age*

Cigarette smoking**

High serum cholesterol**

High blood pressure**

Physical inactivity**

Secondary or contributing risk factors

Diabetes**

Obesity**

Stress**

Race*

*can't be changed
**can be changed

Medicine lists diabetes as a major risk factor and evidence points to the fact that high levels of HDL and the ratio of HDL to total cholesterol are good indicators of risk.

The disease is more common in men than women, those with a family history of the disease, and susceptibility increases with age. The risk factor of coronary heart disease also increases with the number of cigarettes smoked, the degree to which blood pressure is elevated, and the quantity of cholesterol in the blood. In addition, the overall risk factors of coronary heart disease increase with the number of risk factors. It is vital to remember that risk factors interact with each other to increase the overall risk of coronary heart disease.

To determine your risk factor of developing coronary heart disease refer to table 3.2.

High Blood Pressure

High blood pressure, or **hypertension,** is believed to affect approximately sixty million Americans. It is broadly defined as chronically elevated blood pressure above the normal level considered healthy for your age and sex.

A complex system of hormones, nerve signals, and other elements regulate blood pressure by widening or narrowing small blood vessels called arterioles. Blood pressure will normally fluctuate with each heart beat, time of day, anxiety level, and a number of other factors. In some individuals the regulatory system goes awry causing the arterioles to stay constricted, thus increasing blood pressure (see table 3.3 for appropriate levels).

TABLE 3.2   Suggested Lab Exercise: What Is Your Heart Attack Risk?

Physical activity

Choose the column (A, B, or C) that best describes your usual level of physical activity.

A	B	C
Highly active	**Moderately active**	**Inactive**
My job requires very hard physical labor (such as digging or loading heavy objects) at least four hours a day	My job requires that I walk, lift, carry or do other moderately hard work for several hours per day (day care worker, stock clerk or busboy/waitress)	My job requires that I sit at a desk most of the day
OR		AND
I do vigorous activities (jogging, cycling, swimming, etc.) at least three times per week for 30—60 minutes or more	OR	Much of my leisure time is spent in sedentary activities (watching TV, reading, etc.)
	I spend much of my leisure time doing moderate activities (dancing, gardening, walking, or housework)	AND
OR		I seldom work up a sweat and I cannot walk fast without having to stop to catch my breath
I do at least one hour of moderate activity such as brisk walking at least four days a week		

Rating your activity level

If your physical activity is more like:	Circle
Column A	1
Between Column A and B	2
Column B	3
Between Column B and C	4
Column C	5

Scoring

Add your answers for each question to get your total score.

If you total score is:	Your heart attack risk is:
6–13	Low
14–22	Moderate
23–30	High

Your score is simply an estimate of your possible risk. A high score does not mean you will surely have a heart attack, and a low score doesn't mean you're safe from heart disease. Check your individual category scores to see which factors are increasing your risk of heart attack the most. Then go to the end of the table to learn how to lower your risk.

TABLE 3.2   Suggested Lab Exercise: What Is Your Heart Attack Risk? (Continued)

How to find out

Every year about 1.5 million Americans suffer a heart attack. And almost 500,000 of them die. The fact is, **heart attack claims more lives than any other single cause.** Are you at risk? Take the following quiz to find out! If your score is high, don't despair. You can lower your risk by following the steps listed on the next page.

Instructions: In each category, circle the number next to the statement that's most true for you.

Cigarette smoking

I never smoked or stopped smoking three or more years ago.	1
I don't smoke but live and/or work with smokers.	2
I stopped smoking within the last three years.	3
I smoke regularly.	4
I smoke regularly and live and/or work with other smokers.	5

Total blood cholesterol

Use the number from your most recent blood cholesterol measurement.

Less than 160	1
160–199	2
Don't know	3
200–239	4
240 or higher	5

HDL ("good") cholesterol

Use the number from your most recent HDL cholesterol measurement.

Over 60	1
56–60	2
Don't know	3
35–55	4
Less than 35	5

Systolic blood pressure

Use the first (highest) number from your most recent blood pressure measurement.

Less than 120	1
120–139	2
Don't know	3
140–159	4
160 or higher	5

Excess body weight

I am within 10 pounds of my desirable weight.	1
I am 10–20 pounds above my desirable weight.	2
I am 21–30 pounds above my desirable weight.	3
I am 31–50 pounds above my desirable weight.	4
I am more than 50 pounds above my desirable weight.	5

TABLE 3.2 Suggested Lab Exercise: What Is Your Heart Attack Risk? (Continued)

How to lower your risk	Risk factors that you can't control

How to lower your risk

√ **Quit smoking.**
Smoking increases your heart attack risk. The more you smoke, the higher your risk for heart attack, stroke, and cancer. Your risk of heart disease drops dramatically very soon after you quit smoking.

√ **Get your blood pressure and cholesterol levels checked.**
If you don't know your blood pressure, total cholesterol and HDL cholesterol levels, get them measured soon. You may be at risk without knowing it.

√ **Eat a low-fat diet.**
Cutting back on fatty foods will lower your total cholesterol and help you lose weight. And that, in turn, may help you lower your blood pressure and raise your HDL cholesterol.

√ **Exercise.**
Moderate exercise can reduce your risk of heart attack. People who do more vigorous activities have an even lower heart attack risk.

√ **Take medications.**
If lifestyle changes aren't enough to lower your risk, your doctor may prescribe cholesterol and/or blood pressure-lowering drugs.

Risk factors that you can't control

• **Age.**
Your heart attack risk increases as you get older.

• **Sex.**
Men are at greater risk than premenopausal women.

• **Race.**
African-Americans and Cuban-, Puerto Rican- and Mexican-Americans are more likely to have high blood pressure than Anglo-Americans.

• **Personal medical history.**
If you have diabetes or heart disease, you're at greater risk. If you've already had a heart attack, you're more likely to have another one than someone who hasn't.

• **Family medical history.**
If any close blood relative has had a heart attack or stroke, or died of heart disease before age 55, your heart attack risk is increased.

Source: Reproduced with permission: American Heart Association

---

TABLE 3.3 Blood Pressure Readings

Diastolic (sustained readings)		Systolic (sustained readings; diastolic below 90)	
84 or less	normal	139 or less	normal
85–89	high normal	140–159	borderline
90–104	mild hypertension	160 or higher	severe hypertension
105–114	moderate hypertension		
115 or higher	severe hypertension		

Systolic blood pressure is the highest level of pressure exerted against the walls of the arteries from ventricular contraction. **Diastolic blood pressure** is the lowest level of pressure exerted against the walls of the arteries during ventricular relaxation. Systolic blood pressure of 140 to 160 millimeters of mercury (mmHg) or diastolic blood pressure of 90 to 95 mmHg is considered borderline hypertension. Systolic blood pressure of 161 mmHg or greater or diastolic blood pressure of 96 mmHg or greater is diagnosed as absolute hypertension. See table 3.3 for appropriate levels. The higher the blood pressure, the greater the incidence of coronary heart disease.

Hypertension may result from kidney disease or a hormonal imbalance. However, 95 percent of the time, the cause is unknown. Increased blood pressure may result when arteries are narrowed or when the volume of blood that moves through the arteries increases. Most researchers believe that the kidneys are involved in the narrowing of the arteries because the kidneys play a role in the release of renin, which controls arterial wall constriction.

Narrowed arteries tend to resist the flow of blood as it leaves the heart, which places additional pressure on the left ventricle to pump the blood out. If resistance to the flow of blood from the left ventricle continues, the muscle of the ventricle wall enlarges and forms abnormal tissue, which eventually can lead to heart failure. Increased pressure can also lead to stroke and kidney damage.

High blood pressure over a long period of time also results in increased wear and tear on the arteries. Thus, there is always the danger that a weakness in one of the artery walls might rupture, resulting in heart failure, cerebral hemorrhage, or kidney failure.

Many individuals with hypertension may be completely unaware of it. Even mild hypertension (diastolic pressure of 90 to 104 mmHg) may be dangerous. Fortunately, control of hypertension has been aided by a number of effective drugs.

Considerable evidence indicates that continuous, rigorous exercise can reduce resting diastolic and systolic blood pressures in middle-aged people. The reduction, however, is most significant in men and women who are leading sedentary lives, who are in poor physical fitness, and who have high blood pressure. Individuals under thirty years of age probably will see no reduction in blood pressure resulting from exercise.

Individuals with high blood pressure should avoid isometric exercises such as lifting and arm-support types of exercises or exercises where the breath is held during lifting. The sustained muscle contraction required in isometrics causes occlusion of the blood and results in increased pressure in the arteries and the heart. Increases as high as diastolic 20 mmHg during exercise can be very dangerous.

Tips for Regulating Blood Pressure

Keep weight at desirable level.

Exercise regularly.

If you drink, limit alcohol to two drinks a day.

Don't smoke.

Low sodium, low-fat diet.

Eat a diet with adequate amounts of calcium, magnesium, and potassium.

High Blood Cholesterol Levels

While the complex process that produces atherosclerosis is still not well understood, it *is* known that cholesterol is an important component of arterial plaque. **Cholesterol** is a fatty alcohol produced by the body and by eating certain foods, and it is found in all body cells that serve as building blocks for cell components and hormones. Its exact role in plaque formation is not really clear.

Cholesterol is transported in the blood with three special kinds of proteins, called lipoproteins, which are differentiated by their density: **high-density lipoprotein (HDL), low-density lipoprotein (LDL),** and **very low-density lipoprotein (VLDL).** High-density lipoproteins appear to protect against coronary atherosclerosis, while low-density lipoproteins seem to promote the disease process. Yet, paradoxically, both HDL and LDL contain cholesterol. It is theorized that HDL works against the atherosclerosis process by resisting the movement of low-density cholesterol into the arterial wall and/or by promoting the influx of cholesterol from the tissues to the liver, where it is broken down and excreted.

The relative distribution of cholesterol into the three types of lipoproteins may be as important as the overall cholesterol level in the blood. Studies indicate that women, lean people, nonsmokers, moderate drinkers, and people who exercise have relatively higher levels of HDL than men, obese people, smokers, nondrinkers, and sedentary people. The effect of diet on HDL is not clear. It is clear, however, that people vary widely not only in their coronary risk factor but also in their blood composition and their response to diet.

Tips to Lower High Serum LDL Cholesterol

1. Reduce saturated fatty acids and cholesterol intake by 10 percent, and total fat to below 30 percent.
2. Perform regular exercise.
3. Maintain a desirable body weight.
4. Increase intake of soluble fiber.

TABLE 3.4   Your Blood Test: What Do Those Numbers Mean?

Your lipid levels can tell your doctor whether you're a candidate for cardiovascular disease. As you compare your numbers with these, remember: Numbers alone don't tell the whole story. Rely on your physician to interpret your test results.

Test	Your level (in mg/DL)*		
	Desirable	*Borderline*	*Undesirable*
Total cholesterol	Below 200	200–240	Above 240
HDL cholesterol	Above 45	35–45	Below 35
Triglycerides	Below 200	200–400	Above 400
LDL cholesterol	Below 130	130–160	Above 160
Cholesterol/HDL	Below 4.5	4.5–5.5	Above 5.5
LDL/HDL	Below 3	3–5	Above 5

---

*For people without known heart disease
Note: The numbers in this table represent a compilation of informed medical opinions from a variety of sources.

5. Eat fish on a regular basis.

6. Keep all types of coffee consumption to prudent levels, two to three cups per day.

Your cells need cholesterol to make cell membranes and hormones. But when total blood cholesterol is over 150 mg/DL or your LDL cholesterol is over 90 mg/DL, the cells have more cholesterol than they can use and have no way to get rid of the excess. Since the cells cannot bring down or oxidize the cholesterol, the result is a buildup of a waxy cholesterol deposit that can eventually choke the cells. (See table 3.4 for borderline high, low, and high cholesterol levels.)

Your total cholesterol divided by your HDL should be under 4.5. The ideal ratio is under 3.5. If your total cholesterol is over 240 mg/DL, LDL is a better predictor because few people have enough HDL to counteract the high levels of LDLs. When total cholesterol is between 200 mg/DL and 240 mg/DL, the total cholesterol/HDL ratio predicts your risk of heart disease three to four times better than LDL levels and five to six times better than total cholesterol.

Triglycerides are the major form of fat in the body (95 percent) and are made up of one cluster of glycerol and three clusters of fatty acids. Triglycerides are transported in the blood primarily in very low-density lipoproteins (VLDL). According to the Framingham Heart Study, there is a possible subgroup of both men and women with high triglyceride levels of 150 mg/DL or higher who also have very low HDLs—under 40 mg/DL. These people have a kind of VLDL that is very bad for their arteries. The majority of people with this ''bad'' VLDL have triglyceride levels between 190 mg/DL and 210 mg/DL and HDL levels under 40 mg/DL.

If the serum HDL level is greater than 60 mg/DL there is a lower risk. If the HDL is less than 40 mg/DL the risk is increased (see table 3.4). Women generally have higher HDL levels, from 50 to 60 mg/DL, compared to men, from 35 to 40 mg/DL. Estrogen produced by the ovaries in the childbearing years helps keep HDL cholesterol levels high. Regular exercise may raise serum HDL levels a bit (5 mg per 100) by reducing fat. The more exercise the better. (See table 3.4 for appropriate levels of blood cholesterol.)

Evidence indicates that HDL plays an important role in predicting coronary risk. Rather than clogging the arteries, HDL keeps them clean. A low level of HDL cholesterol, typically below 35 mg/DL, raises coronary risks even when the total cholesterol and LDL levels are normal. A high level of HDL decreases the risk posed by elevated LDL levels. Overall, HDL seems to predict coronary heart disease at least as accurately as total cholesterol and LDL.

Some individuals have a genetic predisposition to high serum cholesterol levels. Exercise and low-fat diets may be ineffective in lowering these levels. Medication is generally the last resort for treating high LDL or low HDL cholesterol. Most are quite expensive and all have side effects.

The American Heart Association advises that an individual stay below the limit of approximately 250 milligrams of cholesterol a day, or slightly more than the amount found in one egg. On the average, Americans currently consume approximately 450 milligrams daily, with women consuming roughly 350 milligrams and men consuming 550 milligrams.

If your cholesterol level is over 200 milligrams, health professionals strongly advise that you determine your LDL level. Even though there have been breakthroughs in drug therapy, the best approach in reducing cholesterol is through diet modification. Saturated fats (see chapter 9) raise cholesterol along with increasing the level of triglycerides in the blood. They are found primarily in animal products, such as beef, pork, lamb, and chicken, and in eggyolk; dairy fats of cream, milk, butter, cheese; and coconut, palm oil, vegetable shortening, and hydrogenated margarine.

A food product that is currently getting a lot of attention is fish oil. What makes fish oil important is that it contains a unique kind of polyunsaturated fatty acid called **omega-3,** which the fish obtain by eating certain plants. Omega-3 significantly reduces blood clotting and lessens the chance of a clot forming in the coronary arteries.

Fish oil also aids in lowering total cholesterol and triglycerides in the blood while increasing HDLs (high-density lipoproteins). The general rule is the darker the flesh, the more fat it contains. Fish with the highest fat content, and thus the most omega-3s, include mackerel, lake trout, herring, tuna, and salmon. In addition to eating fish, you can also get the oil from new capsule concentrates or cod liver oil. Fish oil pills, however, do have some drawbacks. Some health-related concerns about these pills include: they may contain pesticides and other contaminants; they contain vitamins A and D, which may be toxic in high doses; and prolonged use may produce a vitamin E deficiency. It is still not clear whether omega-3s by themselves provide all the health benefits of fish oil. It is possible that these fatty acids work with other elements in fish not found in supplements. It is recommended to eat fish rather than supplements until there is more complete research.

Smoking

The American Cancer Society's findings indicate that by the age of eighty-five, only 5 percent of lifetime smokers are still alive, as compared with 37 percent of those who never smoked. In addition, smokers at age thirty can expect to live an average age of 64.8 years if they continue to smoke, while nonsmoking thirty-year-olds can expect to reach the age of 82.7.

Cigarette smoking both increases the smoker's airway resistance and decreases the amount of oxygen carried in the blood. Airway resistance is specifically the result of long-term smoking and is caused by narrowing of the bronchial tubes from smoke particles, tar, and constriction of small blood vessels. If severe enough, airway resistance can lead to decreased endurance since there is reduced oxygen exchange, which ultimately results in a reduced oxygen supply to the heart and muscles.

A reduction in the amount of oxygen carried in the blood also is produced by carbon monoxide—the by-product of cigarette smoking. Carbon monoxide has a greater capacity for combining with hemoglobin (the major component of red blood cells, which carry oxygen) than does oxygen. Therefore, when both carbon monoxide and oxygen are present, carbon monoxide is quicker to combine with hemoglobin. And since oxygen and carbon monoxide cannot be carried simultaneously by hemoglobin, the oxygen-carrying capacity of the blood is sharply reduced.

In addition, the nicotine found in cigarettes causes vasoconstriction of the blood vessels, reducing their surface area and the amount of oxygen that can be absorbed into the blood during respiration.

A reduced amount or abnormally low level of oxygen in the coronary circulation results in reduced oxygen to the heart muscle, which can produce ischemia or possible tissue damage. Smoking also results in narrowing or constriction of coronary arteries, further reducing oxygen supply.

Diabetes Mellitus

Diabetes mellitus is a metabolic disorder of energy metabolism caused by an absolute or relative deficiency of insulin. The major problem of diabetes is that glucose has difficulty getting to the cells of the body. Instead, it remains in the blood and builds up to high levels.

Atherosclerosis tends to develop easily in some diabetics, and the arteries become blocked by the formation of plaque. The diseased arteries not only affect the heart but also the eyes and kidneys.

During rigorous exercise, certain diabetics may need more food since exercise has an insulin-like effect. General guidelines are that no extra food is needed for exercise of short duration and modest intensity. During moderate exercise (for example, playing golf), 10 to 15 grams of carbohydrates are allowed per hour. During vigorous exercise (for example, playing basketball and jogging), 20 to 30 grams of carbohydrates may be needed.

Evidence indicates that regular exercise can reduce the amounts of sugars and fats in the blood of diabetics.

Obesity

Obesity (excessive body fat) ironically is one of the most important and least understood areas in the science of nutrition. Considerable evidence, however, has linked obesity to coronary heart disease. Hypertension occurs about three times as often in obese individuals. Among adults ages twenty through forty-four, over-fat individuals are five to six times more likely than others to have hypertension. Also, high blood cholesterol levels occur more than twice as often in the obese as in the nonobese, and the prevalence of diabetes is nearly three times as high. Fat people also die younger from a host of problems, including strokes, heart attacks, and diabetes. In fact, gaining fat appears to precipitate diabetes. Being overfat can cause blood sugar, blood pressure, and blood lipids to climb upward. Fortunately, obesity is reversible in many cases, and if corrected in time, the risk factors also may be reversed.

Physical Activity and Coronary Heart Disease

Regular physical activity has been found to be an essential ingredient in reducing the risk of coronary heart disease. The Blair study (see chapter 1) showed that a high prevalence of sedentary habits and low physical-fitness levels produce high attributable risk factors for coronary heart disease, and that even moderate levels of physical activity appear to be protective against early mortality from coronary heart disease. Regular exercise may also:

1. Reduce triglyceride levels and increase the levels of high-density lipoproteins that seem to afford some protection against heart disease
2. Affect the pituitary gland, which may, in turn, lower lipid (fat) levels in the blood
3. Result in fat loss, which is a major factor in heart disease

4. Reduce emotional tension, which may increase the body threshold to stress response
5. Result in the regression of atheroma (the blocked portion of the artery) in major arteries

Endurance training may improve metabolic capacity and have a modifying effect on a number of other factors involved in the development of heart disease. Changes in metabolic function, such as decreased resting heart rate, increased myocardial efficiency, peripheral blood distribution, and reduced arterial blood pressure, may all lessen the load on the heart.

The American Heart Association states that, "Exercise training can increase cardiovascular functional capacity and decrease myocardial oxygen demand for any given level of physical activity in normal persons as well as most cardiac patients. Regular physical activity is required to maintain the training effects. The potential risk of vigorous physical activity can be reduced by appropriate medical clearance, education, and guidance. Exercise may aid efforts to control cigarette smoking, hypertension, lipid abnormalities, diabetes, obesity, and emotional stress. Evidence suggests that regular, moderate, or vigorous occupational or leisure time physical activity may protect against coronary heart disease and may improve the likelihood of survival from a heart attack."[1]

There is evidence that much of the improved functional capacity due to exercise is not directly related to the heart. Many times, the improvement in fitness is due to increases in the ability of skeletal muscle cells to extract oxygen more efficiently from the blood. Of course, this phenomenon is also true for heart muscle cells.

Table 3.5 shows the mechanics by which physical activity can reduce the occurrence or severity of coronary heart disease.

Coronary Heart Disease and Stress

Emotional stress may chronically overstimulate a part of the nervous system that can cause spasms in the coronary arteries and produce clumping of the blood platelets (blood cells essential for the clotting of blood). The net effect is a sudden reduction of blood flow to the heart, precipitating irregular beats and a possible heart attack. This condition may result even when there is no severe blockage in the coronary arteries.

Personality factors appear to play a part in catalyzing this problem. Two personality types have been identified: "hot reactors" and "cold reactors." Hot reactors tend to overrespond physiologically under stress, even though they

[1]American Heart Association, "Subcommittee on Exercise and Cardiac Rehabilitation: Statement on Exercise," *Circulation* 64 (1981):1302–04.

TABLE 3.5 Mechanics by Which Physical Activity Can Reduce Occurrence or Severity of Coronary Heart Disease	
Physical activity increases:	**Physical activity decreases:**
Coronary collateral vascularization (?)	Serum lipid levels:
Vessel size	Triglycerides
HDL cholesterol	LDL cholesterol
Myocardial efficiency	Glucose intolerance
Efficiency of peripheral blood distribution and return	Obesity-adiposity
Electron-transport capacity	Platelet stickiness
Fibrinolytic capability	Arterial blood pressure
Red blood cell mass and blood volume	Heart rate
Thyroid function	Vulnerability to dysrhythmias
Tolerance to stress	Neurohormonal overreaction
Prudent living habits	"Strain" associated with psychic "stress"
"Joie de vivre"*	The size of atheroma
Width of coronary artery lumina	Collagen accumulation in coronary arteries
Metabolic turnover of collagen in the heart	

Source: From Fox, S. M., J. P. Naughton, and W. L. Haskell, "Physical Activity and the Prevention of Coronary Heart Disease," in *Annals of Clinical Research* 3:404–432, 1971, Helsinki, Finland.
*Joy of Life

appear calm on the outside. They may suffer increased blood pressure, coronary artery spasms, and increased resistance to blood flow. Cold reactors, on the other hand, have a normal cardiovascular response to stress, with blood pressure, heart output, and blood vessels changing slowly or only slightly, appropriate to demand. Some evidence indicates that, because a hot reactor's response may be the result of learned experience, the possibly dangerous physiological response may be unlearned through appropriate stress-reduction methods.

Age

Generally the older you are, the greater your risk for a heart attack. For example between ages of twenty-five and thirty-four the death rate due to heart attack is about ten in every 100,000 white males. At ages fifty-five to sixty-four this increases one hundred fold to nearly 1,000 deaths in 100,000 males.

Gender

The incidence of coronary heart disease is greater in young males than in young females. The lower death rate due to heart disease among young females is primarily related to the production of estrogen. After menopause the estrogen levels drop sharply, increasing the risk for the older female. By the time women reach age sixty, women develop coronary heart disease at the same rate as men age fifty. This ten-year gap prevails until about the age of seventy-five to eighty, when the difference disappears and the rates become similar.

Race

Some African Americans have an elevated risk of coronary heart disease because they have a higher risk of hypertension and diabetes than white people. Puerto Ricans, Cubans, and Mexican Americans are also more likely to have high blood pressure than Anglo-Americans.

Hostility As a Risk Factor?

The American Heart Association has indicated that there is mounting evidence that hostility (being cynical, angry, easily provoked) may be linked to an increased risk of coronary heart disease. The exaggerated response to everyday stress causes excessive amounts of stress hormones, such as epinephrine, to be dumped into the blood. This increases heart rate and blood pressure. In addition, the strain of the hormone laden blood appears to narrow and injure artery walls and make them more susceptible to blood clots and plaque deposits.

Exercise and Heart Attacks

There is concern that exercise in some individuals may provoke a heart attack, particularly in a person unaccustomed to exercising. Even though exercise may be hazardous for a few people, the lack of exercise is a true danger for most. Individuals who normally exercise infrequently or not at all are at the greatest risk when they exert themselves. It is theorized that heavy exercise increases blood flow and blood pressure, which may dislodge plaque from the wall of the coronary artery, setting up a series of events leading to the blockage of blood flow to the heart. This should not scare people into thinking that exercise is dangerous. The beneficial effects for the majority of people far outweigh the hazardous ones for the minority. Numerous studies have shown that exercise, when performed regularly and over the long term, reduces the risk of coronary artery disease and heart attack by 35 to 55 percent.

Coronary Rehabilitation

Exercise therapy is one intervention in the treatment of individuals who have suffered a heart attack or who are prone to coronary heart disease. Evidence shows that post-heart attack individuals involved in exercise rehabilitation programs show reduced anxiety and depression, improved self-concept, reduced

S.T. depression on an electrocardiogram (which indicates ventricular recovery), reduced blood pressure, reduced resting heart rate, improved exercise capacity, reduced cholesterol and triglyceride levels, and an elevated level of high-density lipoprotein cholesterol.

The primary goal of cardiac rehabilitation is to help patients reach their optimum physiological and psychological condition. Physical activity should be part of a comprehensive program that includes proper diet, weight control, cessation of smoking, and other social and emotional factors.

While heart attack victims are in the hospital, they should have graded physical activity so that when they leave the hospital, they are able to meet the demands of normal activity, for example, dressing, showering, or walking up a flight of stairs. After leaving the hospital, they should participate in outpatient supervised exercise usually three days a week, while being closely monitored by a physician. Evidence indicates that some active physical training can begin as early as three weeks after a heart attack if the exercise is preceded by an intensive physical examination.

The heart attack victim's exercise prescription should be based on careful evaluation with treadmill testing to determine safe parameters, and it should be evaluated periodically. Each individual should maintain a daily training record of intensity, duration, and frequency of exercise. Activities such as walking, jogging, cycling, and swimming are appropriate. Exercising in groups; close, professional supervision; careful evaluation of distress signals; slow warm-ups with gradual increases in the exercise intervals; and periodic heart rate and electrocardiograph monitoring are essential. Cardiac patients involved in any heavy exercise should take some precautions and avoid unnecessary risks.

Fear of exercise is a common problem among those who have suffered a heart attack. Renewed physical exercise, accompanied by physical stress symptoms, may be viewed as dangerous and cause unnecessary anxiety. The anxiety usually decreases, however, as the individual gains confidence through a responsible exercise program.

Key Terms

Atherosclerosis
The most common type of coronary heart disease; caused by the collection of plaque on the inner walls of the arteries

Cholesterol
A fatty alcohol produced by the body and by eating certain foods; elevated levels are associated with an increased risk of heart disease

Coronary Heart Disease
A disease of the arteries that supply blood to the heart muscle

Diabetes Mellitus
A metabolic disorder of energy metabolism caused by an absolute or relative deficiency of insulin

Diastolic Blood Pressure
The lowest level of pressure exerted against the walls of the arteries during ventricular relaxation

High-Density Lipoprotein (HDL)
A class of lipoprotein, high levels of which are thought to provide some protection against coronary heart disease

Hypertension
High blood pressure; chronically elevated blood pressure above the normal level considered healthy for an individual's age and sex

Low-Density Lipoprotein (LDL)
A class of lipoprotein, high levels of which are associated with greater risk of coronary heart disease

Myocardial Infarction (MI)
Death of muscle cells in the heart because of reduced oxygen supply; heart attack

Obesity
Excessive body fat: males—over 20 percent, females—over 30 percent

Omega-3
A unique type of polyunsaturated fatty acid from fish oil that reduces blood clotting

Plaque
Deposits of cholesterol, lipids, blood cells, calcium, and tissue debris on the inner walls of arteries; a primary factor in atherosclerosis

Primary Risk Factor
This factor alone increases the risk of coronary heart disease

Secondary Risk Factor
This factor increases the risk of coronary heart disease only if one of the primary factors is present or that its significance has not been determined

Systolic Blood Pressure
The highest level of pressure exerted against the walls of the arteries from ventricular contraction

Triglycerides
Stored form of free fatty acids

4

Fitness Evaluation

Chapter Concepts

After you have studied this chapter you should be able to

1. describe the importance of fitness evaluation before starting an exercise program;

2. describe cardiorespiratory endurance;

3. describe body composition;

4. explain the tests for cardiorespiratory endurance—the 1.5-mile run, step test, bicycle ergometer test, swimming test, walking test;

5. explain the tests for body composition—skinfold, girth, and body mass index;

6. explain the test for flexibility—modified sit-and-reach test;

7. explain the tests for muscle strength—the bench press, leg press, shoulder press, and biceps curl—and explain the muscle endurance tests—push-ups, head-and-shoulder raise, leg power test; and

8. describe the fitness profile.

Evaluating Your Fitness

The old saying, "You can't get lost if you don't know where you are going," is very appropriate to starting a fitness program. It is vital that an objective evaluation of your present fitness status be made so that the proper intensity, duration, and frequency of exercise can be prescribed. This evaluation enables you to set reasonable fitness goals and prevents unnecessary stress on your body systems.

The tests in this chapter evaluate the four basic components of physical fitness: (1) cardiorespiratory endurance, (2) body composition, (3) flexibility, and

(4) muscle strength and endurance. Norms are provided for each fitness component so that you are able to compare your fitness levels with the prescribed norms for your age and sex.

These tests, which have been used for a number of years, have provided thousands of individuals their first chance to assess their fitness. Because of the many variables found in fitness tests, such as sex, age, height, weight, and flexibility, these tests are not precise measures and are subject to error. With this in mind, don't overemphasize the importance of the test standards. They are to be used as general guides for the outline of your fitness program and as indicators of how you compare with other individuals of your age and sex.

Your physical fitness profile charts (tables 4.16–4.28 and figures 4.18 and 4.19) are found at the end of the chapter. When they are properly filled out, the interpretation of your profile will point out areas in need of improvement and provide the starting levels for your exercise program. You should reevaluate all of the fitness components six to eight weeks after commencing your exercise program.

Tests for Cardiorespiratory Endurance

The chief means of evaluating cardiorespiratory endurance is to determine the body's capacity to consume oxygen at a maximum rate. In other words, determine the greatest amount of oxygen that can be used by the cells per unit of time during maximum exercise, which is referred to as the maximum oxygen uptake ($\dot{V}O_2$ max). The assessment of oxygen uptake through laboratory testing is accurate, but it requires a certain amount of time and sophisticated equipment, which would be impractical for determining your own fitness. Instead, there are a number of cardiovascular tests that indirectly measure the amount of maximum oxygen uptake by determining the heart rate response to certain prescribed exercises.

Five different tests are provided for you to measure your cardiorespiratory endurance: the 1.5-mile run, the step test, the bicycle ergometer test, the swimming test, and the walking test. These tests, which measure the heart's response to various intensities of exercise, are good measures of your cardiorespiratory endurance level.

The 1.5-mile run should be attempted only by those individuals in good enough condition to run this distance. All others should use either the step test, the bicycle ergometer test, the swimming test, or the walking test. The bicycle ergometer and the swimming test, unlike the others, are nonweight-bearing tests, which are more appropriate if you plan to cycle or swim for fitness. You also may wish to take all five tests; in this way, you have a more reliable measure of your fitness. However, you need take only *one* of the following five tests before starting your exercise program.

1.5-Mile Run

The 1.5-mile test can be run on an oval track or on a straightaway. You only should consider this test if you have been conditioned to run this distance or are in good physical condition. If you are over thirty years of age, you should not take this test unless you have had a stress electrocardiogram that was normal or have had a thorough physical examination. If you become overtired while running, shift down to a slow jog or walk. Do not unduly overstress yourself. Keep track of the amount of time it takes you to run the 1.5 miles, and then find your fitness level in table 4.1. Record your score and fitness level on your fitness evaluation form (table 4.16).

Step Test

This five-minute pulse-recovery step test consists of stepping at approximately twenty-three steps per minute for exactly five minutes.

Equipment needed for the test includes (1) a bench that is 15¾ inches (40 centimeters) high for men or 13 inches (33 centimeters) high for women and (2) a metronome or another audible signaling device (for example, a tape-recorded metronome) programmed for ninety beats per minute. Room temperature should be between sixty-eight degrees and seventy-four degrees Fahrenheit (F).

The test directions are as follows:

1. Take your resting heart rate five minutes before the test. Rest five minutes before taking heart rate.
2. Step onto the bench with one foot (tick), then the other (tock), and return to the floor (tick, tock) in a four-count sequence. You should complete one sequence approximately every three seconds.
3. After completing five minutes of exercise, sit down and take your pulse for exactly fifteen seconds, starting exactly at fifteen seconds and ending exactly at thirty seconds after exercise. The pulse is taken by placing four fingertips in the groove directly below the base of the thumb on the underside of the wrist.
4. Weigh yourself in the clothing worn during the test.

The step test should not be given after strenuous activity, immediately after drinking coffee or smoking, or in an extremely warm room (above seventy-eight degrees Fahrenheit).

When properly administered, the step test gives an accurate estimate of your maximum oxygen uptake, or physical fitness. Scores do not fluctuate even with extreme differences in resting heart rates. In addition, this test does not place undue stress on the respiratory and circulatory systems. Therefore, it is especially useful in screening individuals who are at various levels of physical fitness.

TABLE 4.1 Aerobic Fitness Guidelines for the 1.5-Mile Test (Times in Minutes)

Fitness category		Age (years)		
		13–19	20–29	30–39
I. Very poor	(men)	>15:31*	>16:01	>16:31
	(women)	>18:31	>19:01	>19:31
II. Poor	(men)	12:11–15:30	14:01–16:00	14:44–16:30
	(women)	16:55–18:30	18:31–19:00	19:01–19:30
III. Average	(men)	10:49–12:10	12:01–14:00	12:31–14:45
	(women)	14:31–16:54	15:55–18:30	16:31–19:00
IV. Good	(men)	9:41–10:48	10:46–12:00	11:01–12:30
	(women)	12:30–14:30	13:31–15:54	14:31–16:30
V. Excellent	(men)	8:37– 9:40	9:45–10:45	10:00–11:00
	(women)	11:50–12:29	12:30–13:30	13:00–14:30
VI. Superior	(men)	<8:37	<9:45	<10:00
	(women)	<11:50	<12:30	<13:00

Fitness category		Age (years)		
		40–49	50–59	60+
I. Very poor	(men)	>17:31	>19:01	>20:01
	(women)	>20:01	>20:31	>21:01
II. Poor	(men)	15:36–17:30	17:01–19:00	19:01–20:00
	(women)	19:31–20:00	20:01–20:30	21:00–21:31
III. Average	(men)	13:01–15:35	14:31–17:00	16:16–19:00
	(women)	17:31–19:30	19:01–20:00	19:31–20:30
IV. Good	(men)	11:31–13:00	12:31–14:30	14:00–16:15
	(women)	15:56–17:30	16:31–19:00	17:31–19:30
V. Excellent	(men)	10:30–11:30	11:00–12:30	11:15–13:59
	(women)	13:45–15:55	14:30–16:30	16:30–17:30
VI. Superior	(men)	<10:30	<11:00	<11:15
	(women)	<13:45	<14:30	<16:30

*< Means "less than"; > means "more than."

Source: From The Aerobics Program for Total Well-Being by Kenneth Cooper, MD. Copyright 1982 by Kenneth H. Cooper. Used by permission of Bantam Books, a division of Bantam Doubleday Dell, Publishing Corp., Inc.

To determine your cardiorespiratory endurance category, refer to tables 4.2 and 4.3, which are fitness indexes for men and women; to table 4.4 for age-adjusted scores; and to table 4.5 for a fitness rating. Then record your score and fitness level on your fitness evaluation form (table 4.17).

To use the fitness indexes in tables 4.2 and 4.3, locate the number that is in the column directly above your body weight (bottom horizontal column) and that intersects with the row horizontal to your post-exercise heart rate found in the

---

TABLE 4.2 Fitness Index for Men (Step Test)

Fitness score

Postexercise pulse count	120	130	140	150	160	170	180	190	200	210	220	230	240
45	33	33	33	33	33	32	32	32	32	32	32	32	32
44	34	34	34	34	33	33	33	33	33	33	33	33	33
43	35	35	35	34	34	34	34	34	34	34	34	34	34
42	36	35	35	35	35	35	35	35	35	35	35	34	34
41	36	36	36	36	36	36	36	36	36	36	36	35	35
40	37	37	37	37	37	37	37	37	36	36	36	36	36
39	38	38	38	38	38	38	38	38	38	38	38	37	37
38	39	39	39	39	39	39	39	39	39	39	39	38	38
37	41	40	40	40	40	40	40	40	40	40	40	39	39
36	42	42	41	41	41	41	41	41	41	41	41	40	40
35	43	43	42	42	42	42	42	42	42	42	42	42	41
34	44	44	43	43	43	43	43	43	43	43	43	43	43
33	46	45	45	45	45	45	44	44	44	44	44	44	44
32	47	47	46	46	46	46	46	46	46	46	46	46	46
31	48	48	48	47	47	47	47	47	47	47	47	47	47
30	50	49	49	49	48	48	48	48	48	48	48	48	48
29	52	51	51	51	50	50	50	50	50	50	50	50	50
28	53	53	53	53	52	52	52	52	52	52	51	51	51
27	55	55	55	54	54	54	54	54	54	53	53	53	52
26	57	57	56	56	56	56	56	56	56	55	55	54	54
25	59	59	58	58	58	58	58	58	58	56	56	55	55
24	60	60	60	60	60	60	60	59	59	58	58	57	
23	62	62	61	61	61	61	61	60	60	60	59		
22	64	64	63	63	63	63	62	62	61	61			
21	66	66	65	65	65	64	64	64	62				
20	68	68	67	67	67	66	66	65					
Body weight	120	130	140	150	160	170	180	190	200	210	220	230	240

Source: "Step Test," by Brian Sharkey, copyright 1984, Human Kinetics Publ., Champaign, IL 61820.
Obtain your age-adjusted score from table 4.4.

left-hand column. Now locate this number in the top horizontal column of table 4.4. The number that is in the column directly below this number and in the row horizontal to your age is your age-adjusted score. Finally, locate your age-adjusted score in the row horizontal to your nearest age in table 4.5 to determine your fitness rating.

TABLE 4.3 Fitness Index for Women (Step Test)

Fitness score

Postexercise pulse count	80	90	100	110	120	130	140	150	160	170	180	190
45										29	29	29
44								30	30	30	30	30
43							31	31	31	31	31	31
42			32	32	32	32	32	32	32	32	32	32
41			33	33	33	33	33	33	33	33	33	33
40			34	34	34	34	34	34	34	34	34	34
39			35	35	35	35	35	35	35	35	35	35
38			36	36	36	36	36	36	36	36	36	36
37			37	37	37	37	37	37	37	37	37	37
36		37	38	38	38	38	38	38	38	38	38	38
35	38	38	39	39	39	39	39	39	39	39	39	39
34	39	39	40	40	40	40	40	40	40	40	40	40
33	40	40	41	41	41	41	41	41	41	41	41	41
32	41	41	42	42	42	42	42	42	42	42	42	42
31	42	42	43	43	43	43	43	43	43	43	43	43
30	43	43	44	44	44	44	44	44	44	44	44	44
29	44	44	45	45	45	45	45	45	45	45	45	45
28	45	45	46	46	46	47	47	47	47	47	47	
27	46	46	47	48	48	49	49	49	49	49		
26	47	48	49	50	50	51	51	51	51			
25	49	50	51	52	52	53	53					
24	51	52	53	54	54	55						
23	53	54	55	56	56	57						
Body weight	80	90	100	110	120	130	140	150	160	170	180	190

Source: "Step Test," by Brian Sharkey, copyright 1984, Human Kinetics Publ., Champaign, IL 61820. **Obtain your age-adjusted score from table 4.4.**

For example, a twenty-year-old male who weighs 160 pounds and has a postexercise heart rate of 29 (per 15 seconds) would have a score of 50 (table 4.2). A score of 50 for a twenty-year-old male results in an age-adjusted score of 51 (table 4.4). The fitness rating in table 4.5 for a score of 51 is "excellent."

TABLE 4.4 Age-Adjusted Fitness Scores (Step Test)

Enter fitness score
↓

Nearest age	30	31	32	33	34	35	36	37	38	39	40	41	42	43	44	45	46	47	48	49	50
15	32	33	34	35	36	37	38	39	40	41	42	43	44	45	46	47	48	49	50	51	53
20	31	32	33	34	35	36	37	38	39	40	41	42	43	44	45	46	47	48	49	50	51
25	30	31	32	33	34	35	36	37	38	39	40	41	42	43	44	45	46	47	48	49	50
30	29	30	31	32	33	34	35	36	37	38	39	40	41	42	43	44	45	46	47	48	49
35	27	28	29	31	32	33	34	35	36	37	38	39	40	41	42	43	44	45	46	47	48
40	26	27	28	30	31	32	33	34	35	36	37	38	39	40	41	42	43	44	45	46	47
45	25	26	27	29	30	31	32	33	34	35	36	37	38	39	40	41	42	43	44	45	46
50	24	25	26	28	29	30	31	32	33	34	35	36	37	38	39	40	41	42	43	44	45
55	23	24	25	27	28	29	30	31	32	33	34	35	36	37	38	39	40	40	41	42	43
60	22	23	24	25	26	27	28	30	31	32	33	34	35	36	37	37	38	39	40	41	42
65	21	22	23	24	25	26	27	28	29	30	31	32	33	34	35	36	37	38	38	39	40

(*Nearest age* at left; *Age-adjusted score* at right)

Enter fitness score
↓

Nearest age	51	52	53	54	55	56	57	58	59	60	61	62	63	64	65	66	67	68	69	70	71	72
15	54	55	56	57	58	59	60	61	62	63	64	65	66	67	68	69	70	71	72	74	75	76
20	52	53	54	55	56	57	58	59	60	61	62	63	64	65	66	67	68	69	70	71	72	73
25	51	52	53	54	55	56	57	58	59	60	61	62	63	64	65	66	67	68	69	70	71	72
30	50	51	52	53	54	55	56	57	58	59	60	61	62	63	64	65	66	67	68	69	70	71
35	49	50	51	52	53	54	55	56	57	58	59	60	60	61	62	63	64	65	66	67	68	69
40	48	49	50	51	52	53	54	55	55	56	57	58	59	60	61	62	63	64	65	66	67	68
45	47	48	49	50	51	52	52	53	54	55	56	57	58	59	60	61	62	63	64	65	65	66
50	45	46	47	48	49	50	51	52	53	53	54	55	56	57	58	58	59	61	61	62	63	64
55	44	45	46	46	47	48	49	50	51	52	53	53	54	55	56	57	58	59	59	60	61	62
60	42	43	44	45	46	46	47	48	49	50	51	51	52	53	54	55	56	57	57	58	59	60
65	41	42	42	43	44	45	46	46	47	48	49	50	50	51	52	53	54	54	55	56	57	58

(*Nearest age* at left; *Age-adjusted score* at right)

Source: ''Step Test,'' by Brian Sharkey, copyright 1984, Human Kinetics Publ., Champaign, IL 61820.
Now get your step test fitness rating from table 4.5.

TABLE 4.5 Fitness Rating of Men and Women (Step Test)

Physical fitness rating—men

(Use age-adjusted score from table 4.4)

Nearest age							
15	57+	56–52	51–47	46–42	41–37	36–32	31–
20	56+	55–51	50–46	45–41	40–36	35–31	30–
25	55+	54–50	49–45	44–40	39–35	34–30	29–
30	54+	53–49	48–44	43–39	38–34	33–29	28–
35	53+	52–48	47–43	42–38	37–33	32–28	27–
40	52+	51–47	46–42	41–37	36–32	31–27	26–
45	51+	50–46	45–41	40–36	35–31	30–26	25–
50	50+	49–45	44–40	39–35	34–30	29–25	24–
55	49+	48–44	43–39	38–34	33–29	28–24	23–
60	48+	47–43	42–38	37–33	32–28	27–23	22–
65	47+	48–42	41–37	36–32	31–27	26–22	21–
	Superior	Excellent	Very good	Good	Average	Poor	Very Poor

Fitness level

Physical fitness rating—women

(Use age-adjusted score from table 4.4)

Nearest age							
15	54+	53–49	48–44	43–39	38–34	33–29	28–
20	53+	52–48	47–43	42–38	37–33	32–28	27–
25	52+	51–47	46–42	41–37	36–32	31–27	26–
30	51+	50–46	45–41	40–36	35–31	30–26	25–
35	50+	49–45	44–40	39–35	34–30	29–25	24–
40	49+	48–44	43–39	38–34	33–29	28–24	23–
45	48+	47–43	42–38	37–33	32–28	27–23	22–
50	47+	46–42	41–37	36–32	31–27	26–22	21–
55	46+	45–41	40–36	35–31	30–26	25–21	20–
60	45+	44–40	39–35	34–30	29–25	24–20	19–
65	44+	43–39	38–34	33–29	28–24	23–20	19–
	Superior	Excellent	Very good	Good	Average	Poor	Very poor

Fitness level

Source: ''Step Test,'' by Brian Sharkey, copyright 1984, Human Kinetics Publ., Champaign, IL 61820.

Bicycle Ergometer Test

For those of you who have access to a bicycle ergometer (stationary bicycle), this is a simple five-minute test for measuring your aerobic fitness. The test directions are as follows:

1. The bicycle ergometer pedal speed should be set at 60 RPM (revolutions per minute) with a workload of 150 watts (900-kilopound meters per minute) for males and 100 watts (600-kilopound meters per minute) for females. Poorly conditioned individuals or those over forty years of age should exercise at a workload of 50 watts (300-kilopound meters per minute).

2. The exercise duration is five minutes. Warm up one minute with no load on the pedal before commencing the five-minute exercise.

3. Measure your heart rate for fifteen seconds during the latter half of the fifth minute.

Once you have determined your fifteen-second heart rate during the fifth minute of the exercise, find your fitness index score opposite your heart rate and underneath the appropriate workload column in table 4.6. Then locate your fitness level in table 4.7 opposite your age. For example, a twenty-five-year-old woman in good physical condition with a fifteen-second heart rate of 40 would have a fitness index score (from table 4.6) of 32. In table 4.7, a score of 32 opposite the age of twenty-five falls into the "average" category. Shifting one category to the right (female adjustment) gives a fitness level of "good."

Record the results of this bicycle ergometer test on your fitness evaluation form in table 4.18.

Swimming Test

The energy demands for swimming are much greater and subject to more variables than running-type exercises. Wide variations in individual skill levels directly affect energy requirements. For example, a highly skilled swimmer expends much less energy for a given distance than an individual with low-level skills. In addition to differences in swimming abilities, many individuals have difficulty breathing efficiently while swimming (mainly while doing the crawl), which can result in premature fatigue. It also is possible for an unskilled swimmer to score in the "excellent" category on the 1.5-mile run and in the "poor" category on the swimming test. Even individuals with good swimming skills who have not swum in some time may experience premature fatigue until the specific muscles needed for swimming have been properly conditioned. Therefore, the

TABLE 4.6	Bicycle Ergometer Fitness Index			
Fifteen-second heart rate	Men: 900 kpm/min (60 RPM × 150 watts)	Women: 600 kpm/min (60 RPM × 100 watts)	Poorly conditioned men or men over forty: 300 kpm/min (60 RPM × 50 watts)	Poorly conditioned women or women over forty: 300 kpm/min (60 RPM × 50 watts)
28	75	63	32	38
29	72	61	32	37
30	70	59	31	37
31	65	55	31	35
32	60	50	30	32
33	58	47	30	29
34	55	45	26	28
35	52	41	24	26
36	49	39	22	25
37	46	38	21	24
38	45	36	20	24
39	43	33		
40	41	32		
41	39	30		
42	38	29		
43	37	28		
44	35	27		
45	34	26		

Now get your bicycle ergometer fitness level from table 4.7.

specific nature of the swimming test makes it a more appropriate test for evaluating cardiorespiratory endurance if you plan to participate in a swimming program.

The test directions are as follows:

1. Warm up a few minutes by stretching before getting into the water.
2. Start off gradually and swim until you feel fatigued (out of breath). Do not push yourself to the limit.
3. Do not swim more than twelve minutes.
4. Determine the total distance and the total time you swim.

TABLE 4.7 Range of Maximum Oxygen Uptake (ml/kg/min) Values with Age (Bicycle Ergometer Test)

Age group (years)	Very poor	Poor	Average	Good	Very good	Excellent	Superior
10–19	Below 30	30–35	35–38	38–46	47–56	57–66	Above 66
20–29	Below 25	25–31	31–33	33–42	43–52	53–62	Above 62
30–39	Below 23	23–25	25–30	30–38	39–48	49–58	Above 58
40–49	Below 21	21–23	23–26	26–35	36–44	45–54	Above 54
50–59	Below 19	19–21	21–24	24–33	34–41	42–50	Above 50
60–69	Below 18	18–20	20–22	22–30	31–38	39–46	Above 46
70–79	Below 17	17–19	19–20	20–27	28–35	36–42	Above 42

Source: From Fox, E. L., Bicycle Ergometer Test, in *Journal of Applied Physiology.* Copyright 1973 American Physiological Association. Reprinted by permission.
Note: Since females are generally 20 percent lower (on average) compared to males, normal values for females can be obtained by shifting over one category to the right. For example, the "average" category for males would be considered "good" for females.

TABLE 4.8 Swimming Fitness

Distance in yards	Approximate time in minutes	Fitness level
700+	12 min	Superior
600–700	10–12 min	Excellent
500–600	10–12 min	Very good
400–500	10–12 min	Good
300–400	10–12 min	Average
200–300	8–10 min	Poor
0–200	6–8 min	Very poor

Source: From The Aerobics Program for Total Well-Being by Kenneth H. Cooper, MD. Copyright 1982 by Kenneth H. Cooper. Used by permission of Bantam Books, a division of Bantam Doubleday Dell, Publishing Corp., Inc.

Now find your fitness level in table 4.8. If your time falls above the time listed in the table for the distance that you completed, drop down one level to determine your score. Add 50 yards to your distance completed for each ten years over thirty years of age to arrive at an age-corrected fitness level. Record the results of this test on your fitness evaluation form in table 4.19.

Walking Test

To perform the test find a measured track or a flat course where you can measure a mile. Take time to warm up for several minutes first by stretching thoroughly or walking. Your walking shoes should have a roomy toe box, flexible soles with good traction, and a stiff heel cup for stability. Running shoes have too much padding, which makes your feet wobble.

Time yourself as you walk the mile as fast as you can without experiencing signs of exhaustion such as nausea or shortness of breath. When you finish, record your heart rate. (Take your pulse for 15 seconds and multiply by 4.) Cool down by walking slowly for a few minutes.

Table 4.9 will compare your current fitness level to "moderate" fitness. If you walk the mile in less time than the range shown for that heart rate, your fitness level is high. If it takes you longer than that range, your fitness level is low. An older person needs a lower heart rate than a younger person in order to score as equally fit. This is because younger people have a higher maximum heart rate. They can end the test with a faster pulse rate and still have as much cardiac capacity and reserve as an older person who tests at a slower pulse.

If you fall within the moderate fitness range in table 4.9 then you can begin your walking-jogging program (table 7.1) at starting level two to three (average). If your score is two or more minutes over the moderate fitness range for your age, your starting level should be one to two (poor-very poor). If you are two minutes under the moderate fitness range, your starting level is four to five (good-very good). If you are four minutes or more under, your starting level can be five to seven (excellent-superior). Record the results of this test on your fitness evaluation form in table 4.20.

Tests for Body Composition

As discussed in chapter 1, **body composition** refers to the proportion of body fat to lean body tissue. The recommended percentage of body fat for adult males is 12–17 percent; for adult females, 19–24 percent; for preadolescent boys, 5–8 percent; and for preadolescent girls, 10–11 percent.

Approximately 50 percent of the body's fat is located just below the skin. The **skinfold test** for the determination of body fat is based on the relationship of subcutaneous fat (fat just below the skin) to total lean body tissue. Unfortunately, the skinfold test is subject to error. In some cases, a 3 percent error can result when different people evaluate the same individual using skin calipers. In addition, dehydration can affect the skinfold test as much as 10 to 15 percent. Underwater weighing is the most accurate technique for determining body composition. However, it is somewhat complicated and requires expensive

TABLE 4.9 One-Mile Walking Test

Age	Heart rate	Time showing moderate fitness[1]	
		Men (175 lbs.)	Women (125 lbs.)
20–29	110	17:06–19:36	19:08–20:57
	120	16:36–19:10	18:38–20:27
	130	16:06–18:35	18:12–20:00
	140	15:36–18:06	17:42–19:30
	150	15:10–17:36	17:12–19:00
	160	14:42–17:09	16:42–18:30
	170	14:12–16:39	16:12–18:00
30–39	110	15:54–18:21	17:52–19:46
	120	15:24–17:52	17:24–19:18
	130	14:54–17:22	16:54–18:48
	140	14:30–16:54	16:24–18:18
	150	14:00–16:26	15:54–17:48
	160	13:30–15:58	15:24–17:18
	170	13:01–15:28	14:55–16:54
40–49	110	15:38–18:05	17:20–19:15
	120	15:09–17:36	16:50–18:45
	130	14:41–17:07	16:24–18:18
	140	14:12–16:38	15:54–17:48
	150	13:42–16:09	15:24–17:18
	160	13:15–15:42	14:54–16:48
	170	12:45–15:12	14:25–16:18
50–59	110	15:22–17:49	17:04–18:40
	120	14:53–17:20	16:36–18:12
	130	14:24–16:51	16:06–17:42
	140	13:51–16:22	15:36–17:18
	150	13:26–15:53	15:06–16:48
	160	12:59–15:26	14:36–16:18
	170	12:30–14:56	14:06–15:48
60+	110	15:33–17:55	16:36–18:00
	120	15:04–17:24	16:06–17:30
	130	14:36–16:57	15:37–17:01
	140	14:07–16:28	15:09–16:31
	150	13:39–15:59	14:39–16:02
	160	13:10–15:30	14:12–15:32

[1]For every ten pounds over 175 pounds for men or over 125 pounds for women, time must be fifteen seconds faster. For every ten pounds under those weights time can be fifteen seconds slower.
Source: Reprinted by permission of the Cooper Institute for Aerobic Research, Dallas, Texas, 75265.

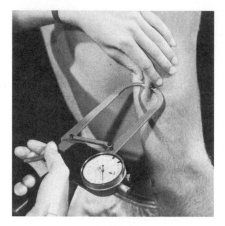

Figure 4.1 Triceps skinfold measurement. Locate a vertical skinfold on the back of the arm halfway between the tip of the acromion process (bony projection on the tip of the shoulder) and the olecranon process (rear point of the elbow), with the arm hanging in a relaxed position.

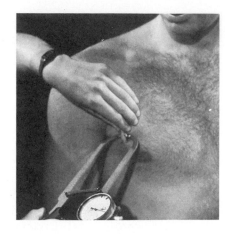

Figure 4.2 Chest skinfold measurement. Locate a point over the outside edge of the pectoralis major muscle just adjacent and medial to the armpit. The skinfold should run diagonally between the shoulder and the opposite hip.

equipment. The skinfold method, even though subject to some error, is an inexpensive, rapid, and easy-to-learn method and gives you a good idea of your present percentage of body fat.

Skinfold Test

The skinfold test requires three skinfold measurements for both male and female: the chest, thigh, and abdomen for the male and the triceps, thigh, and iliac crest for the female. To perform the test, you need a pair of skinfold calipers (or you can use the pinch test described later in the chapter). Hold the skinfold between the thumb and index finger. Release the tension on the calipers slowly so that they pinch the skinfold as close as possible to your fingers. Then simply read the number from the gauge.

Figures 4.1–4.5 illustrate the methods of taking the various skinfold measurements.

After taking the three skinfold measurements appropriate for you, total the measurements. Then, on the nomogram in figure 4.6, use a ruler to connect the point on the left that corresponds to your age with the point on the far right that

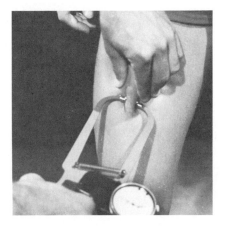

Figure 4.3 Thigh skinfold measurement. Locate a vertical skinfold in the anterior midline of the thigh, halfway between the hip and the knee joint. Place your body weight on the opposite leg while taking the measurement.

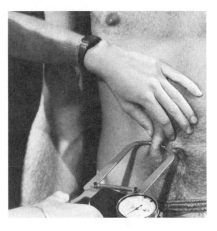

Figure 4.4 Abdomen skinfold measurement. Locate a vertical skinfold adjacent to the umbilicus.

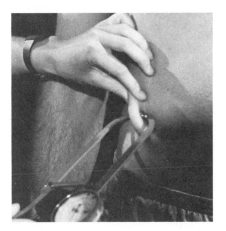

Figure 4.5 Iliac crest skinfold measurement. Locate a vertical skinfold over the iliac crest (point of the hip) in the midaxillary line (middle of the armpit).

corresponds to the sum of your three skinfold measurements. Then read the percentage of body fat from the center male or female scale. Now use your percentage of body fat to find your fitness level in table 4.10, and record the results on your fitness evaluation form (table 4.21).

Suggested Lab Activity

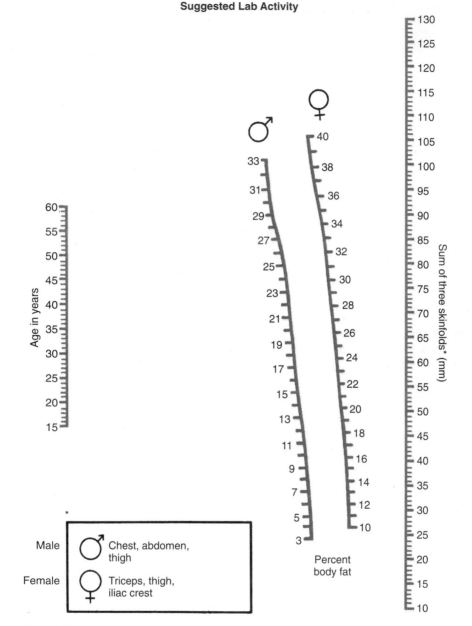

Figure 4.6 Nomogram for the determination of percentage of body fat for the sum of the chest, abdomen, and thigh skinfolds of males fifteen years of age and above, and for the sum of the triceps, thigh, and iliac crest skinfolds of females fifteen years of age and above. Adapted from W. B. Baun, M. R. Baun, and P. B. Raven, "A Nomogram for the Estimate of Percent Body Fat from Generalized Equations," *Research Quarterly for Exercise and Sport* 52(1981): 380–84. Reprinted by permission of the American Alliance for Health, Physical Education, Recreation and Dance, 1900 Association Drive, Reston, Virginia 22091.

TABLE 4.10 Body Fat Score			
Male percentage of body fat	Fitness level	Female percentage of body fat	Fitness level
10	Very lean	13	Very lean
11–12		13–15	
12–14	Lean	17–18	Lean
14–15		18–22	
15–17	Acceptable	22–28	Acceptable
17–18	Fat	28–30	Fat
20+	Obese	30+	Obese

Body Mass Index

If you don't have a skin caliper, **Body Mass Index** offers an alternative way to define obesity. To calculate Body Mass Index, you divide your weight in kilograms by height in meters squared. The nomogram in figure 4.7 does this calculation for you. When the Body Mass Index exceeds twenty-five, obesity-related health risks begin for men and women. Refer to figure 4.7 for your index score. Record your results in table 4.22.

Mark your height and your weight on the corresponding scales, using a ruler or straight edge. Draw a line connecting those two points, then read your BMI from the middle scale and record in table 4.22.

Girth Test

The **girth test** is simply a circumference measure that results in a linear dimension such as inches or millimeters. This method combines waist or hip girth with body weight or height for the prediction of fat in men or women.

Method

The subject is in a standing position while a partner measures the girth. Ideally the measuring tape of reenforced fiberglass or metal tape should be used to insure better accuracy. When applying the tape to the anatomical sites, the partner should avoid any air space between skin and tape. Do not pull tape so tightly that it indents the skin. The tape should be read to the closest 0.25 inches.

Men

1. Body weight to the closest pound.
2. Lower abdominal girth horizontally at the level of the umbilicus (naval). See figure 4.8.

59

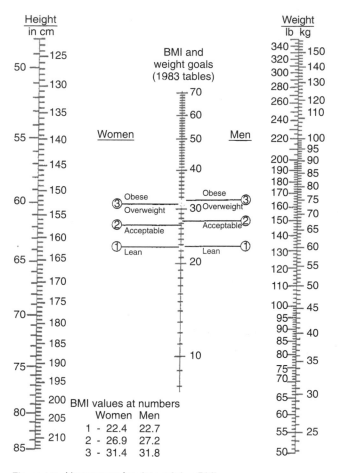

Figure 4.7 Nomogram for determining BMI.
B. T. Burton and W. R. Forster. Health
Implications of Obesity. An NIH Consensus
Development Conference, *Journal of the
Dietetic Association, 85* (1985): page
1117–21.

Women

1. Body height to the closest 0.25 inches.
2. Hip girth—horizontally at the widest point. See figure 4.8.

For men a straight edge is placed on the weight (to the closest pound) of the left vertical axes and then pivoted to the lower abdominal girth (to the closest 0.25 inches) of the right vertical axes. Percent fat is then read where the straight edge intersects the diagonal axes. Refer to figure 4.9a for percent of body fat.

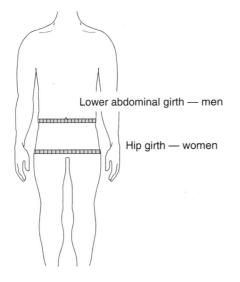

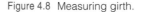
Figure 4.8 Measuring girth.

Lower abdominal girth — men

Hip girth — women

For women a percent of fat is found by placing the straight edge of the hip girth (closest 0.25 inches) of the left vertical axes and then pivoting to the height (closest 0.25 inch) of the right vertical axes. Refer to figure 4.9b for percent of body fat.

Record your percentage of body fat in table 4.23.

Modified Sit-and-Reach Test

The modified sit-and-reach test is an excellent measure of trunk **flexibility** (the extent and range of motion around the joint).

Method

1. Place a yard stick on the floor with the zero mark closest to you. Tape the yardstick in place at the 15 inch mark. See figure 4.10.

2. Ask a partner to help you keep your legs straight during the sit-and-reach test. However, it is important that the partner not interfere with your movement.

3. Warm up properly using the ''Easy Seven'' in chapter 5.

4. Sit on the floor with the yardstick between your legs, your feet 10 to 12 inches apart, and your heels even with the tape at the 15 inch mark.

Suggested Lab Activity

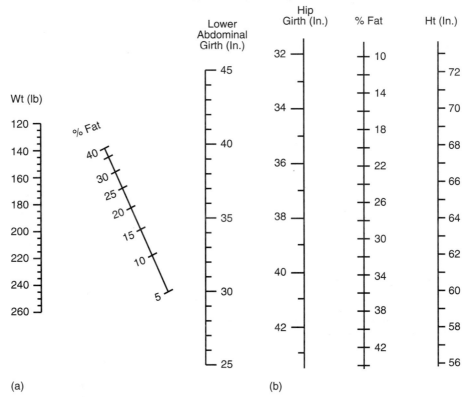

(a)

(b)

Figure 4.9 (a) Men's nomogram for determination of percent body fat (%Fat) from weight (lb) and lower abdominal girth (in.). From *Sensible Fitness* (pp. 30) by J. Wilmore, Champaign, IL: Human Kinetics Publishers. Copyright 1986 by Jack H. Wilmore. Reprinted by permission.

(b) Women's nomogram for determination of percent body fat (%Fat) from height (in.) and hip girth (in.). From *Sensible Fitness* (pp. 31) by J. Wilmore, Champaign, IL: Human Kinetics Publishers. Copyright 1986 by Jack H. Wilmore. Reprinted by permission.

5. Place one hand over the other. The tips of your two middle fingers should be on top of one another.
6. Slowly stretch forward without bouncing or jerking, and slide your fingertips along the yardstick as far as possible. The greater your reach, the higher your score will be.
7. Do the test three times and record your best score to the nearest inch. See table 4.11 for your score. Record your results in table 4.24.

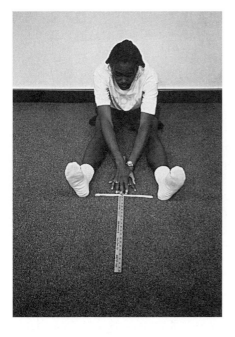

Figure 4.10 The stretched position for the modified sit-and-reach test.

TABLE 4.11 Modified Sit-and-Reach

	Score at age				
	20–29	30–39	40–49	50–59	60+
Men					
High	≥19	≥18	≥17	≥16	≥15
Average	13–18	12–17	11–16	10–15	9–14
Below average	10–12	9–11	8–10	7–9	6–8
Low	<9	<8	<7	<6	<5
Women					
High	≥22	≥21	≥20	≥19	≥18
Average	16–21	15–20	14–19	13–18	12–17
Below average	13–15	12–14	11–13	10–12	9–11
Low	<12	<11	<10	<9	<8

Note: Reprinted by permission from *ACSM Resource Manual for Guidelines for Exercise Testing and Prescription* (p. 165) by S. Blair, P. Painter, R. R. Pate, L. K. Smith, and C. B. Taylor, 1988, Philadelphia: Lea & Febiger, which was adapted from *The Y's Way to Physical Fitness* (pp. 106–111) by L. A. Golding, C. R. Myers, and W. E. Sinning (Eds.), 1982, Rosemont, IL: YMCA of the USA.

Tests for Muscle Strength and Endurance

Muscle Strength Tests

Muscle strength is the amount of force that can be exerted by a muscle group for one movement or repetition. It can be easily assessed by the one-repetition maximum test (1 RM)—the maximum amount of weight you can successfully lift once. Four muscle groups are tested in this section. For each, determine the greatest weight you can lift just once for that particular lift. Begin with a weight you can lift comfortably. Then keep adding weight until you can lift the weight correctly just one time. If you can lift the weight more than once, more pounds should be added until a true 1 RM is reached. Figures 4.11–4.14 illustrate the four lifts used to evaluate strength. Warm up by stretching the appropriate muscle groups before each lift. (See chapter 5.) For each muscle group, divide the total amount of weight lifted by your present body weight in pounds to determine the percentage of weight lifted. Now find your percentages in table 4.12, and record your scores on your fitness evaluation form (table 4.25).

Precaution: 1 RM Maximum Strength Test

Older individuals, those who have been sedentary for some time, or those with a low level of strength should not attempt the 1 RM test for maximum strength until approximately week six of their training program. After six weeks, they will have developed enough skill, flexibility, and familiarization with lifting to reduce the chance of possible injury with the 1 RM test. The 10 RM level, which is 75 percent of maximum strength (see chapter 8 for determining the amount of resistance), should be used in training until the sixth week. Physically active college students may be given the 1 RM test during the second or third week.

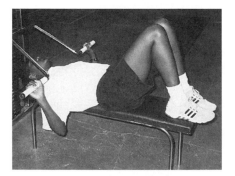
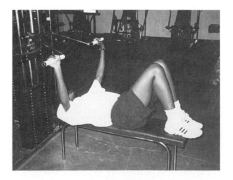

Figure 4.11 Bench press (universal description). From a supine position on the bench, grasp the bar with an overhand grip with the hands approximately shoulder- width apart. Extend the elbows fully, but do not lock them. Progressively increase the weight until you can no longer make the lift.

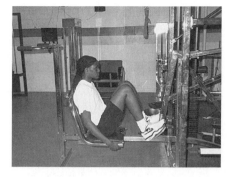

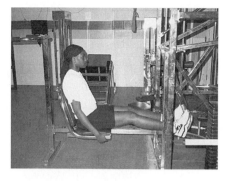

Figure 4.12 Leg press. Place your feet on the pedals and grasp the handles on the seat. Press your feet forward to elevate the weight and return. Inhale while lowering the weight and exhale while lifting it. Progressively increase the weight until you can no longer make the lift. Avoid hyperextending or locking knees.

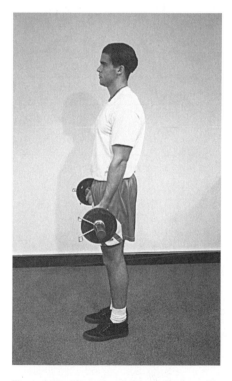

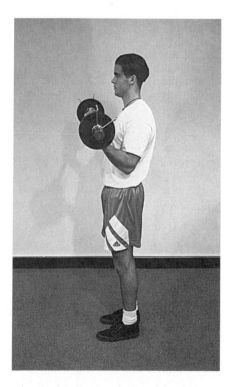

Figure 4.13 Biceps curl. Grasp the bar with your hands shoulder-width apart, using an underhand grip. Bring the bar to a position of rest against your thigh, with your elbows fully extended and your feet spread shoulder-width apart. Using only your arms, raise the bar to your chest and then return to the starting position. Keep your back straight and always return to a position where your elbows are fully extended. Progressively increase the weight until you can no longer make the lift.

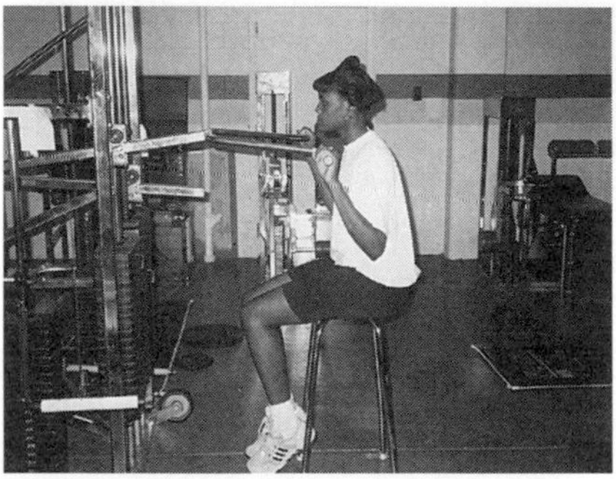

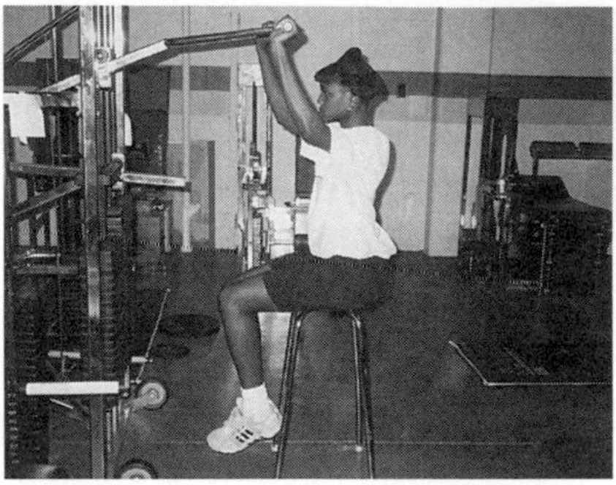

Figure 4.14 Shoulder press (universal description). Sit with your feet resting on the chair. Bend your knees forty-five degrees and grasp the bar with an overhand grip, hands spread approximately shoulder-width apart. With your elbows under the bar, press the bar over your head as you exhale, and return to your starting position. Progressively increase the weight until you can no longer make the lift.

TABLE 4.12 Muscle Strength Scores (1 RM)

Male		**Fitness level**						
	Percentage of weight lifted	Very poor	Poor	Average	Good	Very good	Excellent	Superior
Bench press	______	50	75	100	110	120	140	150
Leg press	______	160	180	200	210	220	230	240
Biceps curl	______	30	40	50	55	60	70	80
Shoulder press	______	40	50	67	70	80	110	120
Female		**Fitness level**						
	Percentage of weight lifted	Very poor	Poor	Average	Good	Very good	Excellent	Superior
Bench press	______	40	60	70	75	80	90	100
Leg press	______	100	120	140	145	150	175	190
Biceps curl	______	15	20	35	40	45	55	60
Shoulder press	______	20	30	47	55	60	60	80

Source: Reprinted with the permission of Simon & Schuster from the Macmillan College text *Health and Fitness through Physical Activity* by Michael Pollock, Jack H. Wilmore and Samuel Fox. (New York: Macmillan College Publishing Company., 1978) All Rights Reserved.

However, the test for muscular endurance can be safely administered during the first weeks of the training program. See "Guidelines for Determining Your 1 RM."

Guidelines for Determining Your 1 RM

Warm up by performing three to four repetitions with 40–60 percent of your perceived 1 RM load for the exercise. Rest for two to three minutes.

Perform three to four reps with 60–80 percent of your perceived 1 RM. Rest for two to three minutes.

Perform a single rep with 95 percent of your perceived 1 RM. Rest for two to three minutes.

Perform a single rep of what you think you can maximally lift. Rest for two to seven minutes.

If you are close to your 1 RM, add more weight in five-pound increments. If you can lift it, this is your 1 RM. If you have dramatically undershot your true 1 RM, increase the weight in larger increments.

Accumulated fatigue from extreme multiple efforts may "undershoot" your true 1 RM. If you take more than three to four maximal 1 RM attempts to find your 1 RM, retest yourself at another session.

Muscle Endurance Tests

Muscle endurance is to some degree dependent on your muscle strength. **Muscle endurance** is the ability of the muscle group to maintain a continuous contraction or repetition over a period of time. You may have enough strength to lift a box of groceries, but muscle endurance is necessary to hold it in your arms for the two or three minutes it takes you to move it from the store to your car. Two tests that are widely used to measure muscular endurance are push-ups (shoulder, arm, and chest muscle endurance) and head-and-shoulder raises (abdominal muscle endurance).

Push-ups

Start in a standard "up" position for a full push-up, with your weight on your toes and hands. (The less fit individuals should perform this test with their knees bent and their weight on their knees and hands.) Your partner should place his or her fist on the floor beneath your chest. Lower yourself down until your chest touches your partner's fist. Keep your back straight while raising to an "up" position (figure 4.15). Count the number of consecutively performed push-ups and then refer to table 4.13 to determine your fitness level. Record your score and fitness level on your fitness evaluation form (table 4.26).

TABLE 4.13 Push-Up Muscular Endurance Test Standards

Age (years)	Standard push-up: fitness level						
	Superior	Excellent	Very good	Good	Average	Poor	Very poor
15–29	Above 54	51–54	45–50	35–44	25–34	20–25	15–19
30–39	Above 44	41–44	35–40	25–34	20–24	15–20	8–14
40–49	Above 39	35–39	30–35	20–29	14–19	12–14	5–11
50–59	Above 34	31–34	25–30	15–24	12–14	8–12	3–7
60–69	Above 29	26–29	20–25	10–19	8–9	5–7	0–4
Age (years)	Modified push-up: fitness level						
	Superior	Excellent	Very good	Good	Average	Poor	Very poor
15–29	Above 48	46–48	34–45	17–33	10–16	6–9	0–5
30–39	Above 38	33–37	25–33	12–24	8–11	4–7	0–3
40–49	Above 33	29–32	20–28	8–19	6–7	3–5	0–2
50–59	Above 26	21–25	15–21	6–14	4–5	2–3	0–1
60–69	Above 20	15–19	5–15	3–4	2–3	1–2	0–

Source: From *Health and Fitness through Physical Activity* by M. L. Pollock, J. H. Wilmore, and S. M. Fox. Copyright © 1978 by John Wiley & Sons. Reprinted with permission of the publisher.

Head-and-Shoulder Raise

Lie on your back with arms across your chest. Your knees should be bent at about ninety degrees with both feet flat and no more than 18 inches in front of the buttocks. See figure 4.16. Don't forget to breathe to assist in muscular contraction. Complete as many raises as possible in one minute. Warm up with a few raises before the test. Curl your neck and upper back until your trunk reaches a 30 to 40 degree angle with the exercise surface, then return to the starting position.

Refer to table 4.14 to determine your fitness level. Record your score and fitness level on your fitness evaluation form (see table 4.27).

Test for Leg Power

Leg power is the ability of your leg muscles to mobilize strength in a short period of time. Lower-body power is the application of strength through the dimension of time.

For the leg power test, a piece of cloth tape or a chalkboard is attached vertically to a wall. With chalked fingertips, stand facing the wall with both arms extended overhead and feet and chin touching the wall. Mark the point where

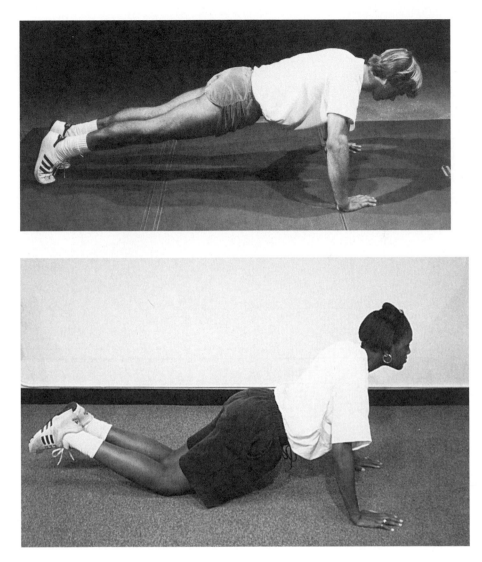

Figure 4.15 Push-ups.

your fingertips touch the tape or chalkboard. Then stand at a right angle to the taped wall. Take a deep squat position with your knees bent at forty-five degrees and your trunk bent forward thirty to forty-five degrees. Jump, touching the tape or chalkboard at the highest point that you can (figure 4.17). Record the difference between the prejump touch mark and the postjump touch mark. Then find your score in table 4.15.

Record your score and fitness level on your fitness evaluation form (table 4.28).

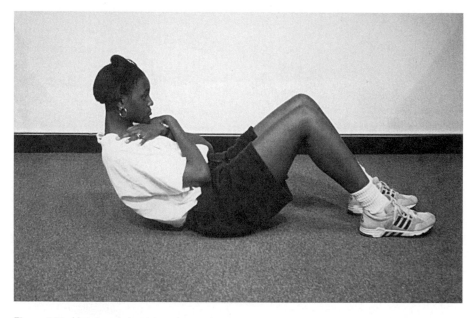

Figure 4.16 Head-and-shoulder raise.

TABLE 4.14	Head-and-Shoulder Raise Score						
Age (years)	**Fitness level**						
	Very poor	Poor	Average	Good	Very good	Excellent	Superior
Males							
17–29	0–17	17–35	36–41	42–47	48–50	51–55	55+
30–39*	0–13	13–26	27–32	33–38	39–43	44–48	48+
40–49	0–11	11–22	23–27	28–33	34–38	39–43	43+
50–59	0–8	8–16	17–21	22–28	29–33	34–38	38+
60–69	0–6	6–12	13–17	18–24	25–30	31–35	35+
Females							
17–29	0–14	14–28	29–32	33–35	36–42	43–47	47+
30–39*	0–11	11–22	23–28	29–34	35–40	41–45	45+
40–49	0–9	9–18	19–23	24–30	31–34	35–40	40+
50–59	0–6	6–12	13–17	18–24	25–30	31–35	35+
60–69	0–5	5–10	11–14	15–20	21–25	26–30	30+

Source: Reprinted by permission of the Cooper Institute for Aerobic Research, Dallas, Texas, 75265.
*The value of ages over thirty is estimated.

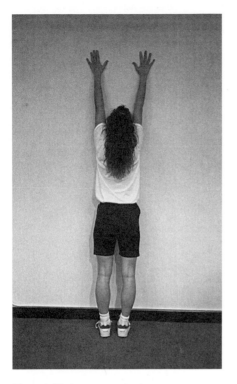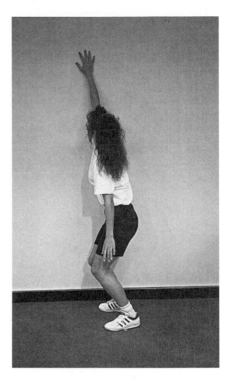

Figure 4.17 Leg power test.

TABLE 4.15 Leg Power Score

Difference between prejump and postjump touch marks	Fitness level	
7 in.	Very poor	_____
10 in.	Poor	_____
16 in.	Average	_____
18 in.	Good	_____
20 in.	Very good	_____
22 in.	Excellent	_____
24+ in.	Superior	_____

Determining Your Fitness Profile

Use figures 4.18 and 4.19 to determine your fitness profile. With figure 4.18, fill in the circles that correspond to your fitness level for each activity and then connect the circles with straight lines. The resulting graph shows your fitness

71

Chapter 4

Suggested Lab Activity

Name _____

Date _____

| Fitness level | Cardiorespiratory | | | Body composition | Flexibility | | Muscle strength | | | | Muscle endurance | | Leg power |
	1.5-mile run	Step test	Bicycle ergometer test	Swimming test	Skin-fold test	Back hyper-extension test	Sit and reach test	Bench press test	Leg press test	Biceps curl test	Shoulder press test	Push-ups test	Bent-knee sit-ups test	Vertical jump test
Superior	0	0	0	0	0	0	0	0	0	0	0	0	0	0
Excellent	0	0	0	0	0	0	0	0	0	0	0	0	0	0
Very good	0	0	0	0	0	0	0	0	0	0	0	0	0	0
Good	0	0	0	0	0	0	0	0	0	0	0	0	0	0
Average	0	0	0	0	0	0	0	0	0	0	0	0	0	0
Poor	0	0	0	0	0	0	0	0	0	0	0	0	0	0
Very poor	0	0	0	0	0	0	0	0	0	0	0	0	0	0

Figure 4.18 Fitness level and progress chart profile.

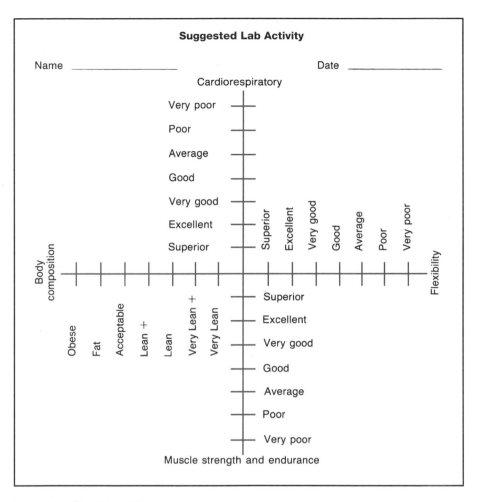

Figure 4.19 Fitness paradigm.

profile. Reevaluate and rescore every six to eight weeks in order to note improvement or maintenance of physical fitness. These scores will assist you in planning your individualized exercise program and setting short- and long-term goals.

With figure 4.19, mark your predominant fitness level for each of the four basic components of physical fitness with a small circle and then connect the four circles with straight lines. The smaller and more symmetrical the square you can draw by connecting the four fitness categories, the better your overall fitness level. Fill out the paradigm every six to eight weeks to chart your progress.

SUGGESTED LAB ACTIVITY—Physical Fitness Evaluation Form

Name _____ Age _____ Height _____ Weight _____ Sex _____

TABLE 4.16 1.5-Mile Run

Time: min _____ sec _____

Estimated $\dot{V}O_2$ max (ml/kg/min) _____

Fitness level

Very poor _____
Poor _____
Average _____
Good _____
Very good _____
Excellent _____
Superior _____
Retest in six to eight weeks.
Date _____

TABLE 4.17 Step Test

Resting pulse count _____
Post-exercise pulse count _____
(per fifteen seconds)
Body weight _____
Fitness score _____
Age-adjusted fitness score _____

Fitness level

Very poor _____
Poor _____
Average _____
Good _____
Very good _____
Excellent _____
Superior _____
Retest in six to eight weeks.
Date _____

TABLE 4.18 Bicycle Ergometer Test

Exercise heart rate _____
(per minute)
Estimated
$\dot{V}O_2$ max (ml/kg/min) _____

Fitness level

Very poor _____
Poor _____
Average _____
Good _____
Very good _____
Excellent _____
Superior _____
Retest in six to eight weeks.
Date _____

TABLE 4.19 Swimming Test

Distance swam _____ (yards)
Approximate time _____ (minutes)

Fitness level

Very poor _____
Poor _____
Average _____
Good _____
Very good _____
Excellent _____
Superior _____
Retest in six to eight weeks.
Date _____

TABLE 4.20 Walking Test

Heart rate at the end of walk _____
(beat/min.)
Time of walk _____

Fitness level:

Very poor   _____
Poor   _____
Average   _____
Good   _____
Very good   _____
Excellent   _____
Superior   _____
Retest in six to eight weeks.
Date _____

TABLE 4.21 Skinfold Test

Male: Female:
Chest   _____   Triceps   _____
Abdomen _____   Iliac crest _____
Thigh   _____   Thigh   _____
Total   _____   Total   _____
Percentage of body fat _____

Fitness level

Very lean   _____
Very lean+   _____
Lean   _____
Lean+   _____
Acceptable   _____
Fat   _____
Obese   _____
Retest in six to eight weeks.
Date _____

TABLE 4.22 Body Mass Index

B.M.I. score _____
Retest in six to eight weeks.
Date _____

TABLE 4.23 Girth Test

Percent of body fat _____
Rctest in six to eight weeks.
Date _____

TABLE 4.24 Modified
                Sit-and-Reach Test

Sit-and-reach score _____

Fitness level

Very poor   _____ Low
Poor   _____
Average   _____ Below average
Good   _____ Average
Very
good   _____
Excellent   _____
Superior   _____ High
Retest in six to eight weeks.
Date _____

TABLE 4.25 Muscle Strength Tests

Male	Percentage of weight lifted	Very poor	Poor	Average	Good	Very good	Excellent	Superior
				Fitness level				
Bench press	_____	50	75	100	110	120	140	150
Leg press	_____	160	180	200	210	220	230	240
Biceps curl	_____	30	40	50	55	60	70	80
Shoulder press	_____	40	50	67	70	80	110	120

Female	Percentage of weight lifted	Very poor	Poor	Average	Good	Very good	Excellent	Superior
				Fitness level				
Bench press	_____	40	60	70	75	80	90	100
Leg press	_____	100	120	140	145	150	175	190
Biceps curl	_____	15	20	35	40	45	55	60
Shoulder press	_____	20	30	47	55	60	60	80

Retest in six to eight weeks.   Date _____

TABLE 4.26 Push-Up Test

Number of push-ups _____

Fitness level

Very poor   _____
Poor   _____
Average   _____
Good   _____
Very good   _____
Excellent   _____
Superior   _____
Retest in six to eight weeks.
Date _____

TABLE 4.27 Head-and-Shoulder Raise

Number of sit-ups _____

Fitness level

Very poor   _____
Poor   _____
Average   _____
Good   _____
Very good   _____
Excellent   _____
Superior   _____
Retest in six to eight weeks.
Date _____

TABLE 4.28 Leg Power Test

Difference between prejump and postjump touch marks _____

Fitness level

Very poor _____

Poor _____

Average _____

Good _____

Very good _____

Excellent _____

Superior _____

Retest in six to eight weeks.   Date _____

Key Terms

Body Composition
The proportion of body fat to lean body tissue

Body Mass Index
Method using body weight and height to determine body fat

Flexibility
The extent and range of motion around a joint

Girth Test
A circumference measure that predicts body fat

Leg Power
The ability of the leg muscles to mobilize strength in a short period of time

Muscle Endurance
Ability of the muscle group to maintain a continuous contraction or repetition over a period of time

Muscle Strength
The force produced by a muscle group

Skinfold Test
The method of estimating body fat by measuring subcutaneous fat with skinfold calipers

5

chapter

Warm-Up and Flexibility

Chapter Concepts

After you have studied this chapter you should be able to

1. describe what is meant by warm-up exercise;
2. explain three basic types of warm-up exercises;
3. describe the importance of flexibility exercise;
4. differentiate between static stretching and ballistic stretching;
5. discuss the importance of stretching;
6. describe the key warm-up principles;
7. describe and demonstrate the "Easy Seven" stretching exercises; and
8. describe contraindicated exercises.

Warm-Up and Exercise

The term **warm-up** has a variety of meanings. To one person, it may mean a few push-ups and jumping jacks; to another, it may mean stretching and flexibility exercises; to someone else, it may mean jogging for fifteen or twenty minutes. Regardless, there is general agreement that warm-up exercises are essential to prepare the heart, lungs, and muscles to adequately meet the demands placed on them during rigorous physical exercise, and that they are an important prerequisite to all physical activity.

Generally, there are three types of warm-up exercises. The first type involves static stretching techniques that stretch the muscles prior to an activity. Stretching increases extensibility and reduces the resistance of the muscles. It also produces more efficient muscle contractions and reduces the chances of injury or soreness.

The second type of warm-up exercise is concerned with general body warm-up. These exercises, such as jogging or calisthenics, are aimed at increasing the body temperature and gradually stimulating the heart. Substantial evidence indicates that when body temperature is increased at least one degree Fahrenheit,

a number of changes that aid physical performance occur in the muscles and circulatory system. General body warm-up also prepares the heart to efficiently meet the stressful demands placed upon it during rigorous exercise and helps to prevent the possibility of heart damage during the initial stages of exercise. Research has shown abnormalities in electrocardiograms of individuals who did not warm up prior to exercise. Subjecting the heart to a sudden overload without a warm-up can result in a reduced flow of blood to the heart muscles, which could lead to serious consequences. It is therefore vital to gradually stimulate the cardiovascular system with a general warm-up activity before engaging in rigorous exercise.

The third type is a specific neuromuscular warm-up where the skill is performed at a less intense level prior to the actual activity to ensure that the proper muscles are being stimulated and that the coordination and skill level are maximized. In other words, the type of warm-up is specific to the type of activity that is to follow. For example, hurdlers generally do not do push-ups before a race but engage in some mild running and practice the specific leg movement involved in hurdling. Many athletes believe that this type of warm-up must precede an activity to produce optimal skilled performance.

Flexibility

Flexibility is generally defined as a looseness or suppleness of the joint. More specifically, flexibility is the range and the extent of the movement of a joint. Some individuals have a wide range of motion; others' range of motion is fairly limited.

Joint flexibility is controlled by a number of factors: the joint capsule contributes approximately 47 percent to the range of motion, the muscles contribute 41 percent, the tendons contribute 10 percent, and the skin contributes 2 percent. Because the joint capsule itself is rigid, the emphasis when attempting to increase or decrease flexibility is placed on the muscle and skin tissue. Stretching exercises enable these tissues to increase the range of the movement. Conversely, strengthening exercises may tighten up the muscles and tendons and can decrease the range of movement if not done correctly through the full range of motion.

Women tend to have a greater range of movement in the joints than men primarily because men have generally larger and bulkier skeletal muscles, which tend to reduce joint movement. However, flexibility is one characteristic of well-developed muscles, regardless of gender.

All activities require varying degrees of flexibility. A competitive tennis player needs good shoulder flexibility. A laborer requires good lower-back flexibility. Even such everyday movements as walking and running require flexibility. Good flexibility reduces the possibility of the aches, pains, and inflammations associated with joints that are stressed through rigorous activity. Running for a long period of time without pre- and poststretching activities may lead to reduced flexibility in the legs and back and may result in lower-back problems.

Excess Flexibility

Too much flexibility may be as dangerous as too little. There is evidence indicating that abnormal looseness may produce joint instability, **hyperextension,** and make you more vulnerable to injury.

The Importance of Stretching

Stretching involves extending and holding muscles for a specific period of time to increase range of movement in a joint. Failure to stretch muscle tissue regularly can lead to a decrease in soft tissue elasticity.

Two kinds of stretching exercises—static and ballistic—increase flexibility. **Static stretching** consists of stretching the muscle slowly and gradually for periods of ten to twenty seconds, followed by several seconds of relaxation. This method is a very effective stretching technique and does not impose unnecessary stress on the muscle. In addition, an integral part of cooling-down is static stretching of the muscles that have been used during exercise. The stretching will increase the exit of lactic acid from the muscles, prevent blood pooling in the muscles, and reduce muscle soreness. **Ballistic stretching,** on the other hand, involves rapid bouncing, jerking movements, which have the potential for injuring soft muscle and joint tissue. The ballistic method of jerking and bouncing actually invokes what is called a stretch reflex, wherein the muscle senses that it is overextended and contracts as a means of protection. The purpose of stretching is to lengthen the muscle not shorten it; therefore, ballistic stretching is counterproductive.

Proprioceptive Neuromuscular Facilitation (PNF)

An alternative method of stretching is to precede a static stretch with an isometric contraction of the muscle group to be stretched. This stretching method is called proprioceptive neuromuscular facilitation (PNF). This method is effective in improving muscle relaxation and leads to increased flexibility. The procedure generally requires two people. A partner moves the limb passively through its range of motion. After reaching the end point of the range of motion, the muscle is isometrically contracted for six to ten seconds against the partner's resistance. The muscle then relaxes and is again stretched using static techniques. This method is also called contract-relax (C-R). It is vital that the partner is adequately trained in the technique so that injury will not result.

81

Key Warm-Up Principles

1. No matter what the nature of the exercise to come, a slow, gradual warm-up consisting of calisthenics, stretching, and slow jogging, always should precede exercise, even if you are highly trained.
2. Be ready to make minor adjustments to your stretching routine. You may be more flexible on some days than others.
3. Your warm-up should last ten to fifteen minutes.
4. Stretching following mild jogging should be slow but thorough.
5. Initial stretching should be gentle and specific to the muscles that will receive the most stress.
6. Jogging should be conducted at an intensity and rate specific to your anticipated activity and level of fitness.
7. Only a few minutes should lapse between the completion of the warm-up and the activity.
8. Experiment with different types of warm-ups. Find the one that best fits your body. The warm-up should feel good.
9. A portion of the warm-up exercise should consist of skill drills and other skilled movements related to the anticipated activity to follow the warm-up.
10. Remember to stretch and cool down following the activity.

Stretching Exercises*

The stretching exercises illustrated and explained in figures 5.1–5.7 include all of the major muscle groups in the body and thus are preparatory for the majority of physical activities in which you might wish to participate. Use record sheets B-1 and B-2 in appendix B at the back of the book to record your progress with these exercises.

The "Easy Seven"

Flexibility in areas that experience particular stress is necessary for specific activities. The "Easy Seven" are a good foundation. These exercises stretch the most commonly used muscles of the body, or those that will experience the most stress.

*Certain flexibility exercises have a greater potential for injury; therefore, caution should be observed when performing such exercises. Proper instruction by a certified professional in an exercise class is recommended if there is any doubt about a specific stretching exercise.

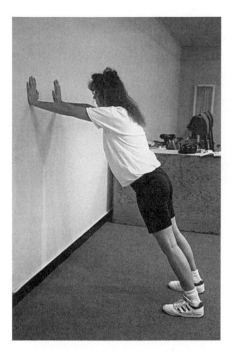

Figure 5.1 Lower-leg and heel stretch. (The Achilles tendon is a large tendon connecting the calf muscle to the heel.) Face a wall and stand approximately three feet in front of it with your feet several inches apart. Place your outstretched hands on the wall while keeping your feet flat on the floor. Gradually lean forward toward the wall. Hold the stretch for ten seconds. Repeat five times. Muscles stretched: Gastrocnemius.

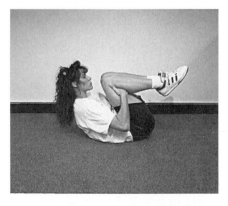

Figure 5.2 Back stretch. While lying on your back, bring both of your knees to your chest. Grasp both of your legs behind the knees and pull the knees toward your chest. Hold for ten seconds. Repeat ten times. Muscles stretched: Lower back, Gluteus, Hamstrings.

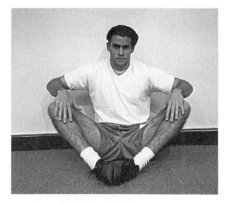

Figure 5.3 Groin stretch. Sit on the floor with the soles of your feet touching in front of you. Gradually push your knees down as far as possible. Hold the final stretched position for ten seconds. Repeat five times. Each day try to push your knees closer to the floor. Muscles stretched: Adductors.

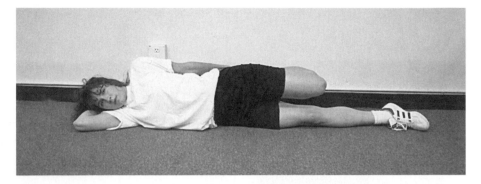

Figure 5.4 Quadriceps stretch. While lying on your right side, flex the knee of your left leg and grab the ankle with your left hand. Gradually move your hip forward until a good stretch is felt on the thigh. Hold for ten seconds. Repeat five times. Repeat for the right leg while lying on your right side. Caution: Do not pull the ankle. Let the hip movement create the stretch. Muscles stretched: Quadriceps.

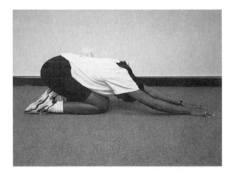

Figure 5.5 Lower-back and hip stretch. Get down on all fours by placing your hands and knees on the floor. Lean back onto your heels. Extend your arms and place your chest on the floor. Hold for ten seconds. Repeat five times. Muscles stretched: lower back, Latissimus dorsi.

Cyclists, runners, and swimmers should engage in other special stretching exercises, in addition to the "Easy Seven" stretching exercises shown in figures 5.1–5.7. Special stretching exercises for cyclists are illustrated and explained in figures 5.8–5.11; figures 5.12–5.16 show stretching exercises for runners; and swimmers' stretching exercises are demonstrated in figures 5.17–5.23.

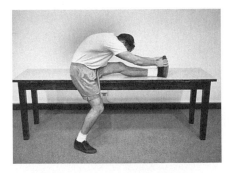

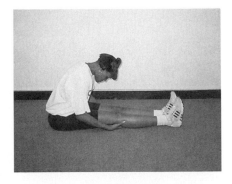

Figure 5.6 Hamstring stretch. (The hamstring is a group of muscles in the upper leg that are important in knee flexion.) Sit on a table with one leg extended across the table and the opposite leg hanging over the side of the table. Bend forward at the waist and reach toward the toes of your extended leg. Bend the knee slightly. Reach gradually; do not bob. Hold for ten seconds. Repeat five times for each leg. Muscles stretched: Lower back, Hamstrings.

Figure 5.7 Lower-back stretch. While sitting on the floor with your legs extended out in front of you, force your knees flat against the floor. Grab behind your knees and slowly pull your head down toward your knees. Move slowly. Hold for ten seconds. Repeat five times. Muscles stretched: Lower back, Hamstrings.

Stretching Exercises for Cyclists

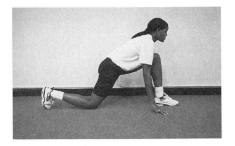

Figure 5.8 Leg and groin stretch. Move one leg forward until the knee of the front leg is directly over the ankle. Rest the back knee on the floor. Without changing leg position, lower the front hip downward to create a stretch. Hold for ten seconds. Repeat five times. Change position and repeat for the other leg. Muscles stretched: Hip flexors, Rectus femoris, Iliopsoas.

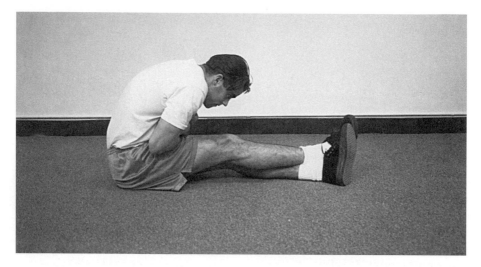

Figure 5.9 Back extensor. Sit with your legs crossed and your arms folded in front of you. Touch your chin to your chest. Roll forward and attempt to touch your forehead to your knees. Roll forward gradually, keeping your hips on the floor. Do not bob. Hold for ten seconds. Repeat five times. Muscles stretched: lower back, Hamstrings.

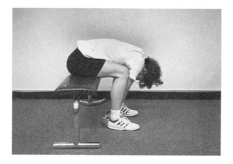

Figure 5.10 Lower-back extensor. Sit on a chair or bench with your feet flat on the floor and about six inches apart. Touch in your chin and curl forward between your knees with your arms hanging toward the floor until you feel resistance in your back. Hold for ten seconds. Repeat five times. Muscles stretched: Lower back.

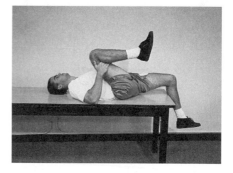

Figure 5.11 Hip flexor. Lie on your back on a table with your legs over the edge of the table. Bring your right knee to your chest. Use both of your hands on your kneecap to gradually press the knee toward your armpit. Hold for ten seconds. Repeat five times for each leg. Caution: Do not apply downward pressure with hand on knee joint. Muscles stretched: Hamstrings, Gluteus.

Stretching Exercises for Runners

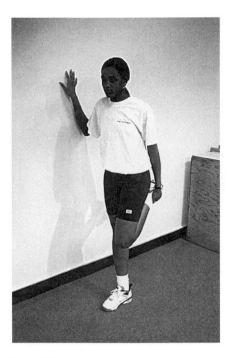

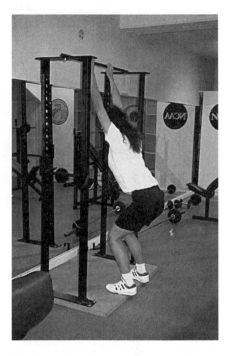

Figure 5.12 Front-leg stretch. Lean against a wall. Bring your left foot up behind you. Grasp the foot with your left hand and touch the foot to your buttocks. Hold for ten seconds. Repeat five times for each leg. Caution: Only grasp ankle. Do not pull toward buttocks. Muscles stretched: Quadriceps.

Figure 5.13 Shoulder and arm stretch. Place both hands shoulder-width apart on a ledge or stationary bar. Bend knees slightly and let upper body drop down. Adjust height of hands and degree of knee bend to increase or decrease stretch. Hold for ten seconds. Repeat five times. Muscles stretched: Shoulder girdle.

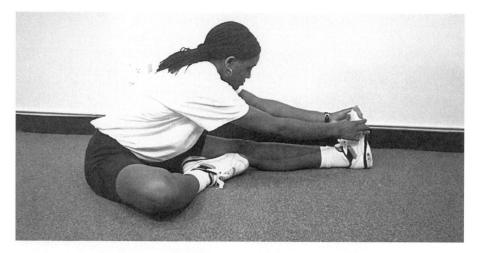

Figure 5.14 Modified hurdler stretch. Sit with your left leg extended and your right leg crossed in front with the heel near your crotch. Reach forward with your left arm as far as possible. Bend knee slightly. Hold for ten seconds. Repeat five times for each leg. Muscles stretched: Hamstrings, Gastrocnemius, Lower back.

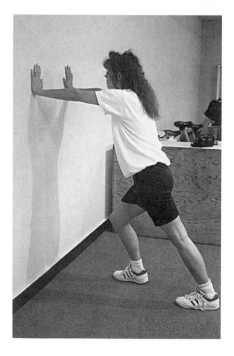

Figure 5.15 Wall lean and heel stretch. Stand about three feet from the wall, with one foot in front of the other. Bend the front knee slightly, and keep the back leg fully extended. Keep heels on the ground. Hold for ten seconds. Repeat for other leg. Muscles stretched: Hamstrings, Gastrocnemius.

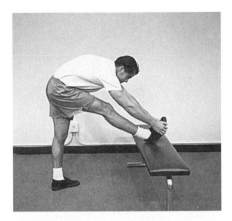

Figure 5.16 Leaning hamstring stretch. While standing, raise one leg with the toes pointing up, and rest the heel of your foot on a solid object, for example, a car bumper or bench. Begin with the leg in a bent position. Lean forward and reach with both arms toward raised foot. Slightly bend knee of the raised foot. Hold for ten seconds. Repeat five times for each leg. Muscles stretched: Lower back, Hamstrings.

Stretching Exercises for Swimmers

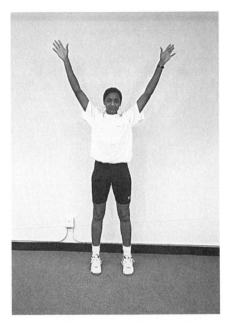

Figure 5.17 Arm and leg stretch. Stand with your feet shoulder-width apart. Raise your extended arms overhead. Place your weight on your toes and stretch to the sky. Hold for ten seconds. Repeat five times. Muscles stretched: Trunk, Shoulder girdle.

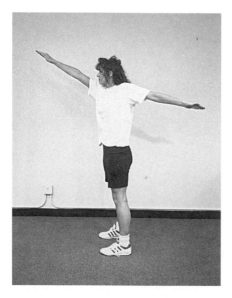

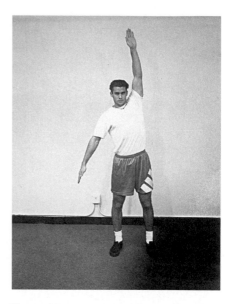

Figure 5.18 Forward-and-back arm stretch. Stand with your feet shoulder-width apart. Bend forward about twenty degrees from the waist. Extend your left arm to the front and your right arm to the rear. Hold your arms shoulder high for ten seconds. Repeat five times. Then reverse arm positions and repeat five times. Muscles stretched: Obliques, Back.

Figure 5.19 High-low arm stretch. Stand with your feet shoulder-width apart. Extend your right arm straight up from your body and extend your left arm straight down. Hold the stretch for ten seconds. Repeat five times. Then reverse arm positions and repeat five times. Muscles stretched: Shoulder, Chest, Obliques.

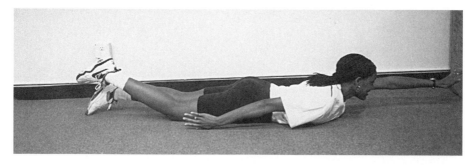

Figure 5.20 Arm and leg stretch. Lie face down with your arms extended above your head. Slowly raise your right arm and left leg simultaneously. Be careful not to arch your back. Hold for six seconds. Repeat five times for each side of body. (Not recommended for people with weak backs.) Muscles stretched: Lower back.

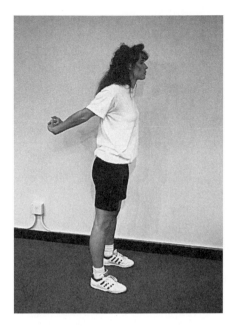

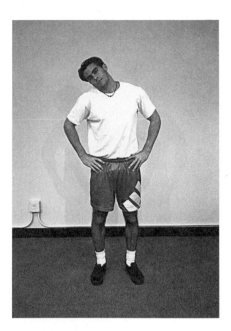

Figure 5.21 Upper-chest stretch. Stand with your feet slightly apart. Grasp your hands behind your back and raise your arms. Hold for ten seconds. Repeat five times. Muscles stretched: Anterior shoulder, Rotators.

Figure 5.22 Neck stretch. Stand with your hands on your hips. Flex your head toward your right shoulder. Hold for ten seconds. Then flex your head toward your left shoulder and hold for ten seconds. Repeat five times. Muscles stretched: Lateral neck.

Lower-Back Problems

Difficulty in straightening up after bending over, stiffness, or mild to crippling pain are common symptoms of lower-back problems. Generally, lower-back problems result from injury to muscles, ligaments, or discs in the lumbar area of the spine. Injuries to these areas are more common when the following factors are present: weak abdominal and back muscles, poor flexibility, a sedentary life-style, and improper sitting or lifting. Weak abdominal muscles lead to hyperextension (increasing the arch of the lower back), which puts added strain on muscles, ligaments, and spinal discs. Acute back strain that does not receive proper treatment can develop into chronic back strain.

Exercises to stretch the spine and enhance the condition of abdominal muscles are essential for prevention and rehabilitation of lower-back problems. Lower-back problems also may be prevented through observance of the following principles:

1. Maintain the strength of your abdominal muscles with conditioning exercises. Head-and-shoulder-raises (see figure 4.14) are excellent abdominal strengtheners.

2. Engage in stretching exercises for the hamstrings, which aid in the prevention of lower-back problems.

3. Avoid standing for long periods of time. This can aggravate the lower back. If you must stand, shift your weight from one leg to the other, and flex one knee so that one leg is supported higher than the other.

4. When lifting, keep your back straight and shoulders up. Lift with your leg muscles, not with your back muscles. Don't bend over without bending your knees, and keep the weight you are lifting close to your body. Avoid lifting objects above your waist, which can increase pressure on lower-back muscles and ligaments.

5. Sleep on your side with your knees bent. Do not sleep on your stomach or lie on your back with your legs straight. If you must lie on your back, bend your knees.

6. Before getting out of bed in the morning, perform a few lower-back exercises, such as single-leg or double-leg pulls (see figures 5.24 and 5.25). Then stand up slowly after leaving the bed.

7. When sitting, try to keep your knees above your hips to reduce lower-back arching and strain.

8. When kneeling down (as when doing gardening), avoid sudden lateral or turning movements with your upper body.

9. When driving, move your car seat forward so that your knees are bent.

10. When carrying a heavy load, don't arch your lower back or twist your body, try to have your arms and abdominal muscles bear the weight.

The exercises illustrated and explained in figures 5.24–5.26 are beneficial in the prevention and rehabilitation of lower-back pain.

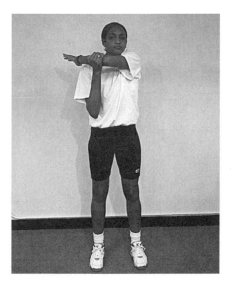

Figure 5.23 Shoulder stretch. Bring arm shoulder high, across the front of the body. Bend the elbow ninety degrees and grab the elbow with the opposite hand. Apply tension for ten seconds, repeat five times with each arm. Muscles stretched: Shoulder girdle.

Lower-Back Exercises

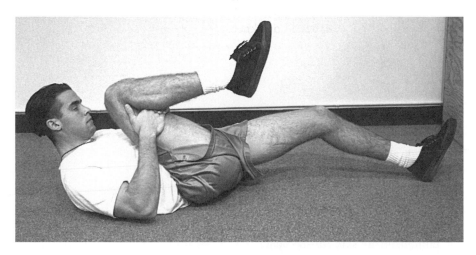

Figure 5.24 Lower-back stretch. Lie on your back with both legs straight. Bring one knee to your chest. Grasp your leg just below the knee with both hands and pull your knee toward your chest. Hold for eight to ten seconds. Then, while still grasping the knee, bring your head and shoulders toward the knee. Hold for five to eight seconds. Return to the original position and repeat the exercise using the other leg. Muscles stretched: Lower back, Hip extensors.

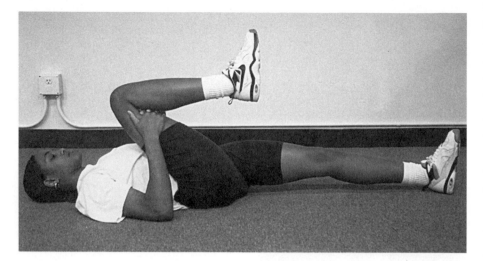

Figure 5.25 Single-leg pull. Lie on your back with both legs straight. Grasp one leg just below the knee and pull the knee to your chest. Hold for eight to ten seconds. Then alternate with the other leg. Repeat five times. Muscles stretched: Lower back, Hip.

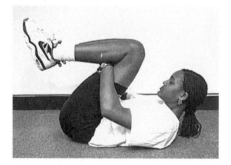

Figure 5.26 Double-leg pull. Lie on your back with both knees bent. Grasp both legs just below the knees and pull the knees to your chest. Hold for ten seconds. Repeat five times. Muscles stretched: Lower back, Hip.

Low-Risk Activities for the Back

Aerobics Low-impact routines in which jarring movements are eliminated are safe for the back.

Cycling Excellent aerobic exercise if you have a back problem; maintain upright position.

Jogging If you are in good condition, have a smooth stride and good shoes, jogging will not put your back at risk.

Swimming The water supports the spine, thus relieving the pressure on it. Back stroke and side stroke are best; avoid butterfly and breaststroke.

Walking Walking puts less strain on the spine than does unsupported sitting and only a little more than plain sitting.

High-Risk Activities

Bowling Lifting a heavy weight while twisting and bending the upper body can put strain on the back. Try to develop smooth delivery and use a lighter ball.

Football, Basketball, Baseball All these activities involve twisting, jarring movements; jumping, bending; and contact with other players.

Golf The twisting in the swing, teeing, removing the ball, and prolonged putting all put strain on your back.

Tennis and Racquetball Sports Twisting, quick stops, and going all out put excessive strain on the back.

Weight Lifting Puts immense stress on lower back; important to learn correct lifting techniques.

Exercises to Avoid

Some exercises that have been popular in the past may be harmful and should be avoided. The general problems associated with these exercises are overflexing a joint, hyperextending the joint, overarching the back or neck, sudden twisting or flexing, bouncing while stretching, and poor body alignment. Figures 5.27–5.37 are examples of such contraindicated exercises.

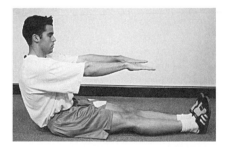

Figure 5.27 Straight-leg sit-ups arch the back and strain it. There's no need to sit up fully. The abdominal muscles work only during the first part of the movement. After that, the hip flexors take over, and the shift to these muscles can further arch the back.

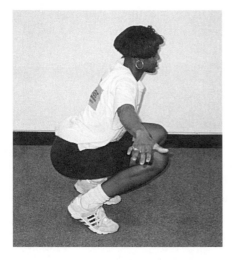

Figure 5.28 Full squats as with deep-knee bends, or squat thrusts, greatly increase stress on the knee joint, stressing ligaments, joint capsule, and cartilage.

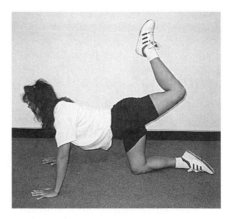

Figure 5.29 Donkey kicks, in which you rapidly lift your leg as high as possible while on all fours, arch the back, and contort the shoulders and neck, can cause compression of intervertebral discs and possible disc herniation.

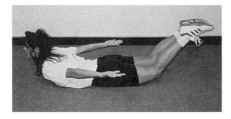

Figure 5.30 Swan stretches—lying on your stomach and lifting your chest and legs—put your back in jeopardy and can cause compression of intervertebral discs.

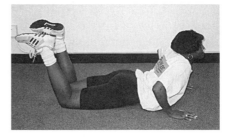

Figure 5.31 Arched push-ups are sloppy push-ups in which you lower your hips and pelvis to the floor. As with any exercise that arches the back, these can injure the discs in the lower spine. They do little for arm and shoulder muscles.

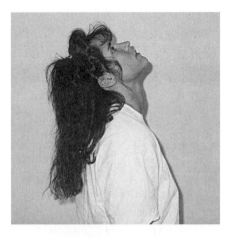

Figure 5.32 Three hundred and sixty degree head rolls, in which you vigorously roll your head around or bend your head back, may injure the disks in your neck.

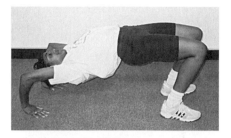

Figure 5.33 Back bend, or pressing up with the feet and hands from a back-lying position, puts the lower back in jeopardy.

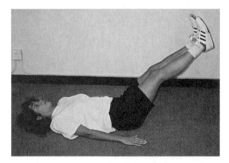

Figure 5.34 Double leg lifts can strain your lower back since raising both legs causes your back to arch. Leg scissors present similar risks, causing compression of intervertebral discs.

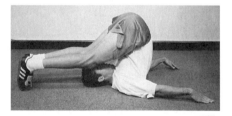

Figure 5.35 Yoga plow can compress disks in your neck area. A shoulder stand (or bicycling position in which you rest on your shoulders and upper back) can do similar damage.

97

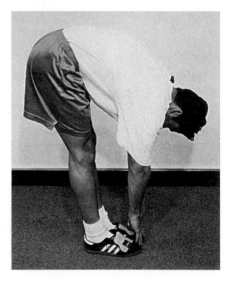

Figure 5.37 Locked-knee toe touches can over-stress the back, knees, and hamstring muscles, especially when done quickly with a bouncing movement.

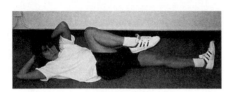

Figure 5.36 Alternating bent-leg sit-ups, in which you pump your legs and hold one straight out, put an asymmetric pull on the pelvis, which can strain the lower back. Also, in your effort to keep both legs off the floor, you may arch your back.

Key Terms

Achilles Tendon
A large tendon connecting the calf muscle to the heel

Ballistic Stretching
Rapid bouncing, jerking types of muscle movements

Flexibility
The range and the extent of the movement of a joint

Hamstring
A group of three muscles in the upper leg that flex the leg at the knee

Hyperextension
Extension beyond the normal range of the joint structure

Static Stretching
A stretching method that consists of stretching the muscle slowly and gradually

Warm-Up
Exercises performed immediately before physical activity to prepare the heart, lungs, and muscles to adequately meet the demands of rigorous exercise

6

Cardiorespiratory Endurance

Chapter Concepts

After you have studied this chapter you should be able to

1. describe the flow of blood through the heart and to the lungs;
2. define maximum oxygen uptake;
3. define stroke volume;
4. describe factors that affect resting heart rate;
5. determine the training effect level for the heart;
6. define a MET;
7. describe perceived exertion;
8. describe anaerobic and aerobic exercise;
9. define intensity, duration, and frequency;
10. describe symptoms that necessitate exercise termination;
11. explain the second wind phenomenon;
12. describe body signals of overexercise;
13. explain the reason for cooling down;
14. describe changes in postexercise heart rate;
15. describe cardiac hypertrophy;
16. describe the effects of cardiorespiratory training;
17. define anaerobic threshold;
18. define aerobic and anaerobic energy systems; and
19. describe preexamine screening.

The Heart

There has been considerable research dealing with the heart and its response to training through exercise. The relationship between exercise and coronary artery disease, which plagues hundreds of thousands of individuals every year, also is being intensively investigated. There is no question that the cardiovascular system is the cornerstone of health-related fitness. A basic understanding of the heart is important for those planning to or actually engaging in physical exercise.

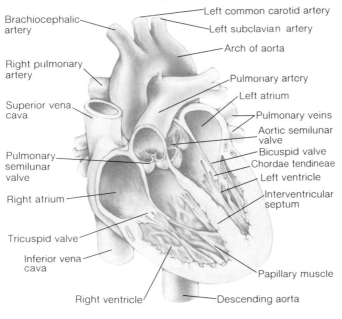

Figure 6.1 Anterior internal view of heart.
From Van De Graaff, Kent M., *Human Anatomy Laboratory Textbook,* 2d ed.
© 1981, 1984 Times Mirror Higher Education Group, Inc., Dubuque, Iowa. All rights reserved. Reprinted by permission.

Structure and Function

The heart weighs less than a pound and is about the size of your fist. This powerful, long-working organ pumps blood through the blood vessels in a closed cycle within the body. The heart begins beating early in embryonic life and continues until death. During an average lifetime of seventy to seventy-eight years, the heart pumps approximately 150 to 200 million liters of blood.

The human heart has four chambers (figure 6.1). The two upper chambers, where the veins empty, are called atria, and the two lower chambers, where the blood leaves the heart, are called ventricles. The muscle walls of the atrias are very thin because, aided by gravity, they only have to pump blood into the ventricles. The ventricles, however, have to pump blood to all parts of the body, a more demanding function that requires a much larger muscle.

Blood circulates through the body in a closed cycle. ''Used'' blood that has given up a large portion of its oxygen and that contains high levels of carbon dioxide is returned to the heart via two large veins—the superior vena cava, which brings blood from the head, arms, and shoulders, and the inferior vena cava, which drains blood from the rest of the body below the heart—into the right atrium. From here, the blood passes through the tricuspid valve into the right ventricle. From the right ventricle, the blood leaves the heart through the pulmonary valve into the pulmonary artery, which travels to the lungs. In the lungs, the blood gives up carbon dioxide and picks up more oxygen. Two pulmonary veins from each lung carry fresh blood back to the left atrium of the heart. From the left atrium, the blood passes through the bicuspid valve into the left ventricle. From the left ventricle, the blood flows through the aortic valve into the aorta, which branches to all parts of the body. Microscopic vessels called capillaries connect the small arteries to the veins. Within the capillaries, oxygen from the blood is transferred to the cells. All of the veins eventually join the superior and inferior vena cava, which lead back to the heart, thus completing the cycle.

The sounds that you hear from a beating heart are caused by the opening and closing of the valves between the chambers of the heart and the valves in the two large arteries leaving the heart.

Maximum Oxygen Uptake and Stroke Volume

The main function of the heart and circulatory system is to provide blood, which is necessary to maintain the proper functioning of all body cells. In terms of exercise, the heart's main concern is its ability to deliver oxygen to the working cells of the body and to rid the cells of waste products. The greatest amount of oxygen used by the cells during maximum exercise per unit of time is referred to as **maximum oxygen uptake.** Maximum oxygen uptake is one of the best indexes of cardiorespiratory fitness. Training may be a 20 percent contributing factor in determining maximum oxygen uptake, whereas the remaining 80 percent is thought to be genetically determined.

The amount of blood pumped out per beat (**stroke volume**) at rest for the average individual is approximately 70 to 90 milliliters. During rigorous activity, the average heart may pump 100 to 120 milliliters per beat. The trained individual, however, may have a stroke volume at rest of 100 to 120 milliliters and a maximum capability during exercise of 150 to 170 milliliters. This gives the trained individual a decided advantage since the more efficient your heart, the greater its ability to maintain exercise levels for long periods of time with less stress. The hearts of some trained individuals may be capable of pumping out as much as 30 to 35 *liters* a minute. This amount is six times the total volume of the blood in the body, which indicates the truly exceptional efficiency of the heart.

Anaerobic and Aerobic Energy Systems

Sports require a great deal of energy. However, among the many different sports, there is a wide variety in the amounts of energy required and in how fast that energy is needed. Activities such as sprinting and weight lifting, **anaerobic**

101

exercises, require large amounts of energy in a very short time. Other activities, such as long-distance running and swimming, **aerobic exercises,** require lower amounts of energy, but the energy must be delivered over a longer period of time.

The body has three basic energy sources during physical exercise. The first two generally are used for anaerobic activities, while the third normally is used for aerobic activities, even though there is some overlapping of the physiological processes.

The first energy source involves two energy-rich compounds—**ATP (adenosine triphosphate)** and **PC (phosphocreatine)**—that are stored directly in the muscle tissue. When the muscle is stimulated through exercise, ATP and PC break down and release immediate energy for muscle contraction. Energy from ATP and PC, however, is only available for a brief period because only very small amounts of these compounds are stored in the muscle. This concept is known as **anaerobic** (without oxygen).

A second energy source during exercise is supported by sugar, which is stored in the muscles in the form of glycogen. When glycogen is broken down, the released energy produces more ATP. However, when glycogen is burned in the absence of oxygen, it gives off an end product called lactic acid, which results in muscle fatigue. For this reason, this energy source is limited to activities that last approximately one to two minutes. If exercise continues beyond this time, the body is required to draw upon oxygen, the third energy source available during exercise.

The oxygen system can use both glycogen and fats as fuel for the production of ATP. Lactic acid, along with the accumulation of calcium 2+ (ions) and heat, are major factors in muscle fatigue. However, when oxygen is used through a complex process that occurs in the muscle cells, the oxygen prevents the buildup of lactic acid and promotes the resynthesis of ATP for energy. This system is referred to as **aerobic** (with oxygen) and is used primarily in endurance activities, such as long-distance running, skiing, and swimming.

Irregular Heartbeats

Irregular heartbeats **(cardiac arrhythmia)** are considered abnormal but not necessarily dangerous. Any type of abnormal beating of the heart, however, should be carefully evaluated by a physician to determine its origin. Extra heartbeats may be caused by caffeine (found in coffee, tea, and chocolate), anxiety, smoking, or heart disease. When there are extra heartbeats, usually one of the lower chambers of the heart (the ventricle) does not have enough time to fill with blood. As a result, a reduced amount of blood is pumped out, resulting in lowered blood pressure and producing a faint or weak feeling.

Heart Murmurs

As blood passes through the heart, it makes a very distinctive noise, called a heart murmur. Some types of heart murmurs may indicate leakage of a valve. Other murmurs, sometimes found in endurance athletes, result from a stronger contraction of the heart muscle and are not important. Valvular leakage or insufficiency are common heart ailments often present in childhood, but they usually disappear as the child grows older. The seriousness of the effects on the body depends upon the valves affected or the degree of defect. It is possible to have a slight heart murmur and still engage in physical exercise, but the intensity and duration of the exercise should be determined in consultation with a physician.

Heart Rate

Normal resting heart rates may range from a low of thirty-five beats per minute to a high of 100 beats per minute. The average for a young adult is around seventy beats per minute. Sedentary individuals usually have higher resting heart rates than physically active individuals. Individuals in excellent cardiorespiratory condition generally have very low resting heart rates. This probably is due to increased efficiency of the heart muscle and changes in the nervous system. Because their hearts have a larger stroke volume, these people are able to deliver the required oxygen to their body cells at a lower heart rate. In addition, after rigorous exercise, the well-conditioned individual's heart generally returns to their resting levels faster than the heart of a sedentary person.

There may be other factors that play an important role in lowering resting heart rate. One finding that supports this contention is that some well-conditioned athletes have been found to have heart rates in the seventies and eighties, whereas we would expect their resting heart rates to be in the forties and fifties.

Measuring Heart Rate

In measuring heart rate, the pulse may be taken either by placing a hand directly over the heart (left breast) or by palpating the radial artery at the base of the thumb (palm side of the wrist) (fig. 6.2) or the temporal artery in front of the ear. Taking the pulse at the carotid artery in the neck is not recommended since the pressure from palpating may slow the heart or cause a cardiac abnormality in some individuals.

Determining the Training Effect

Monitoring your heart rate can be an effective way to determine the exercise intensity that you should strive for. This technique is referred to as the maximal heart rate reserve method. A training heart rate of 70 percent of your maximal

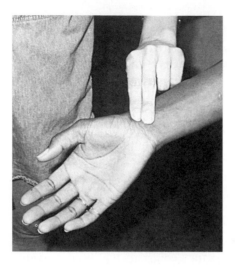

Figure 6.2 Taking the pulse at the radial artery.

heart rate reserve, which is approximately 60 percent of your maximal oxygen uptake level, is considered to be the appropriate level of intensity in order to produce a **heart rate training effect.** This formula predicts rather than assesses maximum heart rate; therefore, there is some error in the measurement.

To determine the heart rate training effect for your heart, it is first necessary to determine your **maximum heart rate.** The direct method of exercising an individual to exhaustion on a treadmill and monitoring heart rate to determine maximum level is difficult and, for some individuals, dangerous. However, a reasonable estimate of your maximum heart rate can be determined by subtracting your age from 220. For example, a twenty-year-old would have a maximum heart rate of 200 (220 − 20).

The next step in determining your training effect level is to find your **resting heart rate** by taking your pulse for one minute shortly after you rise in the morning or after at least five minutes of calm sitting. To arrive at a more reliable measure, take your pulse three mornings in a row and find the average.

Next, subtract your resting heart rate from your maximum heart rate and multiply the difference by 70 percent. Add this product to your resting heart rate, which will give you your training effect level. Approximately two-thirds of all people who use this technique are within ten beats of their predicted heart rate when subtracting their age from 220. It is best to select the lower end of the range if you are sedentary. This method is an estimate; therefore, you must allow for individual differences. It may be necessary to start your exercise at the 60 percent level or lower depending upon your present fitness status and how your body responds to the exercise. If you perceive the exercise as relatively nonstressful, you may increase the threshold level five beats per minute after three to four workouts until you reach your threshold level.

The following is an example of determining the training effect level for a twenty-year-old individual with a resting heart rate of eighty beats per minute:

$$220 - 20 = 200 \text{ beats per minute (maximum heart rate)}$$
$$200 - 80 = 120 \text{ (80 is the resting heart rate in this example)}$$
$$120 \times .70 = 84 \text{ (.70 is the desired intensity of activity)}$$
$$84 + 80 = 164 \text{ beats per minute}$$

The training effect level in this example is 164 beats per minute.

Calculating Your Training Target
Heart Rate (TTHR)

1. Maximum Heart Rate $= 220 \text{ beats/min} - \dfrac{}{\text{age in years}} = \text{beats/min.}$

2. TTHR $= \dfrac{}{\substack{\text{your maximum} \\ \text{heart rate}}} - \dfrac{}{\substack{\text{your resting} \\ \text{heart rate}}} \times .7 + \dfrac{}{\substack{\text{your resting} \\ \text{heart rate}}} = \text{beats/min.}$

The Ten-Second Rate

A convenient technique for counting the heart rate during exercise is determining the ten-second rate. Divide your training effect level by six, since there are six ten-second intervals in one minute. For example, an individual with a training effect level of 164 would have a ten-second heart rate of $164 \div 6 =$ approximately 27.

METS

Another way to determine the intensity of physical activity is through the use of METS (metabolic equivalents). One **MET** is the equivalent of the resting metabolic rate; two METS would be two times the resting metabolic rate; and so on. Resting metabolic rate is approximately 3.5 milliliters of oxygen per kilogram of body weight per minute. If, for example, an individual has a maximum oxygen uptake of 28 milliliters per kilogram of body weight per minute, this would be equivalent to 8 METS (28 milliliters $\div$ 3.5 milliliters $= 8$). If you wanted to determine the MET training level for this individual at a 70 percent capacity, simply multiply 8 METS times 70 percent, which will give you 5.6 METS. Now turn to table 6.1 to determine the appropriate exercise at a 5.6 MET level. As you can readily see, the MET approach for determining the exercise intensity is not as precise as the target heart rate level. Activities vary widely in terms of metabolic cost. Factors such as heat, skill level, altitude, and motivation can all result in a wide variation of exercise intensity.

TABLE 6.1 Selected Activities and MET Values

Activities		MET values
Badminton		4–8
Bowling		2–3
Basketball		8–10
Climbing		8.5–10
Cycling	5.5 mph	3–4
	9.4 mph	5–6
	13.1 mph	9–10
Dancing		4–5
Football		6–7
Golf		3–4
Gymnastics		2–5
Handball		10–13
Rope jumping		10–15
Rowing	51 st/min	4–5
	97 st/min	12–15
Running	1 mile–12 min	7–8
	1 mile–5 min	15–20
Standing		1–1.5
Tennis		5.5
Skating, fast		10–15
Skiing, downhill		6–10
Skiing, cross-country		15–20
Squash		10–15
Soccer		6–12
Swimming	crawl 1 ft/sec	5–6
	3 ft/sec	15–20
Volleyball		4–8
Level walking	1 mile–30 min	2.5
	1 mile–15 min	6.5
Water skiing		4–6

Source: From Jack H. Wilmore and David L. Costill, *Training For Sport and Activity;* 3rd. edition. Copyright 1988, Times Mirror Higher Education Group, Inc., Dubuque, Iowa. All rights reserved. Reprinted by permission.

Anaerobic Threshold

Another more sophisticated method used to determine training intensity for endurance programs is based on the concept of **anaerobic threshold.** This is when the workload intensity or oxygen consumption level reaches a point where anaerobic metabolism is accelerated and lactic acid begins to accumulate in the blood and muscles. Workload levels at or slightly above this threshold are used for endurance athletes. The degree of stress placed on the metabolic system in the muscles is the major factor in determining training intensity. However, this technique requires laboratory measurements of blood lactate and minute ventilation.

Perceived Exertion

It is extremely difficult to get an accurate pulse rate while exercising. In addition, when you stop exercising, your heart rate drops very rapidly, giving you an unreliable reading. Therefore, it is necessary to locate your pulse quickly to determine what level of intensity you have reached during exercise. However, once you are comfortable with your training program, you may want to experiment with an indirect technique of determining heart rate that comes pretty close to actual heart rate. This method is referred to as **perceived exertion.**

Considerable evidence indicates that normal individuals (those with an absence of neurosis or extremely high levels of anxiety) are capable of integrating various body sensations, such as body temperature, breathing intensity, muscle and joint sensations, and heart rate, to arrive at a subjective estimate of exercise intensity that approximates the actual metabolic cost of exercise.

Borg has developed a model that correlates heart rate with perceived exertion (see table 6.2). The model rates perceived exertion on a scale of 6 to 19. Multiplying the perceived exertion factor by a factor of 10 corresponds to actual heart rate at that perceived intensity level. For example, if your work intensity is perceived at an intensity of 17, the predicted heart rate would be 170 ($17 \times 10 = 170$).

When you first begin your exercise program, you may want to use Borg's model to determine your perceived level of exercise. At various times in your exercise program, monitor your intensity level by choosing a number that you think approximates your level of exertion. When rating your perceived exertion, use a combination of all sensations of physical stress, effort, fatigue, and breathing. Don't concentrate on just one sensation, such as shortness of breath or sore leg muscles.

Once you have decided on a level of exertion, take your heart rate for 10 seconds $\times$ 6. Then compare your actual heart rate with the heart rate in table 6.2 that corresponds with the number you have chosen as your perceived exertion

TABLE 6.2 Perceived Exertion Scale	
6	60 beats per minute
7—Very, very light	
8	
9—Very light	
10	
11—Fairly light	
12	
13—Somewhat hard	
14	
15—Hard	
16	
17—Very hard	
18	
19—Very, very hard	

Source: From Borg, G. A. V., "Perceived Exertion: Note on History and Method," in *Medicine & Science in Sports*, 5:90. © 1973 American College of Sports Medicine. Reprinted by permission.

level. With a little practice, you will be amazed how accurate you can be in predicting your heart rate. Borg's model has been found to be approximately 80 percent accurate.

This ability to predict your perceived exertion enables you to monitor your exercise in order to remain at or near the heart rate training effect level to prevent excess stress and assure you of a safe exercise routine.

Anaerobic and Aerobic Exercise

All-out exercise lasting one to two minutes is referred to as **anaerobic** (without oxygen). Such exercises as weight lifting, sprinting, tennis, handball, squash, volleyball, and racquetball train the anaerobic system. Continuous rigorous exercise lasting beyond one to two minutes, such as jogging, long-distance swimming, cycling, and cross-country skiing, trains the **aerobic** system (with oxygen).

The physical demands of the all-out burst of muscle effort in anaerobic exercise require that the heart and the circulatory system be in a high state of fitness. Anaerobic activities often are competitive and may produce overexertion. Thus, even young individuals in good health should be careful not to engage in anaerobic activities until they are aerobically fit and have participated in an aerobic exercise program for several weeks. In general, if your primary concern is maintaining good cardiorespiratory endurance and you are not interested in competitive activities, anaerobic kinds of training can be eliminated from your exercise program with little effect on cardiorespiratory endurance.

Principles of Training Before Starting an Exercise Program

Before starting your cardiorespiratory program, you must be aware of three principles: intensity, duration, and frequency. **Intensity** refers to the degree of overload or "stressfulness" of the exercise; **duration** is the amount of time used for each exercise bout; and **frequency** is the number of exercise bouts per week. Generally, the more intensive, the longer, and the more frequent the training program, the greater the cardiorespiratory benefits.

A preexercise medical evaluation also is advised prior to beginning a cardiorespiratory exercise program. What time of the day would be best for your exercise and exercise precautions are two additional topics you should consider. All of these areas are explored in further detail in the sections that follow.

Intensity

For a training effect to occur within the cardiorespiratory and muscle systems, the exercise program must consist of activities that produce an overload on these systems. As discussed previously, research has shown that the intensity for cardiorespiratory training should be at least 70 percent of the maximum heart rate reserve and that this training effect level must be maintained throughout the exercise period. However, low-intensity programs below the 70 percent level are appropriate for nonactive individuals who are just beginning an exercise program or those interested only in maintaining proper body weight. The American College of Sports Medicine suggests a range of 60 to 90 percent for development and maintenance of cardiorespiratory fitness.

Your desired exercise intensity must be gauged to your age and relative fitness. An exercise pulse rate from 110 to 120 beats per minute for middle-aged individuals may be an effective training stimulus, whereas younger people may have to work at a steady pulse rate from 140 to 160 beats per minute.

Duration

How long you exercise depends primarily on the intensity of the exercise and your long-range goals. Beginners should exercise for a minimum of fifteen to twenty minutes. As fitness level improves, the exercise session can be increased from thirty to sixty minutes. Maintaining your target training effect level during the thirty to sixty minutes of exercise will improve your cardiorespiratory endurance. Longer work periods are only necessary for those interested in competing in such activities as long-distance running or swimming. Strength training should be approximately fifteen minutes in duration. Generally longer exercise sessions over 35 minutes produce greater fitness benefits. However, low-fit individuals should start out with 5- to 10-minute sessions equivalent to approximately 100 kilocalories per session and work up to expenditures of 200 to 300 kilocalories per workout. (A kilocalorie is the amount of heat necessary to raise one kilogram of water one degree Celsius.) Longer duration exercises tend to improve the muscle's ability to use fat. Presently there is no evidence to indicate that additional health benefits are derived from workouts that exceed 60 minutes (600 kilocalories). Therefore it is recommended that low-fit individuals' exercise should last long enough to burn 100 to 200 kilocalories; medium-fit, 200 to 400; and high-fit individuals, 400 or more kilocalories. There is considerable evidence now to indicate that exercise needs to exceed 7.5 kilocalories a minute to reduce the risk of heart disease.

Frequency

You don't have to knock yourself out seven days a week to achieve cardiorespiratory endurance. Workouts three to five days a week are sufficient. It is important to allow yourself twenty-four to forty-eight hours for rest and recovery between exercise bouts.

Overstressing the body is one of the worst things you can do, and one way to do that is by strenuously exercising only once a week. This kind of regimen is worse than no exercise at all. Strenuous exercising once a week can greatly stress your cardiorespiratory system without producing any benefits. If you cannot exercise at least three times a week, then your once- or twice-a-week exercise should be moderate, with the main objectives of relaxation and burning up a few extra calories. In addition it may lower the risk of coronary heart disease.

Another thing to keep in mind is that if you miss a day or two in your exercise routine, you should never try to make it up. This is a dangerous practice, especially for middle-aged people. The important consideration here is not to become obsessive about exercising. Some people, whose main goal in exercising is to avoid having a heart attack, become so rigidly goal-directed that any interference in their exercise schedule results in anxiety. This is not the object of exercise. Your exercise program should be enjoyable and relaxing. Avoid rigidly structured schedules that lead to anxiety and tension. And remember, don't "pile it on" if you miss a day.

When to Exercise

Some individuals experience light-headedness and nausea if they exercise rigorously early in the morning before breakfast. Because they haven't had anything to eat for a number of hours, their blood sugar levels are low, which is the probable explanation for their discomfort. Rigorous exercise too soon after breakfast also can cause physical distress, such as a feeling of fullness or nausea.

Mild stretching and calisthenic exercises in the morning, however, should not cause any physical discomfort.

If the early morning is the only time you have free to exercise, you should get up earlier so that you have an hour or two between breakfast and exercise. If that is not possible, eat a light breakfast of juice and toast before exercising.

Many individuals are not affected by the time of day that they exercise. Many people enjoy exercise late in the afternoon, when they are through with work and when they feel more relaxed. The best time to exercise is when it is convenient and you are motivated.

Preexercise Screening

For many years in the United States, physicians adopted a somewhat restricted approach to exercise prescription, suggesting that a stress electrocardiogram was needed in all men over the age of thirty-five years who wanted to increase their habitual physical activity. This requirement has now largely been discredited. The need for extensive preliminary screening is particularly questionable given that modern exercise decreases rather than increases a person's overall risk of cardiac death. Potential exercisers can be offered some practical advice that will reduce the likelihood of an exercise catastrophe. A review of such incidents by R. J. Sheppard suggests that risks are increased if:

1. There is a history of fainting or chest pain during exercise.
2. There is a family history of sudden death at a young age.
3. The intensity and duration of activity are much greater than the subject has recently experienced.
4. Competition, publicity, or pride encourages persistence with exercise in the face of warning symptoms.
5. The individual exercises while under pressure of time, or when oppressed by business or social problems.
6. The activity involves heavy lifting or prolonged isometric effort.
7. The weather is unduly hot or cold.
8. The participant has a viral infection, senses chest discomfort or cardiac irregularity, or feels ''unwell.''[1,2]

The current U.S. recommendation as adopted by the American College of Sports Medicine (see table 6.3) looks at the age of the subject, the proposed intensity of effort, and associated symptoms or major cardiac risk factors.

1. Sheppard, R. J. "Sudden Death—A Significant Hazard of Exercise?" *British Journal of Sports Medicine.* 8 (1974): 101–10.
2. Sheppard, R. J. *Ischemic Heart Disease and Exercise.* London: Cromm Helm, 1981.

TABLE 6.3 Indications for Preliminary Medical Screening Among Those Who Wish to Increase Their Habitual Physical Activity (Based on the recommendations of the American College of Sports Medicine, 1991)

Variable	Indication for medical screening
Known disease	Yes, if cardiac, pulmonary, or metabolic
Symptoms or signs suggesting disease[a]	Yes, if cardiac, pulmonary, or metabolic
Major cardiac risk factors[b]	Yes, if two or more
Vigorous exercise[c]	Yes, if man >40 yr. or woman >50 yr.

[a]Pain or discomfort in chest, shortness of breath with mild exertion, dizziness or sudden loss of consciousness, shortness of breath while sleeping, swelling of ankles, palpitations or racing heartbeat, pain in the calves on walking, or known heart murmur.
[b]Blood pressure higher than 160 mm Hg systolic or 90 mm Hg diastolic on two occasions, or use of medication to reduce blood pressure; serum cholesterol higher than 6.2 mmol/L (240 mg/DL); cigarette smoking; diabetes mellitus; family history of coronary or atherosclerotic disease in parents or siblings before the age of fifty-five years.
[c]Exercise that represents a substantial challenge; usually higher than 60 percent of maximal oxygen intake, and causing fatigue within twenty minutes or less.

If the subject is planning no more than a moderate increase of habitual activity (an intensity of less than 60 percent of peak aerobic effort, which the person can sustain comfortably for an hour or longer), is symptom free, and has no more than one major coronary risk factor, then a preliminary medical examination is no longer recommended. Indications for medical advice are:

1. The presence of disease.
2. The intent to undertake vigorous exercise above the specified age limit.
3. Two or more major risk factors, or symptoms suggestive of cardiopulmonary or metabolic disease.

This recommendation is very close to the Canadian position. The Canadian Physical Activity Readiness Questionnaire (rPAR-Q) (table 6.4) has proven to be a very safe screening and has shown remarkable success in detecting potential contraindications to exercise. The rPAR-Q is thus the currently recommended method of determining exercise readiness in symptom-free adults with no more than one major cardiac risk factor. A yes answer on one or more of the seven questions indicates the need for medical screening prior to beginning an exercise program.

TABLE 6.4	Suggested Lab Activity—Revised Physical Activity Readiness Questionnaire (rPAR-Q)

Yes	No	
_____	_____	1. Has a doctor said that you have a heart condition and recommended only medically supervised activity?
_____	_____	2. Do you have chest pain brought on by physical activity?
_____	_____	3. Have you developed chest pain the past month?
_____	_____	4. Do you tend to lose consciousness or fall over as a result of dizziness?
_____	_____	5. Do you have a bone or joint that could be aggravated by the proposed physical activity?
_____	_____	6. Has a doctor ever recommended medication for your blood pressure or a heart condition?
_____	_____	7. Are you aware through your own experience, or a doctor's advice, of any other physical reason against your exercising without medical supervision?

NOTE: If you have a temporary illness, such as a common cold, or are not feeling well at this time—POSTPONE.

From Shephard, R. J., Thomas, S., and Weller, I. (1991). "The Canadian Home Fitness Test: 1991 Update." Sports Medicine. 1: page 359. Used by permission.

Exercise Precautions

Be familiar with the following exercise precautions before beginning your cardiorespiratory endurance program:

1. Get a thorough physical examination before starting your conditioning program.
2. If fatigue lasts two hours or more following an exercise session, the program is too rigorous. Reduce your level of exercise.
3. Alcohol and exercise do not mix. Alcohol constricts the coronary vessels of the heart muscle.
4. Cigarette smoking limits oxygen exchange in the lungs, thus preventing a high level of fitness attainment.
5. Always warm up before exercise and cool down after the activity.
6. Remember to use your heart rate as a guide to the intensity of the exercise.
7. Sporadic exercise may be detrimental to your health. Three to five exercise sessions a week are minimal for optimum benefit.

If any of the following symptoms occur while you are exercising, stop exercising, and consult a physician before continuing your exercise program:

1. Fluttering, palpitating, missed, or extra heartbeats, sudden bursts of rapid heartbeats, or a sudden slowing of rapid pulse
2. Pressure or pain in the center of the chest, left arm, fingers, or throat
3. Dizziness, fainting, nausea, cold sweat, or light-headedness
4. Shortness of breath or inability to attain sufficient oxygen

During Exercise

While exercising, you may be fortunate enough to experience the ''second-wind phenomenon,'' or you may have the misfortune of getting a ''stitch in your side.'' During exercise, you must always be aware of how you are feeling and any body signals that may indicate that you are overdoing it.

Second Wind

The **second wind** is a familiar phenomenon to individuals involved in endurance activities, such as long-distance running, cycling, and skiing, and who are in excellent cardiorespiratory condition. It is generally evidenced by a feeling of relief from the effects of fatigue.

While little research has been conducted in the area of second wind, several factors have been evaluated. There appears to be a psychological mental set that many athletes look forward to that gives them relief from the feelings of discomfort produced by high levels of chemical fatigue products and carbon dioxide in the blood. Other factors that may contribute to the second wind are increased efficiency of circulation, better buffering of the acids produced by muscle contractions, better circulation to the extremities, and a higher metabolic efficiency to the cells. Any of these factors could result in some relief from the symptoms of fatigue.

Stitch in Side

A stitch in the side is pain felt in the lower part of the rib cage or in the upper abdominal area. The pain may be caused by a lack of blood supply to the muscles responsible for the breathing movements. Sometimes, the diaphragm will experience reduced blood flow during rapid breathing. The stitch may also be caused by reduced blood supply to the liver during rigorous physical activity. Eating or drinking just prior to rigorous exercise is another possible explanation for stomach or intestinal cramps.

During rigorous physical exercise, the respiratory muscles are contracting very rapidly and have a tendency to fatigue. As a result of reduced blood supply, they may go into spasm, which results in pain. Try to work through it. Rub it, stretch it, breathe deep. If this does not work, you may have to discontinue the activity to reduce the pain. Sometimes lying on your back with feet positioned above the head may bring some relief.

No matter what kind of cardiorespiratory shape you are in, there is always a risk of getting a stitch. Good cardiorespiratory conditioning, however, does give you some protection because the muscles for breathing, like other muscles in the body, can be conditioned through exercise. The stronger and more efficient your breathing muscles, the more ably they can maintain rapid breathing for longer periods of time during exercise.

Body Signals of Overexercise

When you go beyond the normal limits of physical ability and don't give your body a chance to recover—in other words, when you overexercise—you could fall prey to a number of undesirable symptoms, such as dizziness, severe breathlessness, tightness in the chest or a feeling of weight on the chest, nausea, or a loss of muscular control. If any of these symptoms occur, you should stop exercising immediately.

Common problems *after* a session of overexercising include sleeping difficulties, joint pain, soreness, a feeling of heaviness, loss of appetite, a feeling of anxiety or nervousness, an inability to relax, and reduced skill performance. If these symptoms appear, you should reduce your exercise both in intensity and duration until the symptoms disappear. If any of these symptoms persist, it is important to check with a physician.

After Exercise

After exercise, your body needs both a cooling-down period and then a recovery period before any further exercise is undertaken.

Cooling Down

Cooling down may be defined as the continuation of exercise at a low intensity following a rigorous workout, which allows the body to adjust to a resting state. During rigorous exercise, the muscles use over 85 percent of all the blood pumped out of the heart. Even after you stop exercising, the heart continues to provide large amounts of blood until energy has been restored to the muscles. The amount of blood pumped out of the heart is ultimately dependent on the amount of blood returned to the heart by the circulatory system. The blood that is in the lower part of the body below the heart is dependent upon muscle contractions and breathing movements for its return to the heart via the veins. When you stop exercising, blood is still being sent to the muscles. However, if you become sedentary immediately after exercise, the muscle contractions necessary to send blood back to the heart are minimal, thus allowing blood to pool in the lower extremities. This results in a reduced amount of blood returning to the heart and possible interruption to the cardiac cycle, which could lead to dangerous complications. Cooling down also helps to prevent muscle soreness and dizziness and reduces the amounts of biochemical fatigue products in the blood. It is therefore vital to continue slow, relaxed walking after the end of your exercise for approximately five minutes or until your heart rate is below 100 beats per minute.

Generally, the time required for the heart rate to return to normal after exercise depends upon the intensity of the exercise, the length of the exercise period, and your physical condition. Following very rigorous exercise, the heart rate may remain slightly elevated for as long as two hours. If you are in good physical condition, however, recovery will be rapid. Individuals in poor physical condition will have heart rates that tend to return to normal more slowly after exercise.

Recovery Duration

Your body must have a chance to recover from intensive, rigorous physical exercise. Some individuals may take twelve to fourteen hours to recover from exercise; others may take twenty-four hours or more. Periods of recovery from very prolonged exercise, such as marathon running, long-distance running, and skiing, for fit individuals can be anywhere from ten to forty-eight hours before the amount of muscle glycogen returns to normal. Intermittent exercise, such as interval training (running with rest intervals), where exercise is not continuous, may require anywhere from five to twenty-four hours of recovery before a complete supply of glycogen is restored to the muscles. If you don't allow your body time to recover from exercise, you may counteract any training effects that you are trying to achieve.

The best advice is to give your body plenty of time to recover. Especially in the early stages of your exercise program, twenty-four to forty-eight hours between exercise sessions is preferable. If you find yourself waking up in the morning overly exhausted, it is an indication that you should reduce your exercise intensity level and allow more recovery time.

Increase in Heart Size

Physical training over long periods of time results in a dramatic increase in heart size, along with a number of microscopic cellular changes of unknown significance. This increase in the size of the heart muscle is called **cardiac**

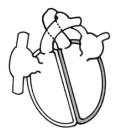 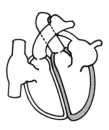 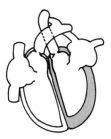

| Endurance athletes | Nonathletes | Nonendurance athletes |

Figure 6.3 Cardiac hypertrophy. From Edward Fox, Richard Bowers, and Merle Foss, *The Physiological Basis for Exercise and Sport,* 5th edition. Copyright 1993, Times Mirror Higher Education Group, Inc. Dubuque, Iowa. All rights reserved. Reprinted by permission.

hypertrophy. In the past, cardiac hypertrophy has been referred to as ''athlete's heart'' to differentiate it from a heart enlarged by disease.

Through training, it is possible for the heart to increase in size as much as 15 percent. This is an obvious advantage to athletes because the stronger contraction from the larger heart muscle results in an increased volume of blood released by the heart. (The cardiac output is how much blood can be pumped out as the result of each stroke from the left ventricle multiplied by the heart rate.) As a result, cardiac hypertrophy is associated with an increased ability to deliver blood to the working muscles.

Evidence suggests that cardiac hypertrophy is manifested in different ways, depending on whether you engage in endurance activities or nonendurance activities. Endurance or aerobic activities, such as long-distance running and swimming, produce an increase in the size of the heart's left ventricular cavity, enabling it to hold more blood, and a slight increase in the thickness of the heart's wall. Nonendurance or anaerobic activities, such as weight lifting or sprinting, produce a greater increase in the ventricular walls' thickness than produced by aerobic training, with no increase in the size of the ventricular cavity (see figure 6.3). In endurance activities, large volumes of blood must be delivered to the working muscles. If a person has a large left ventricular cavity resulting from training, this ensures sufficient blood to sustain the activity. Anaerobic activities, on the other hand, place great stress on the heart and sudden increases in blood pressure. The increased thickness of the heart muscle as a result of training

TABLE 6.5 Cardiorespiratory Training Effects		
Cardiorespiratory training increases	**Cardiorespiratory training produces**	**Cardiorespiratory training decreases**
Tolerance to stress	Lower resting heart rate	Obesity-adiposity
Arterial oxygen content	Physical conditioning of muscles	Arterial blood pressure
Electron transport activity	Greater oxygen use	Heart rate
Efficiency of the heart		Vulnerability to dysrhythmias
Blood vessel size	Greater stroke volume	Stress response
Efficiency of blood circulation	Lower heart rate for submaximal work	Need of heart muscle for oxygen

prepares the heart to deal with these additional stresses and perform more efficiently. Cardiac hypertrophy resulting from exercise should not be confused with asymmetrical hypertrophy, a type of cardiac disease. This abnormal enlargement of the heart muscle is thought to be genetic.

Cardiorespiratory Training Effects

Individuals who participate in regular cardiorespiratory physical activities benefit in a number of ways (see table 6.5). In general, only a few weeks after beginning training, your resting heart rate may decrease. In addition, cardiorespiratory exercise results in an increased supply of red blood cells and hemoglobin, which increases the blood's oxygen-carrying capacity. This enables you to more efficiently supply your working muscles with energy and increases your ability to eliminate metabolic waste products, thus delaying the onset of fatigue.

For physiological changes to occur in the cardiorespiratory system, the oxygen system and the metabolism of the muscle cells must be appropriately stimulated. For example, young individuals who begin an aerobic exercise program three to five times a week for approximately thirty to sixty minutes a day and who train at about 70 percent of their maximum heart rate (140 to 150 beats per minute) can expect a 20 to 30 percent improvement in the oxygen carried in the blood within approximately two months. If you choose to keep constant the amount of time per workout, you can increase the intensity of the workout to ensure improvements in cardiorespiratory endurance.

However, a number of individual genetic and physiological factors contribute to the individual's potential to increase cardiorespiratory endurance.

Key Terms

Adenosine Triphosphate (ATP)
Usable form of stored energy in the muscle

Aerobic Exercises
Continuous, rigorous exercise lasting beyond one to two minutes, such as jogging, long-distance swimming, cycling, and cross-country skiing; exercises using oxygen

Anaerobic Exercises
All-out exercise lasting one to two minutes, such as weight lifting, sprinting, tennis, handball, squash, volleyball, and racquetball; exercises performed in the absence of oxygen

Anaerobic Threshold
When the workload intensity or oxygen consumption level reaches a point where anaerobic metabolism is accelerated and lactic acid begins to accumulate in blood and muscles

Cardiac Arrhythmia
Irregular contractions of the heart muscle

Cardiac Hypertrophy
Increase in the size of the heart muscle

Cooling Down
Continuation of exercise at a low intensity following a rigorous workout, which allows the body to adjust to a resting state

Duration
Amount of time used for each exercise bout

Frequency
Number of exercise sessions per week

Heart Rate Training Effect
The proper intensity level of an endurance training program (approximately 70 percent of maximum heart rate); related to maximum oxygen uptake

Intensity
The level of physiological stress on the body during exercise

Maximum Oxygen Uptake
The greatest amount of oxygen used by the cells during maximum exercise per unit of time

MET
One MET is the equivalent of the resting metabolic rate

Perceived Exertion
An indirect, subjective method of determining heart rate

Phosphocreatine (PC)
A compound found in skeletal muscle used to resynthesize ATP from ADP

Second Wind
General feeling of relief from the effects of fatigue

Stroke Volume
Amount of blood pumped out of the left or right ventricle each time it contracts

7

Starting Your Cardiorespiratory Endurance Program

Chapter   Concepts

After you have studied this chapter you should be able to

1. outline a program for cardiorespiratory endurance for walking/jogging, cycling, rope jumping, and swimming;

2. describe the criteria to judge intensity of exercise;

3. describe the benefits and advantages of walking/jogging;

4. describe the risks involved in cycling and rope jumping;

5. describe water exercises for nonswimmers; and

6. outline a number of indoor exercise options.

Getting Started

Now that you have had a chance to evaluate your fitness level and have shifted your motivation into high gear, you are ready to begin an aerobic fitness program. From the programs presented in this chapter, select an aerobic exercise program that is appropriate for your aerobic fitness level (chapter 4) and your computed heart rate training effect level (chapter 6).

If you have been sedentary for a number of months and are just beginning a program, use 60 percent instead of 70 percent as your heart rate training effect level until you have exercised for four to six weeks. Also, expect a little muscle stiffness and soreness the first few days. This is your body's way of telling you that it has been a long time between workouts. The discomfort should go away in a short time. Follow closely the warm-up principles and procedures presented in chapter 5, and don't take any shortcuts. Remember to cool down after exercise no matter how good you feel.

Make minor modifications to the intensity and duration of the aerobic program you select, depending on how well you respond to the exercise. Time is on your side; don't overstress yourself the first few weeks. Check your heart rate periodically throughout the exercise to make sure that you remain at the proper intensity level. If your heart rate goes over the heart rate training effect level, slow your pace or walk a little farther between repetitions. If, however, you find yourself below your heart rate training effect level, you may want to quicken your pace. After a few weeks of monitoring your heart rate, you will become an expert at determining the proper intensity required to maintain your training effect level.

If you have difficulty completing the repetitions in any of the recommended programs, go back to the previous level until you successfully achieve the new level without undue stress.

At the end of six to eight weeks, reevaluate your cardiorespiratory endurance level and replot your fitness paradigm and profile (figures 4.16 and 4.17).

It is important to remember that the target heart rate intensity and the goals listed in this chapter are only guidelines. Continuing to persevere toward a predetermined intensity when your body is telling you that you are overdoing it is not only foolish but dangerous.

Tune into your body's signals while exercising. You know more or less how you feel and how your body is responding to the exercise. You can tell whether or not you have a feeling of well-being. This is especially important when exercising with a group. Don't let group pressure force you to do things that your body says is too much. You are the best judge as to what your body is capable of doing. Establish your own pace and individualized short- and long-term goals.

If you feel sick or overly fatigued, discontinue your exercise until you are feeling better or the cause of your indisposition has been determined. A general principle is: Don't exercise to the point where you feel exhausted, unduly winded, or have pain or discomfort in your chest area. Appropriate individualized exercises should make you feel good, not sick.

No single exercise can universally meet the needs of all individuals. We all have various levels of skill, motivation, and fitness. You must choose the activity that best meets your interests and capabilities. No matter what exercise program you select, however, it should follow the sequence and fall within the time ranges shown in figure 7.1.

Aerobic Exercise Programs

Four aerobic exercise programs are outlined in this chapter: (1) walking/jogging, (2) cycling, (3) rope jumping, and (4) swimming.

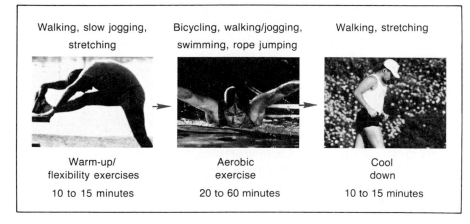

Walking, slow jogging, stretching	Bicycling, walking/jogging, swimming, rope jumping	Walking, stretching
Warm-up/ flexibility exercises	Aerobic exercise	Cool down
10 to 15 minutes	20 to 60 minutes	10 to 15 minutes

Figure 7.1 Sequence and time ranges for basic fitness programs. Photograph by: left and right: Berg & Assoc./Kirk Schlea, middle: Jon Jacobson

Walking/Jogging

Someone once said that the trouble with walking is that it is too easy. Walking is so natural and relaxing that most people don't consider it a form of exercise or understand that it can be beneficial to their health. Walking is appealing because no special equipment is needed, no training is necessary, and you can walk anywhere. Walking uses large muscle groups essential for fitness. It is rhythmic, self-pacing, pleasant, and safe. An average-size woman can walk comfortably at brisk speeds of three and one half to four miles per hour, while the average man can walk four and one half to five miles per hour. Slower walking (two miles per hour) can be advantageous for older people, cardiac patients, and people recovering from illness. Walking at speeds of five miles an hour can burn as many calories as moderate jogging. Even slower walking can burn sixty to eighty calories a mile.

Jogging is a slow run in which the foot hits the ground with the weight centered slightly to the outside of the foot before transferring it to the toes. Avoid running on your toes since this can injure your lower back or joints.

When you first start your walking/jogging exercise program, do not attempt to get yourself in shape in one day. Build up to it gradually. Your intensity and frequency should depend on your individual goals. You might spend two to four weeks walking before you even start to jog. Because this gives your body a chance to gradually accommodate to the exercise load, you probably will have no difficulty when you begin jogging.

Table 7.1 lists recommended walking and jogging regimens that will get you started. For adults whose fitness level falls within the "very poor" to "average" range, the sixteen-week walking/jogging program outlined in table 7.2 is recommended.

Cycling

Long-distance cycling is excellent for building cardiorespiratory endurance and also for increasing the strength and endurance of muscles in the lower extremities. Because cycling is a nonweight-bearing activity, there is less chance of injury to the lower body. Also, those individuals with lower-back and leg problems that prohibit jogging can participate in cycling without fear of further injury.

Safety, however, should be a major consideration when cycling. Accident rates for cyclists have risen sharply. Be sure to wear a helmet and other protective equipment. Try to avoid busy streets and find a bike path or other safe riding areas.

Five miles of cycling at twice the speed of jogging is equivalent to about two miles of jogging. You should aim for a goal of ninety minutes of cycling at approximately 15 miles per hour, three to five days a week. Table 7.3 lists recommended levels of cycling according to your fitness category.

Rope Jumping

Rope jumping does an excellent job of stimulating the cardiorespiratory system. The exercise should be at least twenty minutes long for best results.

A problem with rope jumping, however, is that the continuous stress placed upon the knees and the ankles increases the possibility of injury. Such problems as swollen knees, pain in the lower legs, and stress fractures are not uncommon.

One way to avoid some of these problems is to alternate feet while jumping. Jumping with both feet at once places too much stress on the lower legs. Also, wear a good pair of running shoes with a proper heel support and avoid jumping on very hard surfaces. Another option is to bounce in place on a minitrampoline.

Table 7.4 presents rope-jumping and bouncing in place regimens.

Swimming

Swimming is one of the best cardiorespiratory conditioning exercises. Because swimming is performed in a horizontal position, your body weight is supported by the water, which helps to prevent hip, leg, and back injuries that commonly are associated with running. In addition, swimming is especially appropriate for those who are overweight or handicapped or who have orthopedic problems.

TABLE 7.1 Walking/Jogging Program for Cardiorespiratory Endurance

Fitness category	Starting level
"Very poor" to "poor"	1 to 2
"Average" to "good"	2 to 3
"Very good" to "excellent"	4 to 5
"Superior"	5 to 7

Level	Exercise	Heart rate training effect level (intensity)	Frequency	Duration
1	Walk for 10 to 20 minutes.	60%	3 days	2 to 4 weeks
2	Walk fast for 15 to 20 minutes.	60%	3 days	2 to 4 weeks
3	Jog 100 yards and then walk 300 yards. Repeat four times. Add one repetition for each succeeding exercise session. When you reach eight repetitions, move to level 4 (approximately 30 minutes).	60%	3 days	2 to 3 weeks
4	Jog 200 yards and then walk 200 yards. Repeat four times. Add one repetition for each succeeding exercise session. When you reach eight repetitions, move to level 5 (approximately 28 minutes).	60%	3 to 4 days	2 to 3 weeks
5	Jog 400 yards and then walk 400 yards. Repeat four times. Add one repetition for each succeeding exercise session. When you reach eight repetitions, move to level 6 (approximately 26 minutes).	70%	3 to 4 days	2 to 3 weeks
6	Jog 800 yards and then walk 400 yards. Repeat four times. Add one repetition for every other exercise session. When you reach six repetitions, move to level 7 (approximately 22 minutes).	70%	3 to 5 days	2 to 3 weeks
7	Jog 1,200 yards and then walk 600 yards. Repeat two times. Add one repetition for every other exercise session. When you reach four repetitions, move to level 8 (approximately 22 minutes).	70%	3 to 5 days	2 to 3 weeks
8	Jog 1 mile in 10 minutes and then walk 3 minutes. Then jog 1 mile again in 10 to 12 minutes.	70%	3 to 5 days	2 to 3 weeks
9	Jog 1½ miles in 15 minutes and then walk 6 to 8 minutes. Then jog again 1½ miles in 15 to 18 minutes.	70%	3 to 5 days	2 to 3 weeks
10	Jog 2 miles in 20 minutes.	70%	3 to 5 days	2 to 3 weeks
11	Jog 2 miles in 18 minutes.	70%	3 to 5 days	2 to 3 weeks
12	Jog 2 miles in 16 minutes.	70%	3 to 5 days	2 to 3 weeks
13	Jog 2 miles in 14 minutes.	70%	3 to 5 days	2 to 3 weeks
14	Continue on to 20–40 minutes of aerobic activity.	70%	3 to 5 days a week	

TABLE 7.2 Sixteen-Week Walking/Jogging Program for Adults with Low-Level Fitness

---

Weeks 1 and 2
For the first two weeks, walk at a brisk pace for 10 minutes each day, 3 to 5 days a week. If you become tired after the first 3 to 5 minutes of walking, walk slowly for the remainder of the 10 minutes (50 percent heart rate training effect level).

Weeks 3 and 4
Walk briskly for 15 minutes. If you feel tired after the first 6 to 8 minutes, walk slowly for 3 to 4 minutes and then walk briskly for the remainder of the 15 minutes (60 percent heart rate training effect level).

Weeks 5 and 6
Walk briskly for 10 minutes, then walk slowly for 3 to 4 minutes, and then walk briskly again for the final 10 minutes (60 percent heart rate training effect level).

Week 7
Jog 30 yards and then walk for 2 minutes. Repeat nine times (60 percent heart rate training effect level).

Week 8
Jog 60 yards and then walk for 2 minutes. Repeat nine times (60 percent heart rate training effect level).

Week 9
Jog 110 yards and then walk for 2 minutes. Repeat nine times (60 percent heart rate training effect level).

Week 10
Jog 130 yards and then walk for 2 minutes. Repeat seven times (60 percent heart rate training effect level).

Week 11
Jog 250 yards and then walk for 1½ minutes. Repeat four times (60 percent heart rate training effect level).

Week 12
Jog 500 yards and then walk for 1½ minutes. Repeat three times (70 percent heart rate training effect level).

Week 13
Jog ½ mile and then walk for 300 yards. Repeat two times (70 percent heart rate training effect level).

Week 14
Jog ¾ mile and then walk for 3 minutes. Repeat one time (70 percent heart rate training effect level).

Week 15
Jog 1 mile in approximately 10 minutes and then walk for 3 to 5 minutes. Repeat one time (70 percent heart rate training effect level).

Week 16
Now you are ready for exercise level 9 presented in table 7.1. Within a few weeks, you should be able to jog the 7-minute mile required at level 13. Remember, don't exceed your 70 percent heart rate training effect level. If you find your heart rate going above your training effect level, slow your pace.

Source: Modified from the President's Council on Physical Fitness: Reporting to the President and the Secretary of Health, Education, and Welfare.

TABLE 7.3 Cycling Program for Cardiorespiratory Endurance

Fitness category	Starting level
"Very poor" to "poor"	1
"Average" to "good"	1 to 2
"Very good" to "excellent"	3
"Superior"	3

Level	Exercise	Heart rate training effect level (intensity)	Frequency	Duration
1	Ride for 10 to 25 minutes (10 to 12 MPH).	60%	3 days	4 to 6 weeks
2	Ride for 25 to 30 minutes (12 MPH).	60%	3 days	4 to 6 weeks
3	Ride for 30 to 40 minutes (15 MPH).	70%	3 to 5 days	4 to 6 weeks
4	Ride for 40 to 90 minutes (15 MPH).	70%	3 to 5 days	4 to 6 weeks
5	Continue at level 4 to maintain lifetime fitness.			

Because the entire musculature is involved in swimming, energy expenditure is much greater than walking or jogging the same distance. For example, swimming for thirty minutes may produce cardiorespiratory training effects that would require two to three hours of continuous tennis or badminton. Individuals will have a lower maximum heart rate when swimming than when running. The heart rate is lower because of the body's horizontal position, which helps distribute blood more uniformly. The cool water also helps dissipate heat more rapidly than when you are jogging, thus reducing the workload of the heart. The difference between running and swimming is approximately thirteen beats per minute. This difference must be subtracted from the age-related maximum heart rate if swimming is your means of training. Thus, a forty-year-old swimmer would subtract 40 plus 13 from 220 to get a maximum rate of 167 when computing the training effect. For running, the maximum heart rate would be 180.

Table 7.5 outlines a swimming program for cardiorespiratory endurance.

Aquatic Exercises

The major obvious drawback to swimming is that a moderate level of swimming skill is required. However, even those individuals who are not skilled swimmers or who have disabilities or injuries that prevent them from leg-supported loco-motive movements can improve their cardiorespiratory endurance by performing

TABLE 7.4	Rope Jumping (or Bouncing in Place on a Minitrampoline) Program for Cardiorespiratory Endurance

Fitness category	Starting level
"Very poor" to "poor"	1
"Average" to "good"	2
"Very good" to "excellent"	3
"Superior"	4

Level	Exercise	Heart rate training effect level (intensity)	Frequency	Duration
1	Jump for 30 seconds and then rest for 20 to 40 seconds. Repeat six to eight times (2 to 5 minutes).	50%	3 days	2 to 4 weeks
2	Jump for 60 seconds and then rest for 60 seconds. Repeat six to eight times (4 to 10 minutes).	60%	3 days	2 to 4 weeks
3	Jump for 90 seconds and then rest for 15 seconds. Repeat six to eight times (6 to 12 minutes).	60%	3 days	2 to 4 weeks
4	Jump for 2 minutes and then rest for 30 seconds. Repeat four to eight times (10 to 25 minutes).	70%	3 to 5 days	2 to 4 weeks
5	Jump for 4 minutes and then rest for 30 seconds. Repeat four to eight times (15 to 30 minutes).	70%	3 to 5 days	2 to 4 weeks
6	Jump for 8 minutes and then rest for 30 seconds. Repeat one to two times (15 to 30 minutes).	70%	3 to 5 days	2 to 4 weeks
7	Jump for 10 minutes and then rest for 2 to 3 minutes. Repeat one to two times (30 minutes).	70%	3 to 5 days	2 to 4 weeks
8	Jump for 10 minutes and then rest for 2 minutes. Repeat two times (30 minutes).	70%	3 to 5 days	2 to 4 weeks
9	Continue at level 8 to maintain lifetime fitness.			

water aerobics or the water exercises that follow. The intensity, frequency, and duration of the following exercises should approximate those levels in table 7.5 that are consistent with your fitness category.

1. **Bobbing** Stand in shallow water. Inhale and then duck underwater to a squat position. Blow your air out gradually. Then push off the bottom of the pool to a standing position and inhale.

TABLE 7.5 Swimming Program for Cardiorespiratory Endurance

Fitness category	Starting level
"Very poor" to "poor"	1
"Average" to "good"	1 to 2
"Very good" to "excellent"	2 to 3
"Superior"	3 to 4

Level	Exercise	Heart rate training effect level (intensity)	Frequency	Duration
1	Swim 25 yards. Repeat four times with a 30- to 60-second rest between each repetition. While resting at the end of the pool between laps, move your legs slowly as in a walking movement. Add one to two repetitions for each succeeding exercise session until you can do twelve repetitions. Then move on to level 2.	60%	3 days	2 to 4 weeks
2	Swim 50 yards. Repeat four times with a 30- to 60-second rest between each repetition. While resting at the end of the pool between laps, move your legs slowly as in a walking movement. Add one to two repetitions for each succeeding exercise session until you can do twelve repetitions. Then move on to level 3.	60%	3 days	2 to 4 weeks
3	Swim 100 yards. Repeat four times with a 90-second rest between each repetition. While resting at the end of the pool between laps, move your legs slowly as in a walking movement. Add one to two repetitions for each succeeding exercise session until you can do eight repetitions. Then move on to level 4.	60%	3 days	2 to 4 weeks
4	Swim 150 yards. Repeat three times with a 90-second rest between each repetition. While resting at the end of the pool between laps, move your legs slowly as in a walking movement. Add one to two repetitions for each succeeding exercise session until you can do six repetitions. Then move on to level 5.	70%	3 to 5 days	2 to 4 weeks
5	Swim 200 yards. Rest for 60 seconds and then repeat five times.	70%	3 to 5 days	2 to 3 weeks
6	Swim slowly 400 yards. Rest for 2 minutes and then repeat two times.	70%	3 to 5 days	2 to 3 weeks
7	Swim moderately 600 yards.	70%	3 to 5 days	2 to 3 weeks
8	Swim moderately 800 to 1,400 yards.	70%	3 to 5 days	2 to 3 weeks
9	Continue at level 8 to maintain lifetime fitness.			

2. **Treading** Stand in water that is shoulder deep. Bicycle with your feet and scull with your hands palms down to tread water.

3. **Flutter Kicking** Hold onto the side of the pool while lying on your stomach in the water. Kick your legs using a **flutter kick,** a swimming kick executed with the legs horizontal and the knees straight. The legs are alternately moved up and down in rapid succession. Extend your elbows as far as possible.

4. **Climbing** Stand in the water and hold onto the side of the pool with both hands. Place your feet against the side of the pool and walk up and down the pool side.

5. **Knee Flexion** Hold onto the pool side while lying on your back in the water. Bring your knees up to your chest. Hold for five seconds and then extend your knees.

6. **Running in Place** Stand in water that is chest deep and run in place. Maintain your balance by placing your hands palms down in the water, with your elbows flexed ninety degrees.

7. **Pull-ups** (using side of pool) Place arms on the edge of the pool, raise body weight until arms are extended, then lower in a controlled movement.

8. **Leg Lifts** Using the side of the pool with your back against the wall of the pool, tuck knees to chest and lower slowly. Variation: use straight legs.

Other Exercise Options

The four aerobic exercise programs outlined in this chapter—walking/jogging, cycling, rope jumping, and swimming—are excellent for developing cardiorespiratory endurance. Other exercise options, however, such as jogging in place, dancing, riding a stationary bike, cross-country skiing, and orienteering, can be equally beneficial to the cardiorespiratory system.

Indoor Exercise Options

A number of beneficial exercises can be performed in your home. Jogging in place for around twenty minutes is excellent exercise. If you find it boring, turn on the television set and watch your favorite program or play some music.

If you don't like running in place, purchase a stationary bicycle. Exercising on a stationary bicycle for twenty-five to thirty minutes a day is an excellent method for training the cardiorespiratory system. The pedaling rate for training should average between ten and fourteen miles per hour; however, your best indication of intensity level is your own heart rate response. The stationary bike should be equipped with an odometer and a mechanism for increasing or decreasing resistance to the pedals.

Calisthenics and aerobics (various gymnastic exercises using both aerobic and anaerobic fitness) or dancing to music are other options. Choreograph your own movements to music and exercise continuously for at least thirty minutes. Check out an aerobic dance class for some tips on movement and music, if it is convenient. Minitrampolines, rowing machines, versa climbers, stair masters, and even stair climbing are also effective for maintaining continuous and rhythmic exercise. Low-impact aerobics (floor exercises to music or with aerobic videos) may be another option if you have knee or ankle problems.

Cross-Country Skiing

Cross-country skiing is the most demanding cardiorespiratory exercise in terms of intensity. In addition to the lower body muscles used in running, cross-country skiing requires upper trunk and arm muscles, which add intensity to the cardiorespiratory system. Therefore, before attempting to participate in this activity, you should have already attained a very high level of cardiorespiratory endurance. Needless to say, proper equipment and instruction are also essential.

Orienteering

Orienteering is a combination of cross-country running and land navigation. Competitors use only a map and compass to navigate their way between checkpoints along an unfamiliar course. In some European countries, thousands compete in one race. The main objective is the satisfaction of finishing in the allotted time and enjoying and responding to the challenge. Orienteering incorporates walking, running, and climbing, making it an excellent total body workout.

Cross-Country Ski Simulator

Like real cross-country skiing, a cross-country ski simulator works every major muscle group and puts very little strain on the body. However, if your ankles are not flexible, there may be discomfort or soreness. Cross-country skiing requires good arm and leg coordination.

Jarming

Jarming, invented as a substitute for jogging or cycling, is a series of upper body exercises that can be done sitting in a chair. However, upper body exercise alone is not as efficient in terms of total body exercise and should not be considered a substitute. The best fitness program combines both upper body and lower body exercise. Also, upper body exercise can be dangerous for those individuals with heart problems since the smaller muscles in the arms will raise blood pressure more than larger ones used in total body exercise. Jarming may be useful for the elderly and physically handicapped and can make a difference between a sedentary and an active lifestyle.

Cross-Training

Cross-training is a training method using a variety of complementary exercises to improve performance in a chosen activity. A common example is including the use of resistance training in an exercise program to improve performance in track or swimming and plyometric training for competitive skiers. Cross-training is also effective in extending cardiorespiratory endurance, injury rehabilitation, maintaining motivation, providing variety, and overcoming plateaus in training.

Walking

Of all fitness activities, walking is easiest, safest, and cheapest. It's also easier on your knees, ankles, and back. A long-term program of walking can help you stay healthy and live longer. The American Heart Association now classifies physical inactivity as a risk factor for cardiovascular disease the same as smoking and high blood pressure. A walking program is an easy way to become active. Walking is an excellent way to lose weight and strengthen your bones.

Stationary Bike

A stationary bike allows you to control the intensity of the work-out and with little stress on leg and foot joints and lower back. On the stationary bike, gradually increase the work load to the appropriate heart rate level. Maintain the rate until fatigue begins to set in. As fatigue increases, the intensity can be gradually reduced to keep the heart rate at the appropriate level. Start out with a 1 kp = 300kp-m load with approximately forty revolutions per minute. Work up to seventy to ninety revolutions per minute at the same moderate tension. Peddling slowly at a higher tension (900kp-m's) puts excessive stress on the legs, heart, and lungs. Always adjust the seat to the proper height; your knee should be only slightly bent when the leg is extended.

Water Running

Because of the large number of individuals with lower-back and knee and ankle problems, aerobic activities conducted in the water have become very popular. These activities can provide an excellent training stimulus, and they place much less stress on joints and muscles than similar activities done out of the water. The water and music also provide physical and psychological relaxation. An important benefit is that these exercises do not require swimming skill.

Water running acts as a cushion for weight bearing joints and helps prevent strain, injury, and reinjury so common with running workouts on land. There are two basic methods of water running. Shallow water running entails sprinting in waist-deep water, typically in the shallow end of the swimming pool. Shallow water runners may also use a tether-elasticized tubing secured around the waist and hooked to a pool ladder, a lane marker, or pool furniture that holds them in place and allows them to concentrate on form. For deep water running, a flotation device keeps the head out of the water while the legs hang suspended above the pool bottom. The individual then runs in place.

Bench Stepping

Nothing beats activity like running or aerobic dancing as a good fitness exercise but such activities in some individuals may cause sprains, strains, and stress fractures. Walking and low-impact aerobic dancing, while safer, are less intense, burn fewer calories, and it's harder to get your heart pumping at a beneficial rate. Bench stepping is one way to get a good workout without undo wear and tear on joints and muscles. The exercise involved is stepping on and off a low bench (four to eight inches) while moving your arms. Bench stepping can combine the cardiopulmonary intensity of running and the gentleness of walking. Bench stepping takes, on the average, the same energy as running at seven miles per hour, and about three times as much energy as walking at three miles per hour. Yet the force of the impact from bench stepping is relatively gentle, about the same as the impact from walking. Maximum safe bench stepping height is eight inches.

Treadmill

Treadmills can be an excellent aerobic conditioner. Many models have side or front handrails for maintaining balance. To prevent a mishap, straddle the machine before starting it, and slow it down gradually before getting off.

Stair Climber

This machine provides an easy way to get a strenuous workout. Beginners should be careful not to overexert themselves, since blood pressure and heart rate may rise very quickly. Start with short steps and slow pace, and put your entire foot on the peddle, not just the ball of your foot. Try to keep your knees aligned over your toes.

Rowing Machine

Proper rowing technique and cadence put little strain on the body. If you have a back problem, consult your doctor before using a rowing machine. Make sure your legs, not your back, power your rowing motion. In the early part of the stroke your arms should move forward before you bend your knees. When using a fly wheel model, pull the bar into your abdomen, not your chin.

Ending Exercise

You should never end an exercise period with a wind sprint. Running to exhaustion at the end of an exercise session is unnecessary; can have dangerous consequences to the heart; and can lead to tendon, muscle, and ligament damage. Taper off very slowly at the end of exercise by walking and stretching.

Aesthetic Awareness

An often overlooked factor in exercise, but nevertheless an important one, is the potential for the development of aesthetic awareness. Fortunately, a number of physical activities not only lead to increased fitness, but also allow for creative expression. For example, you can create your own expressive floor exercises, explore different kinds of movements in modern jazz and aerobic dance, and choose your own music. Even though there seem to be fewer ways to catch a pass or hit a tennis ball than there are ways to dance or move to music, the opportunity for creativity exists in all sports. Exercise and staying in shape can develop aspects other than just your cardiorespiratory endurance.

Tracking Your Cardiorespiratory Endurance

Aerobic exercise record sheets are provided for you in appendix B at the back of the book (record sheets B-1 and B-3). Keeping a careful record of your exercise will show you the steady advances you make toward cardiorespiratory endurance. See also appendix E for recording your weekly activity log.

Key Terms

Calisthenics and Aerobics
Various gymnastic exercises using both aerobic and anaerobic fitness

Cross-Training
Combining a variety of complementary exercises to enhance strength, performance, and endurance

Flutter Kick
A swimming kick executed with the legs horizontal and the knees straight—the legs are alternately moved up and down in rapid succession

Orienteering
A combination of cross-country running and land navigation

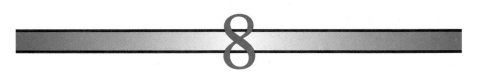

8

chapter

Muscle Strength and Endurance

Chapter Concepts

After you have studied this chapter you should be able to

1. define power;
2. explain the importance of muscle strength and endurance;
3. describe and define the basic principles of weight-resistance training;
4. determine the amount of resistance necessary for strength and endurance training;
5. define the three basic weight-resistance programs;
6. explain advantages and disadvantages of the weight-resistance programs;
7. describe other options for advanced strength training;
8. describe the guidelines for strength training;
9. describe weight lifting complications and potential injuries;
10. describe the physical changes in muscles as a result of weight training;
11. describe red and white muscle fibers;
12. describe the female muscle response to weight training;
13. describe strength and endurance training equipment;
14. define periodization of strength training; and
15. describe circuit training.

Importance of Muscle Strength and Endurance

The terms *muscle strength* and *muscle endurance* are often confused, and it is important to differentiate between them. **Muscle strength** is the amount of force that can be exerted by a muscle group for one movement or repetition (1RM). **Muscle endurance** is the ability of the muscle group to maintain a continuous contraction or repetition over a period of time. The muscle

135

system is at the foundation of all physical exercise. No matter what activity you participate in, your muscle strength and endurance determine your exercise limits.

The American College of Sports Medicine recommends moderate resistance training at least twice a week, with a minimum of eight to ten exercises involving major muscle groups, with each exercise repeated eight to twelve times.

Body motion, the beating of the heart, breathing movements, movements of the bones, balance, and posture are all brought about by the contraction of muscles. Muscles are not independent from the rest of the body systems, and conditioning is not limited solely to the muscles. Your muscles' ability to do work is totally dependent upon the efficiency of the heart, blood vessels, and lungs in providing energy and waste product elimination. Muscles, the heart, blood vessels, and the lungs are simultaneously conditioned because of their interdependence. Weight training has also shown to be of some benefit in maintaining bone density, an important factor in protection from osteoporosis in women.

Your main goal in conditioning the muscle system is not to build big, bulky muscles like the bodybuilders seen on television or the weight lifters in the Olympics. These individuals have trained rigorously for years in highly specialized weight programs to develop their special qualities. Your primary goal is to increase the strength and endurance of your muscles so that they become more efficient in dealing with the everyday demands placed upon them. Whether it's mowing the grass in the backyard, moving the filing cabinet at the office, or meeting the unforeseen physical demands of an emergency situation, well-conditioned muscles enable you to make the necessary adaptations more effectively and without injury.

Power

Strength training by its nature emphasizes the force component of the sport, but not the acceleration component essential in power. Power is basically the product of strength and speed; an increase in either one will increase power. Strength will only play a minor role, however, unless it can be applied explosively over a short period of time. The strongest wrestler, for example, may not be the best if he doesn't have the speed that prevents him from being outmaneuvered. It is important to train at velocities of movement similar to those of the specific sport skill because speed depends upon activating the appropriate neuromuscular patterns involved in a particular skill.

Research on muscles has rapidly advanced in such areas as muscle fatigue, fiber type, weight-resistance training, and injury. Even with these advances, some confusion still exists with regard to the most efficient techniques for increasing strength and endurance. Research indicates, however, that certain training procedures produce greater muscle efficiency than others.

Before discussing the three basic weight-resistance programs, we examine the basic principles of weight-resistance training and how to determine the amount of resistance to use for training.

Basic Principles of Weight-Resistance Training

Four basic principles of weight-resistance training should be followed to derive the maximum strength and endurance gains from the training regimen: (1) overload, (2) progressive resistance, (3) specificity, and (4) allowing for adequate recovery.

Overload

Muscle strength only develops when muscles are **overloaded**—forced to contract at maximum or near maximum tension. Muscle contractions at these tension levels produce physiological changes in the muscles, resulting in strength gains. If muscles are not overloaded to this degree, they do not increase in strength or in size (hypertrophy). Muscles adapt only to the load to which they are subjected. A maximum overload results in maximum strength gains, whereas a minimum overload produces only minimum strength gains.

Progressive Resistance

As muscle strength increases from training, the initial training load no longer provides adequate strength gains. If the intensity of the training load is not increased, only existing strength levels are maintained. Therefore, the intensity of the load must be progressively increased to ensure future strength gains, a concept known as **progressive resistance.**

Specificity

The demands of the exercise must be sufficient to force muscles to adapt, and the subsequent muscle adaptations are specific to the type of training performed, a concept known as **specificity.** For example, aerobic activity develops aerobic capacity, and anaerobic activity develops anaerobic capacity.

Research indicates that muscle adaptations are specific to the type of training performed because exercise not only affects muscles but also nerve control of muscles. The nerve pathways appear to become more efficient with continued exercise. The efficiency, however, is specific only to the particular exercise.

Research also indicates that the joint angle of exercise, the type of exercise (that is, isotonic, isometric, or isokinetic), and the speed and range of movement all produce a variety of specific muscle adaptations.

137

Allowing for Adequate Recovery

Progressive training becomes less effective when muscles become fatigued since the training stimulus cannot be maintained at maximum level. Also, overloading a fatigued muscle may lead to soreness and injury. Therefore, follow four simple rules:

1. Exercise large muscle groups before smaller ones. Movements become fatiguing when the small muscles involved in the movement are fatigued. For example, before performing standing overhead lifts with free weights, first exercise the leg muscles and then the lower arm muscles.
2. Arrange your strength exercises so that successive exercises only minimally affect the muscle groups that were trained previously.
3. Maintain a consistent application of force by raising and lowering the weight in a controlled manner. Generally, the lift phase should take about one to two seconds and the lowering phase approximately three to four seconds.
4. Allow forty-eight hours between strength exercises for complete physiological recovery.

Determining the Amount of Resistance

Muscle strength is most effectively developed when muscles are overloaded—that is, exercised against maximum or near maximum resistance. Heavy resistance forces muscles to contract maximally, thus stimulating the physiological adaptations that lead to increased strength.

Generally, to increase muscle strength, the intensity should be near maximum with a low number of repetitions; to gain muscle endurance, the intensity should be lower with a high number of repetitions. The intensity level for strength gains is believed to be between one and six repetitions maximum; for endurance gains, it is believed to be over six repetitions maximum. One repetition maximum (RM) is the maximum load that you can lift successfully *once* through the full range of movement (100 percent intensity), two repetitions maximum (2 RM) is the amount you can lift successfully *twice* through the full range of movement, and so on.

Weight-training research indicates that weight loads exceeding 75 percent of maximum are necessary for promoting strength gains since the most important factor in strength development is the intensity. A 10 RM weight load usually corresponds to about 75 percent of that maximum.

When beginning a weight-training program, it is best to select an intensity around 10 to 12 RM. This reduces your chance of injury and gives you time to acquire the proper form required for lifting. After several weeks, you may work up to an intensity of 1 to 6 RM, if your goal is muscular strength. As training progresses, you will experience strength gains, and as a result, your original repetition maximum will have to be increased. Therefore, you should determine a new repetition maximum approximately every two weeks. Keep in mind, however, that individuals vary widely in their response to strength programs, and exceptions to these training principles are not uncommon.

Time Between Sets

Muscle fibers will recover to within 50 percent of their innate capacity within three to five seconds after a set. The recovery time will continue to increase in proportion to the rest time allotted. A rest interval may range from thirty seconds to a maximum of one minute. Rest periods longer than two minutes result in pooled blood draining from the muscle, leading to fatigue.

Weight-Resistance Programs

Weight-resistance programs can involve isotonic exercise, isometric exercise, and isokinetic exercise.

Isotonic Exercise

Isotonic exercise is exercise that is performed against resistance while the load remains constant, with the resistance varying with the angle of the joint (for example, lifting free weights [barbells] or weight stacks, such as used on the universal gym). The free weights seem to be the most popular among today's athletes, who are convinced that the way to higher levels of athletic performance is through increases in strength, power, and endurance.

If you are starting your first isotonic weight program, table 8.1 recommends that you start at an intensity load of 10 to 12 RM. To determine your 10 to 12 RM, you must find a weight that you can lift successfully twelve times (using the higher RM) through the full range of movement before you fatigue. For example, using a biceps curl (fig. 8.10), you might find after a little trial and error that you are able to curl thirty pounds twelve consecutive times before fatiguing. Therefore, thirty pounds would be your 12 RM for this exercise. According to table 8.1, you should complete three sets of ten to twelve repetitions for each set with the thirty-pound (12 RM) load. Remember, you must determine your repetition maximum (intensity) for each specific isotonic exercise. Table 8.1 recommends specific intensity and repetition levels for increasing strength and endurance through isotonic exercise.

Variations of isotonic exercise include speed loading, eccentric loading, and plyometric loading.

139

TABLE 8.1	Recommendations for Increasing Strength and Endurance Through Isotonic Exercise		
Frequency	Three to five days per week		
Duration	Six weeks minimum		
Rest	One to two minutes between sets		
	Intensity	*Repetitions**	*Sets*
Beginners	10–12 RM	10–12 rep.	3 sets per exercise
Strength	1–6 RM	1–6 rep.	3 sets per exercise
Endurance	12–14 RM	12–14 rep.	3 sets per exercise
Sports training	8–12 RM	8–12 rep.	3 sets per exercise

*Repetition—the number of continuous contractions per set or group.

Speed Loading

Speed loading occurs when the resistance is moved as rapidly as possible. This technique is believed to be inferior to the more commonly practiced constant resistant isotonic exercise for gaining strength since not enough tension is produced for a training effect. However, many athletes use this technique during competition when maximum power is desired. For example, a football lineman may train by moving a heavy weight as rapidly as possible in an attempt to approach movement velocities similar to those in blocking.

Eccentric Loading

Eccentric loading is sometimes referred to as a negative contraction because the muscle lengthens as it develops tension. Eccentric contraction is frequently a naturally occurring part of the normal range and motion of many exercises and movements. Examples would be letting yourself down slowly from a chin-up or extending your elbow slowly from a flexed position while holding a weight in your hand. This type of exercise tends to produce more muscle soreness than other techniques. It is not superior to other isotonic methods and is used mainly as an addition to other training techniques.

Plyometric Loading

Plyometric loading requires that the muscles be loaded suddenly and then forced to stretch before the contraction for movement occurs. This type of exercise has gained some popularity among volleyball players, skiers, discus throwers, and shot-putters. An example would be to jump from a bench to the floor and then immediately back onto the bench. This exercise has been shown to increase strength and jumping ability. Anyone who attempts this exercise should be aware of the possibility of injury to the ankles and knee joints.

Skeletal Muscles and Structural Design

Figures 8.1 and 8.2 indicate the major muscle groups important in resistance training. Refer to figure 8.3 for the structural design of human skeletal muscles.

Exercise Stations

Figures 8.4–8.7, and 8.12–8.13 illustrate isotonic exercises that can be used on weight training machines.

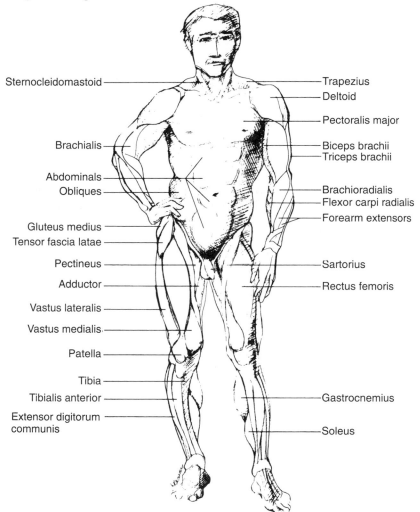

Figure 8.1 Muscles of the Body: Front. From Wayne L. Wescott, Strength Fitness, 2nd. edition. Copyright 1989, Times Mirror Higher Education Group, Inc., Dubuque, Iowa. All rights reserved. Reprinted by permission.

Prescribed Strength Exercises Using Free Weights

Figures 8.8–8.11 and 8.14–8.18 illustrate isotonic exercises for increasing strength with the use of free weights. If you do not have access to free weights, the exercises illustrated in figures 8.19–8.21 can be very useful in increasing muscular strength and endurance.

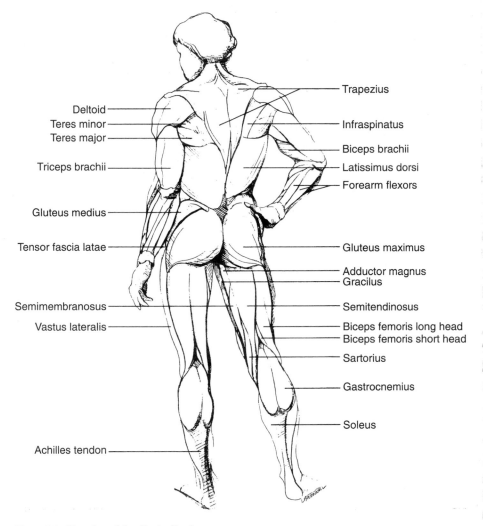

Figure 8.2 Muscles of the Body: Back.
From Wayne L. Westcott, Strength Fitness,
2nd. edition. Copyright 1989, Times Mirror
Higher Education Group, Inc., Dubuque,
Iowa. All rights reserved. Reprinted by
permission.

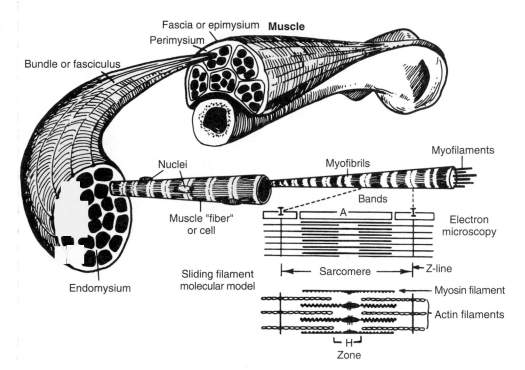

Fascia or epimysium **Muscle**
Perimysium
Bundle or fasciculus
Myofilaments
Nuclei
Myofibrils
Bands
Muscle "fiber"
or cell
A
Electron
microscopy
Sliding filament
molecular model
Sarcomere
Z-line
Endomysium
Myosin filament
Actin filaments
H
Zone

Figure 8.3 Structural design of human skeletal muscle. From Jack H. Wilmore and David L. Costill, Training for Sport and Activity; 3rd. edition. Copyright 1988, Times Mirror Higher Education Group, Inc., Dubuque, Iowa. All rights reserved. Reprinted by permission.

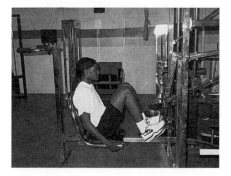

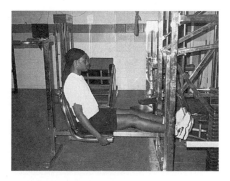

Figure 8.4 Leg press. Push the leg pedal away from you by extending your knees. Caution: Do not lock knees in extended position. Muscles used: Primary—Quadriceps; Additional—Hamstrings, Gluteals.

143

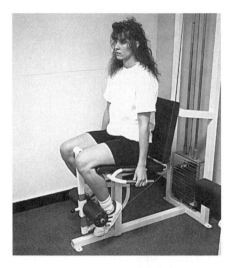
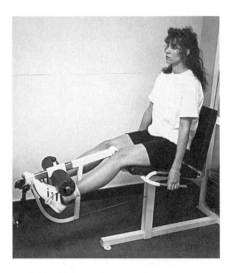

Figure 8.5 Knee extension. Grasp the bench with both of your hands while in a sitting position. Hook the top of your ankles behind the lower bars. Pull the lever up by straightening your knees. Lift up two seconds and lower four seconds. Do not swing or use momentum. Muscles used: Quadriceps.

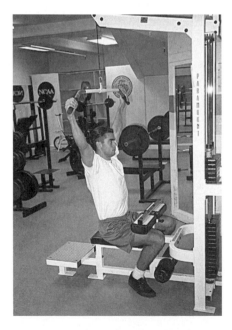
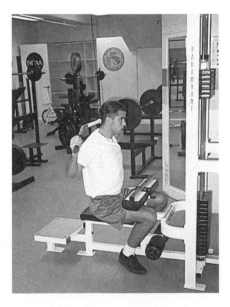

Figure 8.6 Pulldown. Start in a kneeling or sitting position. With your hands palms down, pull the bar down behind your neck to tip of shoulder and then slowly return it to the starting position. Muscles used: Latissimus dorsi.

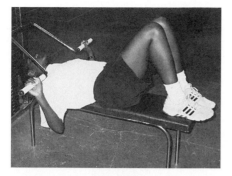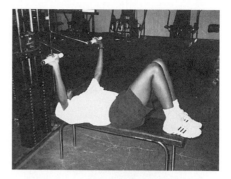

Figure 8.7 Bench press (chest). From a supine position on the bench, grasp the bar with an overhand grip, hands shoulder-width apart, elbows fully extended. Lower the bar to your chest and then return to your starting position. To protect the lower back, place feet on bench or pull knees up toward stomach. Muscles used: Primary—Pectoralis major; Additional—Anterior deltoid, Biceps brachii, Triceps brachii.

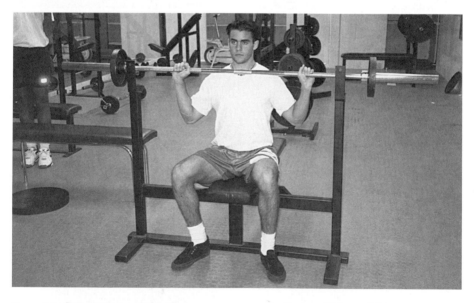

Figure 8.8 Shoulder press (shoulders, upper arms). Sit with your feet shoulder-width apart on the floor. Then bend your knees to forty-five degrees and grasp the bar with an overhand grip, hands spread shoulder-width apart. With your elbows under the bar, lift the weight over your head and return to your starting position. Muscles used: Primary—Trapezius, Deltoid; Additional—Supraspinatus, Levator scapulae.

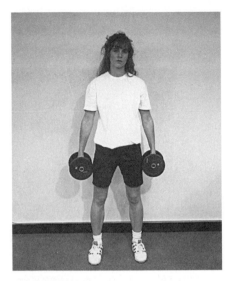

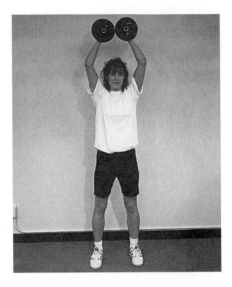

Figure 8.9 Lateral arm raise (shoulder). With one dumbbell in each hand, arms hanging down to your sides, raise both of your arms out to the side of your body and then to an overhead position, keeping your elbows slightly bent. Then return to your starting position. Muscles used: Deltoids, Trapezius.

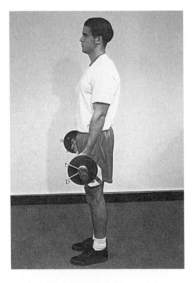

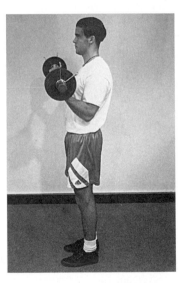

Figure 8.10 Biceps curl (upper, lower arm). Grasp the bar with your hands shoulder-width apart, using an underhand grip. Bring the bar to a position of rest against your thigh, with your elbow fully extended and your feet spread shoulder-width apart. Using only your arms, raise the bar to your chest and then return to the starting position. Keep your back straight and always return to a position where your elbows are fully extended. Muscles used: Primary—Biceps brachii, Brachialis; Additional—Coracobrachialis, Anterior deltoid, Brachiodialis.

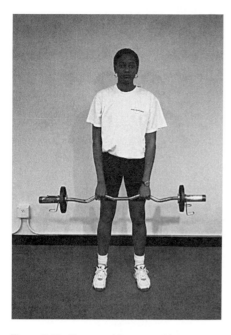 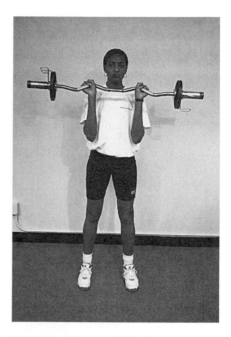

Figure 8.11 Reverse biceps curl (upper and lower arm). Grasp the bar with your hands shoulder-width apart, using an overhand grip. Bring the bar to a resting position against your thighs with your elbows fully extended and your feet spread shoulder-width apart. Using only your arms, raise the bar to your chest and then return to your starting position. Keep your back straight and always return to a position where your elbows are fully extended. Muscles used: Biceps brachii, Brachialis.

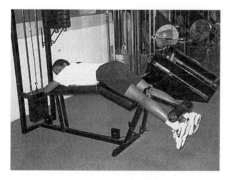 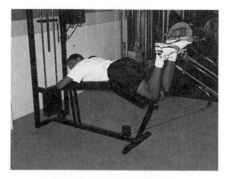

Figure 8.12 Knee flexion. Lie on your abdomen on the leg machine bench. Hook the back of your ankles behind the upper bar. Pull the lever up by bending your knees as far as possible. Muscles used: Hamstrings.

Chapter 8

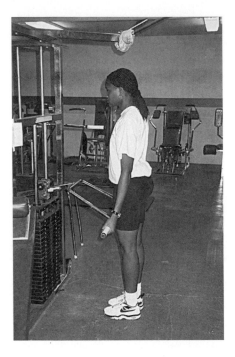

Figure 8.13 Shoulder elevation. Stand with your head and back straight. Grip the bar with your hands palms down. Lift the bar with straight arms. Contract your thighs and rotate the points of your shoulder forward and up, then back in a circular fashion. Muscles used: Triceps brachii, Levator scapula, Deltoid.

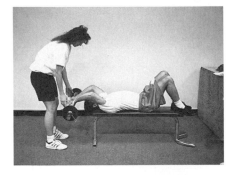

Figure 8.14 Bent-arm pullover (chest). Lying supine on a bench, with the barbell overhead in an overhand grasp, hands shoulder-width apart, lower the barbell slowly over and behind the head as far back as possible and then return to the starting position. Muscles used: Primary—Triceps brachii, Additional—Pectoralis major, Latissimus dorsi.

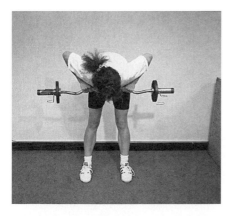

Figure 8.15 Bent-over rowing (shoulder, girdle). Flex your knees at a forty-five-degree angle and bend over from your hips until your back is parallel to the floor. With your arms extended, grab the barbell with your hands pronated. Lift the barbell to your chest and then return. **Caution:** This exercise may cause strain to lower back if not done prudently. Also, avoid locking knees. Muscles used: Primary—Upper-back musculature, Rhomboid major and minor, Teres major and minor.

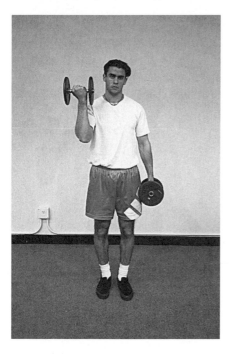

Figure 8.16 Zottman curl (upper arm, forearm). With a weight in each hand, curl your hands alternately, palms up, above the shoulder, and then extend to the rear. When extending to the rear, rotate your forearm so that the palm faces the front. Muscles used: Same as curl (fig. 8.10), with greater use of Anterior deltoid.

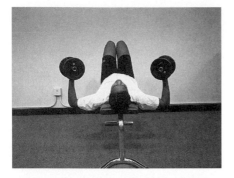

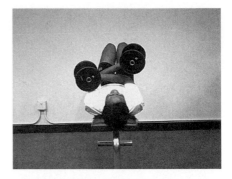

Figure 8.17 Bent-arm lateral (chest and arms). With your elbows bent and your hands palms up, bring the weights from a lateral position and cross them in front of your body. Muscles used: Primary—Pectoralis major; Additional—Anterior deltoid, Biceps brachii, Triceps brachii.

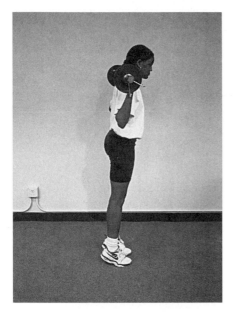

Figure 8.18 Heel raise (calf muscles). Rest the barbell on your shoulders, with the palms of your hands facing forward. Shift your body weight to the balls of your feet and then raise your heels off the floor. Muscles used: Primary—Gastrocnemius, Soleus; Additional—Tibialis posterior.

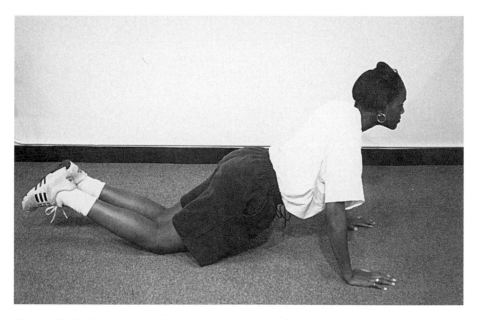

Figure 8.19 Modified push-up. If you have limited upper-body strength, start with the modified push-up. Lie flat on your stomach with your hands in a position to push the trunk upward and with your legs bent upward at the knees. Keeping your back straight and in line with your buttocks, raise your trunk until your arms are fully extended at the elbows. Lower your body to a position where your chest just touches the floor and then push back up to the fully extended position. This exercise is to be done with the arms only, so immobilize the rest of your body. Start with ten repetitions. Muscles used: Biceps brachii, Triceps brachii, Anterior deltoid, Pectoralis major.

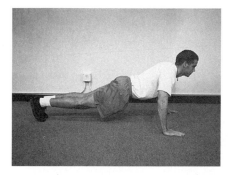

Figure 8.20 Full push-up. Once you have mastered thirty repetitions of the modified push-up, you have the strength to perform the full push-up. Perform this exercise exactly as you did the modified version, except now use your toes—not your knees—as the point of support. This forces you to lift a greater percentage of your body weight. Start with ten repetitions and increase to thirty. Muscles used: Same as modified push-up (fig. 8.19).

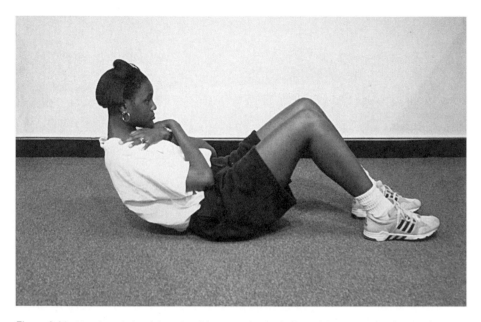

Figure 8.21 Head-and-shoulder raise. Lie on your back with your knees bent to a ninety-degree angle, feet flat on the floor. Place your hands across your chest. Slowly curl the head and shoulders up to a forty-five-degree angle. Hold this position for five seconds and then return to the starting position. Start with ten repetitions and increase to thirty. Muscles used: Primary—Rectus abdominus; Additional—Internal obliques, External obliques, Transverse abdominus.

Body Building

Many individuals lift weights to improve body shape and form and have little interest in athletic performance. Muscle size and definition take priority over strength and endurance gains. Body building refers to the body's morphology or form and structure that depend mainly on inherited or genetic factors. While your body type or build can be altered only slightly, substantial changes can take place in body composition by decreasing body fat and adding muscle mass. When you exercise you burn more calories than when you are sedentary; therefore you start to lose weight provided your food intake remains the same. A strength and endurance program results in an increase of muscle tissue with a decrease in stored fat. Your body dimensions will change resulting in a slimmer waist, trimmer hips and thighs, and improved overall appearance.

Many body builders will use a strength (power lifting) program during portions of the year and then switch to the endurance (body building) for the competitive portion of the year.

TABLE 8.2	Recommendations for Increasing Strength Through Isometric Exercise
Frequency	Three to five days a week
Duration	Six weeks minimum
Intensity	Maximum force held for five to seven seconds
Repetitions	Five to ten

Isometric Exercise

An **isometric exercise** is a contraction performed against a fixed or immovable resistance, where tension is developed in the muscle but there is no change in the length of the muscle or the angle of the joint. This also is referred to as a static contraction. An example would be holding a heavy weight in one position for a fixed amount of time.

It appears that with isometric exercise, strength development is specific only to the joint angle stimulated during training. As a result, isometric exercise does not increase strength throughout the range of movement. Isometric exercise also may inhibit the ability of the muscle to exert force rapidly, as is necessary in the shot put and discus events. In addition, isometric exercise increases pressure in the chest cavity, which results in reduced blood flow to the heart, lungs, and brain, along with increased blood pressure. Consequently, isometric exercises are not recommended for individuals with cardiorespiratory problems.

Isometric exercise can be used by those individuals unable to find free weights or other equipment. It also can be used in conjunction with other weight programs. Unless there are specific reasons for you to limit joint movement or engage in isometric exercise, isotonic exercise is preferred.

Table 8.2 shows the recommended frequency, duration, intensity, and repetitions for increasing strength through isometric exercise. Allow two to three minutes recovery between repetitions if the same muscle group is involved.

Isokinetic Exercise

An **isokinetic exercise** is a contraction in which the muscle contracts maximally at a constant speed over a full range of the joint movement against a variable resistance. Isokinetic means equal motion, which is interpreted to mean equal rate of motion or equal speed. An isokinetic contraction can only be accomplished with the use of special equipment, such as a Cybex 6000 or Merac that uses "accommodating resistance." In other words, the harder you pull, the harder the dynamometer resists you—the resistance is always related to the applied force.

153

TABLE 8.3	Recommendations for Increasing Strength Through Isokinetic Exercise
Frequency	Three to four days per week
Duration	Six weeks
Intensity	Maximum
Repetitions	Eight to fifteen (three sets for each muscle group)
Speed	Sixty to 300 degrees at one second. The exercise should be similar to the skill being trained for. The training speed should be as fast or faster than the speed involved in the actual athletic event.

Isokinetic exercise has become popular because it provides a speed-specific indication of the absolute strength of the muscle group being trained, thus enabling one to more closely replicate specific athletic skills. The most effective strength gains have come from slower training speeds of approximately sixty degrees (measure of distance) at one second or less. Research, however, indicates that training at fast speeds of movement generally increases strength at all speeds of movement. Also, isokinetic training at fast speeds of movement increases muscular endurance for movements that require fast speed. Further, isokinetic exercise produces a little less soreness and is considered safer than isometric and isotonic exercise. The refined dials and gauges on isokinetic equipment make it easier to keep track of your load levels and strength gains. Additional research is needed, however, to develop more precise regimens for isokinetic exercise.

Table 8.3 shows the recommended frequency, duration, intensity, repetitions, and speed for increasing strength through isokinetic exercise.

Refer to figures 8.1 and 8.2 for a proper designation of the skeletal muscles used in your strength and endurance program. Figure 8.3 presents the structural design of a human skeletal muscle.

Advantages and Disadvantages of Weight-Resistance Programs

Isotonic, isometric, and isokinetic exercise have their advantages and disadvantages. As long as the muscle is overloaded, however, it will gain in strength.

Isotonic Exercise

Advantages

1. Generally produces strength gains throughout the full range of movement.
2. Progress in strength gains is easy to evaluate because of numbered free weights and stacked weights.

3. Strength exercises can be developed to duplicate a variety of sports skills.

Disadvantages

1. The equipment is cumbersome.
2. Produces more muscle soreness and greater risk of injury than isometric and isokinetic exercises.
3. Most strength gains occur at the weakest point of the movement and are not uniform throughout.

Isometric Exercise

Advantages

1. Little time is required for training.
2. Expensive and cumbersome equipment is not needed.
3. Exercise can be performed anywhere—in home or office or while on vacation.

Disadvantages

1. Strength gains are not produced throughout the full range of movement.
2. Strength gains are difficult to evaluate; that is, generally, no numbered weights or gauges are used.
3. Increases the pressure in the chest cavity, causing reduced blood flow to the heart, lungs, and brain.
4. Not as efficient in producing strength gains as isotonic and isokinetic methods.
5. Not effective in producing increases in skilled movements.
6. Motivation is difficult to maintain.

Isokinetic Exercise

Advantages

1. Produces maximum resistance at all ranges of movement.
2. Increases strength throughout the full range of movement.
3. Results in less injury and soreness than isometric and isotonic exercise.
4. The uniqueness of the equipment increases motivation.
5. Strength gains are easy to determine.
6. Permits quantification of torque, work, and power.

Disadvantages

1. The equipment is very expensive, with limited availability.
2. Research is still incomplete with regard to motor patterns and force-velocity relationships.

Other Options for Advanced Strength Training

For advanced strength training, you might want to consider using the Pyramid method, the rest/pause method, the wipeout method, or the burnout method.

Pyramid Method

In this procedure you start with a high number of repetitions, using a low weight to warm up and decreasing the repetitions as you add weight. Then you work your way back down, taking off weight and adding repetitions. You can do any number of repetitions for the desired number of sets as long as you follow the high repetition-low weight progression to heavier weights and less repetitions. Scale the weight down or up, according to your ability. The following is an example of a Pyramid Program.

Sets	Reps	Weights
1	14	100
1	10	130
1	6	160
1	4	200
1	2	230
1	1	275

Rest/Pause Method (Muscular Strength)

With the rest/pause method, you first determine your 1 RM for the muscle group to be trained. Perform a single repetition and then rest one to two minutes. Complete a second repetition and then rest again. Continue in this fashion until the muscle group is fatigued. Train with a partner.

Wipeout Method (Muscular Endurance)

The wipeout method requires that you determine your 1 RM for the muscle group to be trained and then halve that amount. Using ½ RM, complete as many consecutive repetitions as possible until fatigued. Train with a partner in case of premature fatigue and for spotting and motivation.

Burnout Method (Continuous Set)

With the burnout method, you determine your 1 RM for the muscle group to be trained and then take three-fourths of that amount. Using ¾ RM, complete as many consecutive repetitions as possible until fatigued. Then immediately remove ten pounds and complete as many repetitions as possible until fatigued. Again remove another ten pounds and complete as many repetitions as possible until completely fatigued. Allow no rest periods between repetitions. Train with a partner in case of premature fatigue.

Guidelines for Strength Training

No matter what strength-training program you select, follow these important guidelines:

1. Warm-up should precede all resistance exercise.
2. Muscles must be overloaded—that is, exercised against near maximum resistance—to increase strength and endurance.
3. The overload must be progressive throughout the duration of the program.
4. Larger muscle groups should be exercised before smaller ones.
5. No two successive lifts or exercises should involve the same muscle group.
6. Avoid holding your breath while lifting. Exhale during main contraction; inhale during return to starting position.
7. Make your exercise interesting. One of the major difficulties of fitness programs—particularly strength programs—is maintaining a high level of motivation. Poorly designed programs lead to boredom and high dropout rates. Be creative in setting up your sequence of exercises; that is, set individual goals, rotate types of strength exercises, and vary the progression of the various exercises.
8. Train with others for spotting and motivation.

Weight Lifting Complications and Potential Injuries

When one is involved in lifting maximum weight, there is a possibility of injury. Common problems are hernia (rupture) and injuries to the lower back and joints. In addition, injuries to the bones, muscles, and other tissues are possible. Also, a maximum lift requires a great deal of strength and effort, and sometimes this can put a terrific load upon the heart, requiring it to beat very rapidly. This, however, is a common response and should not be cause for worry.

Three major weight lifting problem areas are the spinal column, the Valsalva maneuver, and muscle soreness.

Spinal Column

The human spinal column is not well-suited for bearing heavy loads unless the back is kept in a very straight position and a normal curvature is maintained. Some movements, such as a two-hands clean military press, where the barbell is lifted over the head, can increase the curvature of the spine and put extreme pressure on the vertebrae and the spinal discs. This type of movement is condemned by many physicians and is considered dangerous in both long- and short-term exercise programs. It is especially dangerous for individuals who are still growing.

Before beginning a weight-resistance program, you should be well aware of the mechanical principles and precautions involved in lifting weights. You should at least lift under supervision to safeguard against possible injury. Also, use a weight belt as a preventive measure.

Valsalva Maneuver

The epiglottis is a piece of cartilage that closes over the top of the windpipe when we swallow so that food does not pass into the windpipe. During weight-resistance training, an individual often exhales against a closed epiglottis, a process called the **Valsalva maneuver.** This type of strain increases pressure within the chest cavity. Because this pressure is placed against the heart and the large veins, it impedes blood flow into the heart (resulting in lowered blood pressure) and increases pressure in the veins going to the extremities and to the head. To counteract the reduced blood flow, the heart rate increases. As soon as the individual relieves the pressure by breathing out, the accumulated blood in the veins rushes into the right ventricle, causing the heart to increase its output and increasing arterial pressure. When this pressure jumps up, the heart rate briefly declines until the resting conditions are reestablished.

For a young person, these sudden increases in pressure and decreases in blood flow to the heart are not dangerous. However, for a person who suffers from heart disease, they could have serious consequences. Individuals involved in weight-resistance training that requires continuous heavy lifting can modify this response by normal breathing while lifting, especially by exhaling during the main contraction.

Muscle Soreness

Muscle soreness after exercise is a very common phenomenon. There are basically two kinds of muscle soreness. One type occurs immediately after exercise and is due partially to the reduced blood supply to the muscles and in some cases to a loss of minerals and increased lactic acid levels. This soreness goes away after a short while.

The other kind of muscle soreness, which has been the subject of considerable research, occurs approximately twenty-four to forty-eight hours after exercise. You no doubt have had that unpleasant experience of waking up in the morning barely able to move after a previous day of exercise. This is usually the result of engaging in either a new exercise or one that you have not participated in for a long time. The exact cause of this kind of muscle soreness is not known.

One theory is that there are minute tears in the muscle that may be caused by eccentric contractions. During this type of contraction, connective tissue associated with the muscle and tendon is stretched. Overextending the muscle can result in damage to the connective tissue of the muscle and to the ends of the muscle (tendons), producing soreness. It is believed that there is less soreness in concentric (shortening) and isometric contractions because only the connective tissue associated with tendons is stretched.

Another theory of muscle soreness is referred to as the spasm theory. When a muscle contracts forcefully during bouncing and ballistic types of movement, the resulting local muscle spasm reduces the blood supply to the muscle (ischemia). Ischemia produces muscle pain, pain produces more spasm, and the cycle continues. A good way to break this cycle and reduce soreness is through stretching exercises. The stretching decreases the spasm and allows blood to flow through the muscle.

Generally, muscle soreness after exercise can be avoided if there is good pre- and post-warm-up exercise, such as stretching. Stretching also can bring some relief from present pain in the muscle. It is also important to continue light aerobic work until completion of cool-down.

Physical Changes in Muscles as a Result of Weight Training

A number of important physical changes occur as a result of weight training. First, muscle strength, especially around the joints, increases the efficiency of joint action and helps to prevent injury during physical activity.

Second, strength training also increases the integrity of muscle fibers. For example, individual muscle fibers, which are about the size of a human hair, start to increase in thickness because increased muscle tension is resulting in more protein being deposited in the muscle. There also may be increases in muscle glycogen and energy-rich compounds such as adenosine triphosphate (ATP) and phosphocreatine (PC). Some research indicates that muscle fibers actually split (hyperplasia) as a result of training, but these findings are still highly controversial.

One final physical change that results from weight training is that you look a lot better. Muscle training increases your proportion of fat-free muscles and thereby enhances your aesthetic appearance.

Red and White Muscle Fibers (Endurance and Strength)

Human muscles contain three types of muscle fibers: a slow-twitch type I **red fiber** and two types of fast-twitch type II **white fibers.** Each fiber type is structurally and chemically equipped to perform work for long or short periods of time. For example, fast-twitch fibers are preferentially used for short-term, high-intensity exercise (such as sprinting), while slow-twitch fibers are used during longer, less-intensive exercise (such as long-distance running).

Exercise cannot change the types and numbers of fibers in your muscles since this determination is inherited. However, the efficiency of both red and white muscle fibers can be increased through proper training methods. A specific type of exercise must be used to improve the efficiency of a given fiber type. For example, to increase the metabolic potential of fast-twitch fibers, high-intensity exercise must be used with low repetition. Conversely, exercises of longer duration with lower intensities increase the metabolic potential of slow-twitch fibers. This is one reason why the training sessions of most athletes closely resemble the actual competition. For example, the training of marathon runners primarily involves continuous running, while the training of football players primarily involves shorter running intervals that are interrupted by rest and recovery periods. Research indicates that successful performers in aerobic activities, such as marathon runners, generally have a higher percentage of red fibers and that those engaged in anaerobic events, such as sprinters, have a higher percentage of white fibers. The higher percentages are believed to result from a process of selectivity made by the demands of the activity rather than training. Evidence also indicates that individuals engaged in simultaneous programs of strength and endurance training may have more difficulty gaining strength than those engaged only in a strength program.

Female Muscle Response to Weight Training

Research indicates that, when a woman engages in rigorous weight training, her muscles do not respond in the same way as a man's. Women who use the same weight-training techniques and who work to the same weight capacity as men evidence gains in strength and endurance, but the degree of muscle hypertrophy (the increase in muscle size) is smaller than it is in men. The explanation for this is that women's levels of testosterone (a hormone important in building muscle tissue) are twenty to thirty times less than men. Thus, women do not have to fear that they will develop bulky muscles from weight training. They will increase their strength and endurance, but they will not develop the degree of muscle definition that men do. However, some women have higher testosterone levels than others and may develop some muscle definition.

Research also has shown that women who engage in weight-training programs tend to lose body fat but maintain their weight because of small gains in lean muscle. This loss in subcutaneous fat may give their muscles increased definition.

Strength and Endurance Training Equipment

A variety of strength and endurance training equipment is available:

1. **Free Weights**   Barbells and dumbbells provide exercise to produce both positive and negative phases of muscle contraction.
2. **Universal Gym**   This device is designed mainly to duplicate most free-weight exercises. It provides variable resistance in both positive and negative phases of muscle contraction.
3. **Nautilus or Cybex Eagle**   This device provides single muscle group training through the full range of movement with variable resistance in both positive and negative phases of muscle contraction.
4. **Cam II**   This device provides variable resistance with air pressure generated by a central compressor. Specific muscle groups can be trained together or bilaterally through a full range of movement in both positive and negative phases of muscle contraction.
5. **Polaris**   With this device, the weight to be moved is drawn over an oval-shaped plate. Muscles can move through a full range of movement in both positive and negative phases of muscle contraction.
6. **Hydra-Fitness and Eagle Performance**   These two methods combine both isokinetic and isotonic principles. The equipment automatically adjusts to the strength and speed of the individual.
7. **Cybex 6000 and Merac**   These devices provide for accommodating resistance or isokinetic contraction. The resistance is directly related to the force applied. Variable resistance is provided throughout the entire range of movement.

8. **Exer-Genie** This device allows for both isometric and isotonic movement. A cylinder controls the amount of resistance in a braided nylon line.

When using free weights and Nautilus equipment, the following guidelines are important:

1. Use spotters when executing bench presses and squats with free weights.
2. Wear rubber-soled shoes for proper traction.
3. Make sure that metal weights are secured by collars.
4. Chalk your hands with carbonate of magnesium when using free weights.
5. Exhale during lifting phase, inhale during lowering phase.
6. Avoid locking joints when lifting.

Periodization of Strength Training

The majority of high-level athletes strength train approximately three to four days a week during the period of strength building and one to three days a week during competition periods. Major lifts, such as pulls and squats, seldom are executed more than two days per week to help prevent the possibility of injury and subsequent reduced performance.

Russian athletes have developed a unique cyclic training program, called **periodization,** that prepares athletes for maximum performance during peak cycles. Periodization involves four training cycles of different intensities: the load cycle, the recovery cycle, the peak cycle, and the conditioning cycle.

Load Cycle

The load cycle consists of a high number of sets (five to seven) and a moderate number of repetitions (four to seven) at 80 percent of repetition maximum. Within each load cycle are microcycles of about two weeks duration that consist of an intensity progression of heavy to light to moderate workloads. Then the microcycle is repeated using more weight.

The load cycle usually is used during the off-season, in the precompetition period for building strength. This cycle should not be practiced for more than two to three months because of its exhausting nature.

Recovery Cycle

The recovery cycle is a transition period of active rest that separates the strength-building period (load cycle) from the competitive period (peak cycle). The cycle consists of a low to moderate number of sets and repetitions at light to moderate intensity. This cycle generally lasts for two to three weeks.

Peak Cycle

The peak cycle is aimed at producing maximum strength while at the same time allowing for skilled movement. A low number of sets and repetitions and high resistance (80 to 100 percent of repetition maximum) characterize this cycle. Duration is approximately two to three months (equal to that of the load cycle). This cycle is used during or immediately preceding competition. Also, as with the load cycle, it consists of microcycles that last two to three weeks, during which time maximum resistance is employed only once.

Conditioning Cycle

The conditioning cycle is a period of active rest following a competitive season. The cycle consists of a moderate number of sets (four to six) and repetitions (eight to ten) at low intensity (60 to 70 percent of repetition maximum). Approximately every three weeks, a slightly higher intensity is employed to maintain strength. The conditioning cycle prevents deconditioning and allows for a mental and physical break from training.

Circuit Training for Weight-Resistance Programs

Circuit training involves a combination of strength and endurance exercises performed in sequence at various stations. This extremely efficient technique can be specifically designed for a variety of different sports activities. For example, the circuit can emphasize strength activities, cardiorespiratory activities, or a combination of the two.

The circuit should consist of between eight to fifteen stations, with a total circuit completion time of five to twenty minutes. The circuit may be performed more than once during each training session, and you should allow for as many repetitions as possible during the time allotted at each station.

Table 8.4 presents an example of a muscle strength circuit. In this example, ten stations have been selected. The activity at each station depends upon the purpose of the circuit, in this case, building muscle strength. Each task time is

TABLE 8.4	Example of Muscle Strength Circuit			
Station	Exercise	Alloted task time	Pretest repetitions	One-half of pretest repetitions
1	Vertical jumps	60 sec	40	20
2	Push-ups	30 sec	10	5
3	Arm curl	30 sec	15	8
4	Leg press	60 sec	20	10
5	Back hyperextension	60 sec	10	5
6	Upright rowing	60 sec	4	2
7	Bent-knee sit-ups	45 sec	12	6
8	Bench press	30 sec	6	3
9	Leg curl	45 sec	8	4
10	Standing overhead press	30 sec	8	4
	Total circuit time	7½ min × 3 = 22½ min		

set between thirty and sixty seconds. A pretest establishes standards for the circuit. During the pretest, as many repetitions as possible are completed during the allotted task time, with a short period of recovery allowed after each task. The number of repetitions for each circuit task then is determined by taking one-half of those completed in the pretest. The overall circuit time is determined by adding the total time allowed for each task and multiplying by three.

When developing a circuit, try to make the strength exercises as specific as possible to those used in the particular sport for which you are training. Also, for each weight-resistant task in your circuit, periodically increase the intensity to ensure overload. Another important guideline is to separate tasks so that two consecutive stations do not include the same muscle group. Finally, remember to monitor your heart rate to maintain your target heart rate training effect level.

Table 8.5 presents an example of a muscle strength and cardiorespiratory circuit-training program.

Tracking Your Muscle Strength and Endurance

Appendix B at the back of the book provides record sheets for tracking your progress in increasing your muscle strength and endurance (record sheets B-1, B-4, B-5, and B-6). Keeping records of your advances is a great way of maintaining your motivation.

TABLE 8.5	Muscle Strength and Cardiorespiratory Circuit-Training Program
Duration	Ten weeks
Frequency	Three days per week
Circuits/session	Circuit A: 3; Circuit B: 2
Time/circuit	Circuit A: 7½ min; Circuit B: 15 min
Total time/session	Circuit A: 22½ min; Circuit B: 30 min
Load	40 to 55 percent of 1 RM
Repetitions	As many as possible in thirty seconds
Rest	Fifteen seconds between stations

Muscle strength		Cardiorespiratory	
Circuit A		Circuit B	
Station	Exercise	Station	Exercise
1	Bench press	1	Running (440 yd)
2	Bent-knee sit-ups	2	Push-ups or pull-ups
3	Knee (leg) extension	3	Bent-knee sit-ups
4	Pulldown-lat machine	4	Vertical jumps
5	Back hyperextension	5	Standing (overhead) press
6	Standing (overhead) press	6	Bicycling (3 min)
7	Dead lift	7	Hip stretch
8	Arm curl	8	Rope jumping (1 min)
9	Leg curl (knee flexion)	9	Bent-over rowing
10	Upright rowing	10	Hamstring stretch
		11	Upright rowing
		12	Running (660 yd)

Source: From Edward Fox, Richard Bowers, and Merle Foss, The Physiological Basis for Exercise and Sport, 5th edition. Copyright 1993, Times Mirror Higher Education Group, Inc., Dubuque, Iowa. All rights reserved. Reprinted by permission.

Key Terms

Circuit Training
A combination of strength and endurance exercises performed in sequence at various stations

Eccentric Loading
When the muscle lengthens as it develops tension

Isokinetic Exercise
A contraction in which the muscle contracts maximally at a constant speed over a full range of the joint movement against a variable resistance

Isometric Exercise

A contraction performed against a fixed or immovable resistance, where tension is developed in the muscle but there is no change in the length of the muscle or the angle of the joint

Isotonic Exercise

Exercise against resistance while the load remains constant, with the resistance varying with the angle of the joint

Muscle Endurance

The ability of a muscle group to maintain a continuous contraction or repetition over a period of time

Muscle Soreness

Muscle pain resulting possibly from chemical or physical changes in the muscle tissue

Muscle Strength

The amount of force that can be exerted by a muscle group for one movement or repetition

Overload

Forcing a muscle to contract at maximum or near maximum tension

Periodization

A training program that involves varying degrees of training cycles throughout the year

Plyometric Loading

When the muscle is loaded suddenly and then forced to stretch before the contraction for movement occurs

Progressive Resistance

The progressive increase in load intensity

Red Fiber

Slow-twitch muscle fiber physiologically adapted for endurance activity with a high capacity to use oxygen

Specificity

The concept that exercises are specific to the type of training performed

Speed Loading

When the resistance is moved as rapidly as possible

Valsalva Maneuver

Exhalation against a closed epiglottis, which increases pressure in the chest cavity

White Fiber

Fast-twitch muscle fiber physiologically adapted for short-term, high-intensity exercise

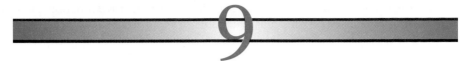

9

Nutrition

Chapter Concepts

After you have studied this chapter you should be able to

1. define and describe the major nutritional constituents: carbohydrates, fats, proteins, vitamins, minerals, and water;

2. describe the aerobic and anaerobic energy systems;

3. discuss special nutritional needs during pregnancy;

4. describe problems associated with eating fast foods;

5. describe common nutritional problems of teenagers;

6. discuss the special concerns of high-fat diets;

7. describe the effect of rigorous exercise on digestion;

8. describe the recommended eating pattern for competitive running;

9. explain the problems associated with fad diets;

10. describe carbohydrate loading;

11. describe the effect of aging, caloric needs, and importance of exercise;

12. discuss cholesterol levels and the association with heart disease; and

13. describe food labels.

Need for Accurate Nutritional Information

Not many years ago, the subject of nutrition was of little interest to the American public. With research showing relationships between diet and such health problems as heart disease, obesity, diabetes, and cancer, however, interest in nutrition and in research on nutrition surged. Unfortunately, along with this increased interest has come widespread misinformation and new myths about nutrition. It is often difficult to determine the validity of statements made by a number of so-called experts. There are a number of major nutritional controversies concerning cholesterol, vitamin C, fiber, sugar, food additives, and various diets. As a result, a continuous need to separate fact from fiction and to educate the public exists in this most vital area.

The college years are a time when most young adults decide for themselves what to eat. At this time there is also the tendency to reject tradition in search of a new identity, which may lead to changes in eating habits. Environmental factors such as part-time jobs, increased mobility, attending classes, and extra-curricular activities disrupt normal eating habits. As a result, young people depend more on vending machines, fast foods, and snacks for keeping their energy levels up.

Eating disorders that are common during this period of life may be the result of fears of becoming fat, uncertainty about physical and social development, and problems concerning hair and skin. Physical appearance is also a topic of great concern to young adults. The desire, for instance, of girls to be thin and boys to be strong may make them more susceptible to fad diets. Rather than relying on a balanced diet and regular exercise, they may turn to inappropriate foods or supplements in order to achieve their desired body image. Many young people realize that their diet may not be ideal, but they figure they can put off acquiring good eating habits until a later date when it is more convenient and they have more time. What they don't realize is that they are presently laying the physical foundation for years to come.

Many Americans have made major changes in their lifestyles and are more health conscious in making food selections in order to live longer and become healthier. They view nutrition as part of the broader context of health, fitness, and physical well-being. They are aware that a proper diet may help prevent chronic and degenerative diseases such as cancer, heart disease, and osteoporosis. Many are modifying their diets in order to reduce calories, fats, cholesterol, and sodium and to increase complex carbohydrates.

Figures from the U. S. Department of Agriculture show that we are eating less eggs and beef and drinking less whole milk than in the 1980s. Avoiding foods with saturated fat and cholesterol has played a major part in reducing death by heart disease, which has dropped by 29 percent since 1978. However, problems still remain. Instead of replacing saturated fats with complex carbohydrates, we are replacing them with unsaturated fats. In addition, we are consuming more sugar than before and downing more soft drinks than milk. On the positive side, the consumption of fresh fruits and vegetables has risen.

Over the past two decades Americans have dramatically changed their eating habits, both at home and away. Busy schedules force many people to "eat on the run," resulting in more snacking and smaller, more frequent meals throughout the day.

The most dramatic development in the away-from-home diet is the increasing dependence on fast foods and take-out establishments. The Food Marketing Institute found that 81 percent of the households in the United States bought take-out foods in a four-week period.

Fast Foods

The kinds of foods most commonly sold in fast-food restaurants are very popular with most Americans: hamburgers, french fries, pizza, fried chicken, milk shakes, and cola drinks. Unfortunately, fast foods often provide excess calories, fat, and sodium and limited complex carbohydrates, dietary fiber, and vitamins A and C. Though most fast foods are high in protein, this is an area where the average American rarely has a deficiency. However, fast foods high in protein are usually high in fat, and fat contains more than twice the number of calories per gram than either protein or carbohydrate. (One gram of fat is nine **kilocalories;** a gram of carbohydrate equals four kilocalories; and a gram of protein is four kilocalories.) Consequently, fast foods contribute additional calories and increase body fat. Furthermore, fast-food meals tend to have an excess of sodium. Salt is used in the batter in which fast food is prepared and also on french fries. (See table 9.1.)

Special Nutritional Needs for Young Adults

A rapidly growing active boy of fifteen may need 4,000 calories or more a day just to maintain weight. Consequently, the potential problems for boys are increased intakes of saturated fat and cholesterol by way of hamburgers, fried chicken, and milk shakes, which may lead to an early onset of coronary heart disease. At the same time, most girls at age fifteen have stopped growing and may need fewer than 2,000 calories, if they are not to become obese. If overeating occurred during the formative years (ages four to thirteen), it may become a habit during adolescence.

Young women need to know that increased hunger and carbohydrate craving that precede menstruation are natural and not a sign of incompetence, inadequacy, or neuroticism. Rather than rigidly fixing daily calorie amounts, if appetite is affected, it is recommended that calories be increased during the two weeks before menstruation and reduced the two weeks after. "Go with it," instead of becoming fixated on rigid amounts.

Between the ages of eighteen and twenty-three, low nutritional intake is common among females, particularly iron, calcium, magnesium, and vitamin B6. Missing meals, especially breakfast, can also significantly decrease some important requirements such as iron, calcium, thiamine, and vitamin C. Folacin, which is necessary for the blood during periods of rapid growth, is hard to achieve without adequate fruits and vegetables.

Along with having sound nutritional knowledge, it is also important to know how to change your behavior toward improved eating habits. Tables 9.2 and 9.3 list important nutritional guidelines to follow for a healthy diet.

TABLE 9.1 Fast Foods

	Calories Kcal	Fat/ (g)	Sodium (mg)	Cholesterol (mg)
Arby's Beef and Cheese	402	18	1634	77
Arby's Roast Beef Sandwich	370	15	869	52
Burger King Double Cheeseburger	483	27	851	100
Burger King Whopper	630	36	990	104
Hardee's Big Country Breakfast—Sausage	850	57	1980	340
Jumbo Jack	551	29	1134	80
Kentucky Fried Chicken—thigh	406	30	688	129
McDonald's Big Mac	560	32	950	103
McDonald's Filet-O-Fish	383	18	613	50
McDonald's Vanilla Frozen Yogurt	100	1	80	3
Pizza Hut Pizza (half 10")	506	15	1281	*
Subway—Ham and Cheese	673	22	2508	73
Taco Bell—Burrito Supreme	457	22	1053	126
Wendy's Double Hamburger	540	27	791	122
Wendy's Tuna Salad	100	6	290	0
Chocolate Shake—"Low Fat"	360	10	273	10
Cola Beverage	151	0	14	0
French Fries	330	16	324	16

*Not Available

Teenagers, Nutrition, and Pregnancy

Every year, in the past few years, about one million teenagers have become pregnant. Of those teenagers, about 600,000 have given birth (one in ten teenaged girls). About 250,000 of the girls who have given birth are under seventeen and about 13,000 are under the age of fifteen. One of the major problems of these pregnancies is that the adolescent girl has not yet achieved her own full physical growth, and then superimposed upon her own nutritional needs are the additional nutritional requirements of the pregnancy. In addition, many young girls have poor eating habits and are poorly nourished. They often skip meals, eat snack foods of low nutrient density, and pursue unwise weight-reduction regimens. Their intake of calories, calcium, iron, vitamin A, and folacin, and sometimes even protein, is frequently inadequate to meet the growth needs of their own bodies let alone those of the developing fetus.

Among the frequent undesirable consequences for the nutritionally deficient mother are anemia, **preeclampsia, toxemia,** premature labor, prolonged labor, and an increased rate of maternal death. For the infant, consequences may be increased premature birth, low birth weight, and neonatal death.

TABLE 9.2 Nutritional Guidelines

1. Keep nutrient-dense appealing foods convenient.
2. Dairy products should be emphasized to ensure sufficient calcium (lowfat yogurt, lowfat cheese, lowfat and nonfat milk, and ice milk).
3. Select whole and fresh foods over refined and processed ones.
4. Choose whole wheat products over white and refined.
5. Reduce intake of high-fat foods: hamburgers, whole milk, shakes, and ice cream.
6. Reduce dietary cholesterol by lowering intake of eggs, red meat, liver, and animal fat.
7. Choose fish and fowl over red meat.
8. Remove fat prior to making sauces and gravy.
9. Avoid commercial snacks such as salted peanuts, chips, and pretzels.
10. Avoid salted or smoked meats.
11. Avoid commercially prepared foods containing butter, eggs, palm oil, and animal fat.
12. Select nonfat dairy products such as nonfat milk, cheese, and yogurt.
13. Select fresh fruits and uncooked vegetables.
14. Substitute fruit juices, nonfat milk, and mineral water for sugared fruit and soft drinks.
15. Select whole grain products for breakfast.
16. Become aware of your daily caloric intake.
17. Vary your selections from the basic four food groups.
18. Reduce intake of simple sugars: cookies, cakes, candies, and sugared cereals.
19. Plan and prepare a meal for family or friends to make you more aware of nutritional balance.
20. If you must snack, make it nutritious.

Major Nutritional Constituents

The major nutritional constituents are carbohydrates, fats, protein, minerals, vitamins, and water. All are essential for life.

Except for pizza, fast-food meals are likely to be low in calcium; choose milk or a milk shake for the beverage. Hamburgers and french fries are low in vitamin A and folacin. Your next meal should be a large salad or include dark green vegetables, which have been added to the menus in fast-food chains.

Carbohydrates

All **carbohydrates** are composed of simple sugars and come in three sizes: sugars with a single ring, like glucose (monosaccharides); pairs of single-ring carbohydrates (disaccharides); and those with long chains of single-ring carbohydrates (polysaccharides). Grain products, fruits, sugar, vegetables, and milk are excellent sources of carbohydrates. Carbohydrates are the major energy sources that enable muscles to do work. When carbohydrates are broken down, they take the

TABLE 9.3 The Basic Four, Revisited

Food Group	Servings per Day	Anytime	Sometimes	Seldom
Grain	6–11	Whole-grain bread*, rolls*, bagels*, Whole-grain crackers*[3], tortillas*, Brown rice* Bulgur Whole-grain breakfast cereal* Pasta*	Muffins*[6] Waffles, pancakes*[3] Heavily-sweetened cereals[6] Granola cereals	Croissants[3] Doughnuts[1,6] Danish[6] Bread stuffing from mix[1,3]
Fruit & vegetable	5–9	All fruits and vegetables (except those at right) Applesauce, unsweetened Potatoes, white or sweet	Avocado[2], guacamole[2] Dried fruit Canned fruit[6] Fruit juice Vegetables, canned with salt[3] French fries, fried in vegetable oil[2]	Coconut[1] Pickles[3] Scalloped or au gratin potatoes[1,3] French fries, fried in beef fat[1] (McDonald's, Burger King, Wendy's)
Milk & milk products	Children 3–4 Adults 2	1% lowfat cottage cheese[3] Dry-curd cottage cheese Skim milk 1% lowfat milk Nonfat yogurt	2% lowfat or regular cottage cheese[3] Reduced-fat or part-skim cheeses[3] 2% lowfat milk Lowfat yogurt, plain or fruit[6] Ice milk[6] Frozen nonfat or lowfat yogurt[6]	Hard cheeses (like cheddar)[1,3] Processed cheeses[1,3] Whole milk[1] Whole-milk yogurt[1] Ice cream[1,6]

Servings are quite small (1 slice of bread, 1 piece of fruit, ½ cup of rice, pasta, or vegetable, 1 cup of milk.)
*refined-grain versions have less fiber, vitamins, and minerals.
[1]high in saturated fat   [2]high in unsaturated fat   [3]may be high in salt or sodium   [4]high in cholesterol   [5]may be rich in omega-3 fats   [6]high in added sugar
Source: Nutrition Action, Center for Science in the Public Interest, Washington D.C., 1 June, 1990.

TABLE 9.3 The Basic Four, Revisited (*Continued*)

Food Group	Servings per Day	Anytime	Sometimes	Seldom
Fish, poultry, red meat, eggs, beans, and nuts	2 Fish 5 oz. roasted	All finfish[5] Salmon, canned[3,5] Sardines, in fish oil[3,5] Tuna, water-pack[3] Shellfish, except shrimp	Fried fish[2] Sardines, in vegetable oil[3] Tuna, oil-pack Shrimp[4]	Fried chicken thigh[2] or wing[2] Chicken hot dog[3]
	Poultry 4 oz. roasted	Chicken breast (without skin) Turkey breast, drumstick, thigh Ground turkey (without skin)	Chicken breast (with skin) Chicken drumstick, thigh Fried chicken, except thigh[2] Ground turkey (with skin)	
	Red meat 3 oz. trimmed and roasted	Pork tenderloin	Round steak, sirloin steak Lean ham[3] Pork or lamb loin chop Leg of lamb, veal sirloin Veal loin or rib chop	Chuck blade[1], rib roast[1] Extra-lean or lean ground beef[1] Pork or lamb[1] rib chop, bacon Bologna[1,3], salami[1,3], Hot dog[1,3] Any untrimmed red meat[1]
	Eggs	Egg white		Whole egg or yolk[4]
	Beans, peas, & nuts	Beans, peas, lentils	Tofu[2], peanut butter[2], nuts[2]	

Servings are quite small (1 slice of bread, 1 piece of fruit, ½ cup of rice, pasta, or vegetable, 1 cup of milk.)

*refined-grain versions *have less fiber, vitamins, and minerals.*

[1]high in saturated fat [2]high in unsaturated fat [3]may be high in salt or sodium [4]high in cholesterol [5]may be rich in omega-3 fats [6]high in added sugar
Source: Nutrition Action, Center for Science in the Public Interest, Washington D.C., 1 June, 1990.

form of sugar in the blood and are supplied to various brain and nervous system tissue. Carbohydrates are stored in the liver and in muscles in a complex form called **glycogen.** It is recommended that 50 percent of the total kilocalories per day come from complex carbohydrates (starch and fiber) and only 10 percent from simple sugars. Too much carbohydrate in the diet may play a major role in the development of such conditions as coronary heart disease, increased fat levels in the blood, cancer, and dental caries.

If you take in a large amount of carbohydrates and the carbohydrates are not fully used, the excess can be converted into fat and stored in fat tissue. If your carbohydrate intake is very low, fat cannot be used efficiently. As a result, fatty acids (organic compounds composed of a carbon chain with hydrogens attached and an acid group at one end) form ketone bodies (a condensation product of fat **metabolism** produced when carbohydrates are not available), making it difficult for the body to maintain a proper balance between acidity and alkalinity. Also, when carbohydrate intake is low, protein is broken down and used for energy, rather than for building tissue and performing other important functions.

Fats

When we speak of **fats,** we are actually talking about a subset of a class of compounds called lipids. Lipids include triglycerides (fats and oils), phospholipids, and sterols. Triglycerides make up approximately 95 percent of our fat intake.

Fats help maintain the structure and health of all cells, protect body organs, provide a continuous fuel supply, maintain body temperature, and help keep the body's lean tissue from being depleted. Fats also promote the absorption of the fat-soluble vitamins A, D, E, and K. Good sources of fats are nuts, meats, and dairy products. The fat that you consume in your diet is carried by the blood to your muscles, where it is used for energy. It also can be stored in fat cells as adipose tissue.

During exercise, both carbohydrates and fats are burned to provide energy for muscle contraction. Generally, fat is the major energy source for moderate physical activity, while carbohydrates usually provide energy during rigorous, exhaustive activity. Highly conditioned individuals participating in endurance-type activities are able to shift to fat metabolism and burn fat, rather than the sugar (glycogen) that is stored in the muscle cells. As a result, greater amounts of the energy required for an activity can be derived from fat than from carbohydrates.

Fatty acids may be saturated or unsaturated. The type of fat you consume is important because **saturated fats** (fatty acids carrying the maximum possible number of hydrogen ions) tend to raise blood cholesterol while **polyunsaturated**

fats (fatty acids that lack four or more hydrogen atoms and have two or more double bonds between carbons) lower it. It is important to be concerned not only about the amount of fat consumed, but the source and composition of that fat because of the possible relationship between dietary fat and the incidence of several degenerative diseases. Dietary lipid has been shown to be related to coronary heart disease, cancer, and obesity.

There is clear evidence that the total amounts and types of fats and other lipids in the diet influence the risk of coronary heart disease and to a less well-established extent certain forms of cancer and possibly obesity. High fat intake is associated with an increased risk of certain cancers, especially cancers of the colon, prostate, and breast. Eating a diet high in fat, especially saturated fatty acids and cholesterol, causes elevated blood cholesterol levels in many people. High blood cholesterol levels increase the risk of heart disease. Reducing fat is an especially good idea for those people who are limiting calories. Not only do fats provide more than twice the calories of protein and carbohydrates but also contain few vitamins and minerals. Eliminating all fats is not a good idea either. For example, milk, meat, poultry, fish, and eggs all contribute fat and chosterol to your diet. They also provide essential nutrients such as calcium, iron, and zinc. The key is moderation. Focus on a balanced overall diet, and avoid too much fat where possible by using lower fat dairy products and lean meats and reducing the amount of fats added at the table. See table 9.4 for tips on avoiding saturated fat and table 9.5 to evaluate your daily fat intake.

The National Heart, Lung and Blood Institute recommendations:

1. Less than 30 percent of total calories should come from fat.
2. Less than 10 percent of calories should come from saturated fat.
3. No more than 10 percent of calories should come from polyunsaturated fat.
4. 10 to 15 percent of calories should come from monosaturated fat.
5. 50 to 60 percent of daily calories should come from carbohydrates.
6. A daily diet should contain less than 300 milligrams of cholesterol.

Unsaturated fats (polyunsaturated and monosaturated) seem to lower blood cholesterol levels, and when they make up less than 30 percent of a day's calories, they are healthy substitutes for saturated fat. Vegetable oils, such as safflower, canola, corn, soybean, cottonseed, sesame, and sunflower are good sources of polyunsaturated fats. However, a few vegetable oils also are naturally high in saturated fat—especially coconut oil (84 percent) and palm kernel oil (79 percent).

TABLE 9.4 Tips for Avoiding too Much Fat and Saturated Fat

---

1. Steam, boil, or bake vegetables. For a change, stir-fry in a small amount of vegetable oil. Consider buying an insert for a pot so you can easily steam your vegetables.
2. Season vegetables with herbs and spices rather than with sauces, butter, or margarine.
3. Try lemon juice on salad or use limited amounts of oil-based salad dressing.
4. To reduce saturated fat, use small amounts of tub margarine instead of butter or stick margarine. In baked products, when possible, use vegetables oil instead of either of these more solid fats or hydrogenated shortenings.
5. Limit baked goods made with large amounts of fat, especially saturated fats: croissants, doughnuts, muffins, biscuits, and butter rolls.
6. Try whole-grain flours to enhance flavors when you bake with less fat and cholesterol-containing ingredients.
7. Replace whole milk with skim or low-fat milk in puddings, soups, and baked products.
8. Substitute low-fat yogurt, blender-whipped low-fat cottage cheese, or buttermilk in recipes that call for sour cream or mayonnaise.
9. Choose lean cuts of meat. Limit bacon, ribs, and meat loaf.
10. Trim fat from meats before and after cooking.
11. Roast, bake, or broil meat, poultry, and fish so fat drains away as the food cooks.
12. Remove skin from poultry before cooking. This eliminates the temptation to eat it along with the meat.
13. Use a nonstick pan for cooking so added fat will be unnecessary; use a vegetable spray for frying.
14. Chill meat or poultry broth until the fat solidifies. Spoon off the fat before using the broth.
15. Eat a vegetarian main dish at least once a week. Include fish (cooked without too much fat) in the diet about two times a week.
16. Choose ice milk, low-fat frozen yogurt, sorbets, and popsicles as substitutes for ice cream.
17. Try angel food cake, fig bars, and ginger snaps as substitutes for commercial baked goods high in saturated fats.
18. Limit high-fat cheese intake.
19. Read labels of commercially prepared foods to find out what type of fat or how much saturated fat they contain.
20. Think about the balance of fats in your menu. If your meal contains whole milk, cheese, ice cream, a higher fat meat, or poultry with skin, use tub margarine and unsaturated vegetable oils for your spreads and dressings. Small amounts of butter, sour cream, or cream cheese can be included if other menu items are low in saturated fat.
21. Use jam, jelly, or marmalade on bread and toast instead of butter or margarine.
22. Buy whole-grain breads and rolls. They have more flavor and do not need butter or margarine to taste good. The dietary fiber present is an added bonus.

Source: From Contemporary Nutrition, Issues and Insides. Wardlaw, G., Insel P. Marolas. Mosby-Yearbook Inc., 11820 Westline Drive, St. Louis, Missouri.

TABLE 9.5 How Does Your Diet Score?

Do the foods you eat provide more fat than is good for you? Answer the questions below, then see how your diet stacks up.

How often do you eat:	seldom or never	1–2× per week	3–5× per week	almost daily
Fried, deep-fat fried or breaded foods?	☐	☐	☐	☐
Fatty meats such as bacon, sausage, luncheon meats and heavily marbled steaks and roasts?	☐	☐	☐	☐
Whole milk, high-fat cheeses and ice cream?	☐	☐	☐	☐
High-fat desserts such as pies, pastries and rich cakes?	☐	☐	☐	☐
Rich sauces and gravies?	☐	☐	☐	☐
Oily salad dressings or mayonnaise?	☐	☐	☐	☐
Whipped cream, table cream, sour cream and cream cheese?	☐	☐	☐	☐
Butter or margarine on vegetables, dinner rolls and toast?	☐	☐	☐	☐

Take a look at your answers. Several responses in the last two columns mean you may have a high fat intake. Perhaps it's time to cut back.

Source: From *Nutrition Annual Editions* "How Does Your Diet Score? A Basic Primer on Fats in Your Diet" Nestle World View.

Proteins

Proteins are compounds made up of carbon, hydrogen, oxygen, and nitrogen. The building blocks of protein are called amino acids, twenty-two of which are recognized as important nutritional requirements. Nine of these proteins cannot be synthesized by the body and are referred to as essential proteins. Individuals on strict vegetarian diets must choose their food source carefully to ensure that they receive these essential proteins. Lacto-vegetarians (milk and milk products) and lacto-ovo vegetarians (eggs, milk, and milk products) have greater opportunities in meeting protein needs.

Proteins help maintain the body's fluid balance, form the basis of antibodies, transport vital substances such as calcium, glucose, and potassium, aid in blood clotting, and form connective tissue. They are an energy source only when fats and carbohydrates are not available. Excellent sources of protein are eggs, meat, fish, poultry, dry beans, peas, nuts, milk, and cheese. Protein needs of sedentary and most active people are about the same. The adult requirements are approximately 12 percent of total daily caloric intake. The Food and Nutrition Board recommends a daily intake of 0.8 grams of protein per kilogram of body weight. Protein supplements are unnecessary and expensive. Excess protein will not build muscles, only exercise will. Extra protein will be stored as fat.

Minerals

Approximately 4 percent of a person's body weight is made up of as many as sixty different **mineral** elements. Twenty-one of these have been proven essential in human nutrition (see table C–5 in appendix C). An essential mineral is one that performs functions vital to life, growth, and reproduction. Its absence results in physical dysfunction and illness. The essential mineral elements are often grouped as macronutrients (those present in relatively high amounts) and micronutrients or trace elements (present in less than .005 percent of the body weight).

Minerals regulate body processes and maintain body tissue. Minerals are found in all foods except sugar, alcohol, and highly refined fats and oils. They are inorganic compounds smaller than vitamins and are found in very simple forms in foods. Some minerals are used as building blocks for such structures as bones and teeth. Calcium, phosphorus, potassium, sodium, iron, and iodine are a few of the more important required minerals (see table C–5 in appendix C).

Vitamins

Vitamins are organic compounds that are needed in only small amounts by the body. They regulate a number of body processes, including the release of energy from food, and also are used in the metabolism of carbohydrates and fats. All foods, except sugar, alcohol, and highly refined fats and oils, contain vitamins.

Vitamins are classified as either water-soluble or fat-soluble. The water-soluble C and B complex vitamins are not stored in the body and therefore must be continuously supplied by the diet. The fat-soluble A, D, E, and K vitamins are stored in the body. As a result, excessive ingestion of fat-soluble vitamins can have toxic effects. See table 9.7.

Vitamin deficiency may result from a restricted diet, lack of absorption in the intestines, loss of vitamin content in food, and conditions such as surgery, alcoholism, fever, and serious illness. Except in unusual circumstances, vitamin supplements are unnecessary. Most individuals can learn to adjust their diets and meet their nutritional needs much better from foods than from pills and with a more solid guarantee that they are getting a proper balance of nutrients. See tables C–3 and C–4 in appendix C for a list of major characteristics of water- and fat-soluble vitamins.

Vitamin C and the Arteries

One way that vitamin C may help prevent cardiovascular disease is by improving cholesterol levels. Several studies have found that people with high levels of vitamin C in their blood tend to have more of the "good" cholesterol (HDL or high-density lipoprotein) than people with low blood levels. Vitamin C may also keep "bad" cholsterol (LDL or low-density lipoproten) from turning bad in the first place; apparently LDL promotes clogged arteries only when its molecular structure has been oxidized or damaged by renegade molecules known as free radicals. Vitamin C is an **antioxidant** that can destroy free radicals before they can do any harm. More will be said on the role of antioxidants later in this chapter. Vitamin C actually surrounds the LDL molecules in the blood shielding them from oxidation. Other evidence indicates that high levels of vitamin C make the blood less sticky, which could reduce the risk of heart attack and stroke and also possibly lower blood pressure. The recommended daily allowance is 60 mg.

Water

Water transports nutrients, regulates body temperature, participates in chemical reactions, and removes waste materials. Although water is indispensable for survival, its importance as a vital nutritional constituent is often taken for granted. The body may be able to survive for weeks without food under certain circumstances, but it can survive without water for only a few hours, especially in hot climates. (See chapter 13 for special needs during exercise in hot weather.)

Nutritional Assessment

In order to determine if you are meeting your current nutritional needs, you must first determine your nutritional status. This can be accomplished by clinical observation, determination of body composition, dietary evaluation, or biochemical evaluation. An assessment of your nutritional status through clinical observation can be accomplished by using table 9.6. This table lists a number of overt indicators of your present nutritional status that you can assess yourself. Body composition (or skinfold measurements), which was covered in chapter 4, will give you a fairly accurate measure of your percentage of fat to lean body weight. This information will also enable you to determine your appropriate weight goals. For a dietary evaluation of your nutritional status, you need to fill out the food intake record, listing all of the food you have eaten over a period of three days. See record sheets B–8 and B–9 in appendix B and tables 9.1, 9.3, 9.4, 9.6, 9.7, and 9.8. A biochemical evaluation of your nutritional status is achieved by

179

TABLE 9.6 Current, Recommended, and High-Energy Nutritional Allowances

	Current	Recommended by American Heart Association	Recommended for high-energy needs
Fats	42%	30%	10 to 20%
Protein	12%	12%	10 to 12%
Complex carbohydrates	22%	48%	60 to 80%
Sugar	24%	10%	5 to 10%

doing a chemical analysis of your blood and urine. This sort of analysis indicates the levels of such substances as serum albumin, hemoglobin, and cholesterol in your body.

Basic Four Food Groups

The Center for Science in the Public Interest has divided the major foods into four groups (table 9.3). Each of the four groups contains foods that are similar in origin and nutrient content. The four food group plan specifies that a certain quantity of food be consumed from each group every day. The U. S. Department of Agriculture has also organized six food groups into a pyramid model. See figure 9.1.

Eating and Exercise

Before rigorous exercise, you should be careful about not only *what* you eat but also *when* you eat it. Your diet and your meal-timing could affect your performance.

Digestion and Rigorous Exercise

There are a number of reasons why you should avoid eating just prior to rigorous exercise. First, when you go from rest to exercise, a large amount of blood is shifted away from the stomach and intestines to other exercising muscles. Therefore, if you have food in your stomach and intestines during exercise, there will be insufficient blood to digest the food properly and you may experience digestive distress, such as nausea and vomiting. Second, rigorous exercise reduces gastric juice secretion, which plays a major role in breaking down food for digestion. Third, lactic acid levels increase during exercise, which can affect the ability of

TABLE 9.7 Symptoms of Nutritional Deficiency

Abnormal signs	Some possible nutrient lacks
Attendance	
Frequent absence from school or work	
Growth failure (children)	
Failure to increase in stature or weight	Energy, protein, zinc
Behavior	
Easily fatigued; listless; apathetic; depressed; nervous; irritable; inability to concentrate; complaints of insomnia; poor work capacity	Multiple deficiencies including energy, protein, B complex
Skin	
Dry, flaky, rough	Vitamin A, essential fatty acids
Bed sores, poor wound healing, edematous	Protein, vitamin C
Excessive bruising	Vitamin K
Keratinization	Vitamin A
Pinpoint, purplish hemorrhagic spots	Ascorbic acid
Symmetrical dermatitis	Niacin
Hair	
Thin, sparse, dry, lusterless, easily plucked out, change in pigments with distinct bands	Protein, energy
Face	
Pale	Iron, vitamin B-6, B-12, folacin
Scaling around nose	Riboflavin, niacin, vitamin B-6
Swollen (edema)	Protein
Eyes	
Pale	Iron
Dry and scaly at corners	Riboflavin, vitamin B-6
Sensitive to bright light, itching	Riboflavin
Increased vascularity	Riboflavin, niacin, vitamin B-6
Nightblindness, Bitot's spots, soft cornea, xerophthalmia	Vitamin A
Lips	
Fissuring at corners	Iron, riboflavin, niacin, vitamin B-6
Swollen, puffy	Riboflavin, niacin
Tongue	
Pale	Iron, vitamin B-12, folacin
Swollen	Niacin, vitamin B-12, folacin
Raw, scarlet red	Niacin
Magenta red	Riboflavin
Atrophy of papillae	Iron, B complex

TABLE 9.7 Symptoms of Nutritional Deficiency (*Continued*)

Abnormal signs	Some possible nutrient lacks
Teeth	
Mottled enamel	*Excess* fluoride
Caries	*Excess* sugar; poor dental hygiene
Gums	
Spongy, swollen, bleeding	Ascorbic acid
Nails	
Brittle, ridged, spoon shaped, pale nail beds	Iron
Glands	
Enlarged thyroid	Iodine
Muscles	
Wasted	Protein, energy
Sore, painful	Ascorbic acid, potassium
Weak	Ascorbic acid, potassium, magnesium
Skeletal	
Poor posture, delayed closing of fontanelles (infant), knock knees, bowed legs, beading of ribs, enlarged joints	Vitamin D, calcium
Fleeting joint pains	Ascorbic acid

the stomach to break down food. Fourth, even light exercise has been shown to negatively affect digestion in the small intestines. Finally, the feeling of fullness after eating may have a psychological effect on your performance during rigorous exercise. All of these factors are good arguments for allowing at least four hours to pass between a heavy meal and rigorous exercise.

As an example of how food and digestion can affect rigorous exercise, let us consider the precompetition eating regimen you would follow if you were a long-distance runner.

For long-distance competitive running, carbohydrates are your main source of energy, and it is therefore imperative that you have a sufficient amount of carbohydrates available before you run. If you are going to compete on a Saturday, for example, you should undergo only a moderate workout on Thursday and a light workout on Friday. This prevents you from depleting your stored glycogen. Your prerunning meal should be fairly light and at least four hours before you run. The two meals preceding your prerunning meal should be high in carbohydrates, such as oatmeal, toast, jam, and honey.

Before a competitive run, keep the following eating guidelines in mind:

1. Avoid foods that are distasteful to you and that you simply don't enjoy eating. They could have a negative psychological effect on your performance.
2. Avoid spicy foods and roughage that might irritate your gastrointestinal tract.
3. Avoid fatty foods for at least four hours before competition since they can slow down your digestive process.
4. Carbohydrates can be eaten two hours before competition with generally no problems.
5. On very hot days, drink some water thirty minutes before the competition.
6. Keep your protein foods to a minimum because an excess of protein may cause an increase of acidosis in the blood, which may increase your chances of fatigue.
7. Derive your fluids from soups, such as bouillon, and fruit juices.

High-Energy Foods for Rigorous Exercise

Considerable evidence indicates that all of us should increase the proportion of complex carbohydrates in our diets while reducing the percentages of fats and proteins. Good sources of complex carbohydrates are brown rice, whole wheat breads, oatmeal, beans, peas, potatoes, pasta, and a number of fresh fruits and vegetables. Complex carbohydrates are especially important for those individuals involved in rigorous exercise requiring high levels of energy expenditure. When carbohydrates are broken down, they produce high levels of energy with relatively small amounts of harmful waste products. If you consume excessive amounts of fats and protein, your body becomes overloaded with their toxic by-products of metabolism, which may result in decreased physical performance. For example, excessive amounts of protein (over 15 percent of daily diet or in excess of 85 to 90 grams) results in increased mineral and water loss and acidosis (excessive acid in blood and body fluids).

Table 9.6 shows current and recommended nutritional allowances, as well as nutritional allowances recommended for the high-energy needs of rigorous physical exercise.

Caffeine and Exercise

A number of individuals are experimenting with the use of caffeine as a means of delaying fatigue during rigorous activity. This use is based on evidence indicating that caffeine may enable the body to more efficiently use fatty acids for

TABLE 9.8 Recommended Daily Dietary Allowances (RDA)[a] (Designed for the Maintenance of Good Nutrition of Practically All Healthy Persons in the United States)

Category	Age (years) or condition	Weight[b] (kg)	Weight[b] (lb)	Height[b] (cm)	Height[b] (in)	Protein (g)	Fat-soluble vitamins Vita-min A (μg RE)[c]	Vita-min D (μg)[d]	Vita-min E (mg α-TE)[e]	Vita-min K (μg)
Infants	0.0–0.5	6	13	60	24	13	375	7.5	3	5
	0.5–1.0	9	20	71	28	14	375	10	4	10
Children	1–3	13	29	90	35	16	400	10	6	15
	4–6	20	44	112	44	24	500	10	7	20
	7–10	28	62	132	52	28	700	10	7	30
Males	11–14	45	99	157	62	45	1000	10	10	45
	15–18	66	145	176	69	59	1000	10	10	65
	19–24	72	160	177	70	58	1000	10	10	70
	25–50	79	174	176	70	63	1000	5	10	80
	51+	77	170	173	68	63	1000	5	10	80
Females	11–14	46	101	157	62	46	800	10	8	45
	15–18	55	120	163	64	44	800	10	8	55
	19–24	58	128	164	65	46	800	10	8	60
	25–50	63	138	163	64	50	800	5	8	65
	51+	65	143	160	63	50	800	5	8	65
Pregnant						60	800	10	10	65
Lactating	1st 6 months					65	1300	10	12	65
	2nd 6 months					62	1200	10	11	65

[a]The allowances, expressed as average daily intakes over time, are intended to provide for individual variations among most normal persons as they live in the United States under usual environmental stresses. Diets should be based on a variety of common foods in order to provide other nutrients for which human requirements have been less well-defined.
[b]Weights and heights are actual medians for the U.S. population of the designated age. The use of these figures does not imply that height-to-weight ratios are ideal.

energy production. The studies in this area, however, are fairly limited and should be viewed with caution.

It is important to remember that caffeine is a stimulant. Large amounts of caffeine can have a variety of effects on the body, such as increased urine output, constriction in the circulatory system, and stimulation of the heart (which may result in irregular heartbeats). Also, research has associated frequent coffee drinking in middle-aged men with high levels of cholesterol and low-density lipoprotein, which are associated with a greater risk of coronary heart disease.

Water-soluble vitamins							Minerals						
Vita-min C (mg)	Thia-min (mg)	Ribo-flavin (mg)	Niacin (mg NE)[f]	Vita-min B$_6$ (mg)	Fo-late (μg)	Vitamin B$_{12}$ (μg)	Cal-cium (mg)	Phos-phorus (mg)	Mag-nesium (mg)	Iron (mg)	Zinc (mg)	Iodine (μg)	Sele-nium (μg)
30	0.3	0.4	5	0.3	25	0.3	400	300	40	6	5	40	10
35	0.4	0.5	6	0.6	35	0.5	600	500	60	10	5	50	15
40	0.7	0.8	9	1.0	50	0.7	800	800	80	10	10	70	20
45	0.9	1.1	12	1.1	75	1.0	800	800	120	10	10	90	20
45	1.0	1.2	13	1.4	100	1.4	800	800	170	10	10	120	30
50	1.3	1.5	17	1.7	150	2.0	1200	1200	270	12	15	150	40
60	1.5	1.8	20	2.0	200	2.0	1200	1200	400	12	15	150	50
60	1.5	1.7	19	2.0	200	2.0	1200	1200	350	10	15	150	70
60	1.5	1.7	19	2.0	200	2.0	800	800	350	10	15	150	70
60	1.2	1.4	15	2.0	200	2.0	800	800	350	10	15	150	70
50	1.1	1.3	15	1.4	150	2.0	1200	1200	280	15	12	150	45
60	1.1	1.3	15	1.5	180	2.0	1200	1200	300	15	12	150	50
60	1.1	1.3	15	1.6	180	2.0	1200	1200	280	15	12	150	55
60	1.1	1.3	15	1.6	180	2.0	800	800	280	15	12	150	55
60	1.0	1.2	13	1.6	180	2.0	800	800	280	10	12	150	55
70	1.5	1.6	17	2.2	400	2.2	1200	1200	320	30	15	175	65
95	1.6	1.8	20	2.1	280	2.6	1200	1200	355	15	19	200	75
90	1.6	1.7	20	2.1	260	2.6	1200	1200	340	15	16	200	75

[c]Retinol equivalents.
[d]As cholecalciferol.
[e]α-Tocopherol equivalents.
[f]Niacin equivalents.
Adapted from National Reasearch Council, National Academy of Sciences, 1989 *Recommended Dietary Allowances,* 10th Edition, Washington DC, National Academy of Sciences.

(One cup of coffee may contain approximately 100 to 150 milligrams of caffeine; tea contains a little less.) Caffeine intake prior to physical activity is *not* recommended.

Special Diets

Special diets have been suggested for all kinds of reasons—for losing weight, for increasing physical well-being, and for improving physical performance. Some of these diets are fads and are potentially dangerous. The others must be

Chapter 9

| TABLE 9.8 | Recommended Daily Dietary Allowances (RDA)[a] (Designed for the Maintenance of Good Nutrition of Practically All Healthy Persons in the United States) (*Continued*) |

Estimated safe and adequate daily dietary intakes of selected vitamins and minerals[g]

		Vitamins	
Category	Age (years)	Biotin (μg)	Pantothenic Acid (mg)
Infants	0–0.5	10	2
	0.5–1	15	3
Children and adolescents	1–3	20	3
	4–6	25	3–4
	7–10	30	4–5
	11+	30–100	4–7
Adults		30–100	4–7

[g]Because there is less information on which to base allowances, these figures are not given in the main table of RDA and are provided here in the form of ranges of recommended intakes.

undertaken cautiously and only with complete knowledge of what is required to meet all daily nutritional requirements and to avoid any of the diet's possible side effects.

Fad Diets

A number of fad diets with varying combinations of nutrients unfortunately have found wide acceptance because of media misinformation and public ignorance. Be very wary of these diets because they may have a number of dangerous consequences. For example, individuals on diets that do not allow for protein or that are low in protein may suffer a loss of muscle tissue and severe weakness. A high-fat diet, sometimes advocated in combination with high protein and very little carbohydrates, may produce a loss of nutrients and electrolytes, very high cholesterol levels, and diarrhea. A high-protein and high-fat diet with low carbohydrates may produce kidney problems, dizziness, weakness, dehydration, irritability, and uric acid formation. Low-fat diets may lead to dry skin, constipation, irritability, stiff joints, and a number of other problems.

Other fad diets that have enjoyed unwarranted popularity include the low-carbohydrate diet, ''super-protein'' diets, and vitamin and mineral supplemental diets. ''Diet foods'' and using drugs to lose weight also are discussed in this section. See the defensive dining list (table 9.18) for tips on proper diet.

186

Estimated safe and adequate daily dietary intakes of selected vitamins and minerals[g]

Category	Age (years)	Trace Elements[h]				
		Copper (mg)	Manganese (mg)	Fluoride (mg)	Chromium (μg)	Molybdenum (μg)
Infants	0–0.5	0.4–0.6	0.3–0.6	0.1–0.5	10–40	15–30
	0.5–1	0.6–0.7	0.6–1.0	0.2–1.0	20–60	20–40
Children and adolescents	1–3	0.7–1.0	1.0–1.5	0.5–1.5	20–80	25–50
	4–6	1.0–1.5	1.5–2.0	1.0–2.5	30–120	30–75
	7–10	1.0–2.0	2.0–3.0	1.5–2.5	50–200	50–150
	11+	1.5–2.5	2.0–5.0	1.5–2.5	50–200	75–250
Adults		1.5–3.0	2.0–5.0	1.5–4.0	50–200	75–250

[h]Since the toxic levels for some trace elements may be only several times usual intakes, the upper levels for the trace elements given in this table should not be habitually exceeded.

Low-Carbohydrate Diet

The oldest and the most popular reducing diet is the low-carbohydrate diet. Although it is advertised as new and revolutionary, it actually is a very old regimen that resurfaces every few years, generally under a new name. A low-carbohydrate diet involves cutting your carbohydrate intake to around sixty grams a day or less, while eating all of the protein and fatty foods that you want.

As you might suspect, there are a number of problems with the low-carbohydrate method of losing weight. The major indictment of the diet is that it is dangerous. Even though some physicians still prescribe this diet, a majority of the medical profession do not consider it medically safe. While restricting carbohydrates in the diet can sometimes produce a dramatic weight loss, no experimental evidence indicates that fat loss occurs if the dieter consumes more calories than he or she is expending, as can happen with the low-carbohydrate diet. Also, whatever fat loss *does* occur as a result of a low-carbohydrate diet appears to come from the toxic effects of ketones (end products of fat breakdown), which produce nausea and thus suppress the appetite. These ketone bodies can cause severe injury to the body tissue, in particular to the blood vessels. The low-carbohydrate diet can also produce weight loss because of a loss of salt. Since water follows salt, much of the weight loss seen on the bathroom scale may be due to the excretion of salt and water. It is dangerous to upset the water and electrolyte balance, and this ''weight loss'' will be regained as soon as the dieter resumes a normal carbohydrate intake. The low-carbohydrate diet's high fat content also tends to contribute to atherosclerosis.

"Super-Protein" Diets

Some athletes ingest large amounts of protein supplements, believing that doing so will help them build up their muscles and energy level, even though there is no scientific justification for the use of these supplements. Athletes generally do not need additional protein but additional calories in the form of complex carbohydrates to provide energy for muscle activity. Most athletes already consume twice as much protein as they can possibly use and probably are wasting about half as much as they eat.

It is impossible to force extra amounts of protein into the muscles just by eating more. For muscle cells to accept additional protein, additional demands have to be made upon the muscles. To make a muscle grow, you have to overload it. The muscle generally responds by taking in more nutrients and subsequently accelerating its growth.

The so-called ''super-protein'' diets are unnecessary, expensive, and in some cases harmful. For example, with large amounts of protein, the blood level of uric acid may increase and damage the kidneys and make the joints more susceptible to injuries. As for energy derived from protein, you burn up as much protein reading a book as running track at top speed. The body burns protein for energy only in starvation.

Vitamin and Mineral Supplemented Diets

Supplementing your diet with vitamins and minerals above the minimum daily requirement does not improve physical performance. In fact, excessive intake of vitamins A, D, and K can cause toxic effects. Minimum daily vitamin and mineral requirements are met easily through a normal, well-balanced diet.

The one exception to this may be the iron requirement of females engaged in rigorous physical activity, particularly after menstrual blood loss. These women have been found to have significantly decreased levels of iron in their blood. Since overdoses of iron can be toxic, however, these women should take iron supplements only after consulting with a physician.

Antioxidants

There is mounting evidence that antioxidants may provide some protection against oxidative stress (breaking down of the cell membranes by oxidizing compounds). Vitamins A, C, and E and beta carotene, which are the major antioxidants, may play some role in protection against certain cancers and heart disease.

As evidence accumulates showing that beta carotene may protect against cancer, scientists are starting to find that other members of the carotenoid family may have some similar beneficial effects. There are more than 500 carotenoids that give fruits and vegetables their characteristic yellow, orange, and red coloring. They also abound in dark leafy vegetables, but hidden by the green color of the chlorophyll. Of the fifty or sixty other carotenoids in our food supply, most research has focused on the carotenoid in carrots; red fruits and vegetables, such as tomatoes and red peppers; oranges; broccoli, and leafy greens, especially kale. Ten carotenoids have been identified so far in broccoli alone, along with six in apricots and five in tomatoes.

More has to be learned before recommending antioxidant supplementation. The best advice now is to obtain antioxidants by eating in moderation a variety of healthy food.

The top ten antioxidant-rich fruits and vegetables are: broccoli, cantaloupe, carrots, leafy greens, mangos, pumpkin, red bell peppers, spinach, strawberries, and sweet potatoes. Running close behind are brussels sprouts, all citrus fruits, tomatoes, potatoes, berries, cauliflower, asparagus, peas, and beets.

Nutrition and Cancer

A comprehensive review by the Committee on Diet and Health, Food and Nutrition Board, National Research Council, of evidence to date indicates that diet influences the risks of several major chronic diseases. The evidence is very strong for cardiovascular disease and hypertension and is highly suggestive for certain forms of cancer especially cancers of the esophagus, stomach, large intestines, breast, lung, and prostate. See table 9.9 for ways to cancer proof your eating.

Calcium

Most people consume far too little calcium. The average woman gets one-third to one-half of her recommended intake (1200 mg), the average man gets three-quarters of his recommended amount. Those meager intakes may have serious health consequences. It is well known that calcium helps prevent osteoporosis (see chapter 14), the brittle bone disease that afflicts many older women and some older men. Now mounting evidence suggests that calcium can also reduce the risk of developing several other chronic ailments, including two major killers: coronary heart disease and colon cancer.

Vegetarian Diets

For years, Americans have had a love affair with meat. For a variety of reasons, however, many individuals have decided to reduce, and in some cases eliminate, meat from their diet. There are many degrees of meat exclusion among vegetarians. Individuals who exclude all foods of animal origin and eat only raw fruits,

TABLE 9.9 Cancer-Proofing Your Eating

In 1991, the American Cancer Society updated its guidelines on dietary measures that may lower cancer risk. In the seven years since the first guidelines were released, there has been a plethora of new research on diet and cancer. Findings from that research have been incorporated into the new recommendations—but very few specific changes have resulted. The new guidelines only further affirm the old, since more evidence backs them up now than when they were first published in 1984. In addition, they have proven to be heart-healthy and to help prevent diabetes. As noted in the guidelines, "The dietary advice in this report can be epitomized in two words—variety and moderation. A varied diet, eaten in moderation, offers the best hope for lowering the risk of a disease that yearly claims a half-million lives in this country, together with untold pain and grief."

Substance	Associated cancers	Comments	Steps to take
Fiber	May **decrease** risk of colorectal cancer.	Different types of fiber may affect cancer risk differently. Benefits may also be due to lower fat intakes usually associated with high-fiber diets.	Eat 4 to 5 servings a day of a variety of vegetables, fruits, whole-grain cereals, and legumes. Maximize fiber in vegetables and fruits by eating them unpeeled.
Fruits and vegetables	May **decrease** risk of colorectal and breast cancers.	Good sources of fiber (see above). Cruciferous vegetables, such as broccoli, cabbage, and Brussels sprouts, also contain indoles—nitrogen compounds which, in some studies, have knocked out carcinogens that can lead to breast cancer.	To maximize indole intake, eat vegetables raw, steamed, or microwaved—boiling leaches up to half the indoles.
Fat	May **increase** risk of breast, colon, and prostate cancers.	Lowering fat intake will almost automatically lower caloric intake and boost fiber intake—steps that will also lower cancer risk.	Decrease calories from fat to 25 to 30% of total daily calories. (Current average intake is 40% of total calories.)
Alcohol	Heavy use **increases** risk of cancers of the oral cavity, larynx, and esophagus; moderate use may **increase** breast cancer risk.	Cigarette smoking in conjunction with alcohol drinking greatly increases cancer risk. Alcohol use also can cause liver cirrhosis, which may lead to liver cancer.	Drink only occasionally and sparingly.

TABLE 9.9 Cancer-Proofing Your Eating (*Continued*)

Salt-cured, smoked, barbecued and nitrite-preserved foods	May **increase** risk of stomach, esophageal, and lung cancers.	Smoking and charcoal-grilling foods produces tars that are similar to those in cigarette smoke, and are absorbed by the food. Manufacturers have substantially decreased nitrites used in meat preservation.	Opt for other cooking methods; limit intake of salt-cured and nitrite preserved foods.
Beta carotene and antioxidant vitamins (A, C, and E)	Inconclusive	Vitamin E and beta carotene have been associated with lower rates of cancer in humans; a lesser effect has been noted with the other antioxidant nutrients. More research is needed.	Eat a balanced and varied diet to insure you get the RDA for all vitamins; do not take megadose vitamin supplements.
Selenium	Inconclusive	Limited evidence shows this trace element may protect against breast and colon cancer—however, it is very toxic in high doses.	Taking selenium supplements can be very dangerous; you get all the selenium you need from a varied diet.
Artificial sweeteners	Inconclusive	High levels of saccharin cause bladder cancer in rats, but no evidence of this in humans. Long-term effects of aspartame are unknown.	Moderate use poses no risk.
Coffee and caffeine	None	Both coffee and caffeine have received a clean bill of health.	Moderate use of coffee and caffeine is fine.
Food additives	None	Chemical additives found to be carcinogenic in animals have been banned; insufficent evidence that additives currently in use have any cancer risk or benefit.	None

Source: American Cancer Society

seeds, and nuts are called pure vegetarians. Individuals who include milk, eggs, and cheese, as well as vegetables, fruits, and grains in their diet are called ovo-lacto vegetarians. Other individuals modify these vegetarian diets to suit their own beliefs.

There are a number of important health considerations related to a vegetarian diet. For example, ovo-lacto or pure vegetarians generally have a lower serum cholesterol count and reduced heart disease, as well as a lower incidence of certain types of cancer. The reduced heart disease may be the result of the lower fat and cholesterol intake. The higher fiber intake of the vegetarian may offer some protection against cancer of the colon. In addition, individuals on vegetarian diets tend to have a greater bone density in older age and fewer incidents of osteoporosis, a disease that degenerates the bones.

As with any kind of diet, the more foods or types of foods that are excluded, the more likely that a nutritional deficiency will occur. The main concern with a vegetarian diet is ensuring sufficient amounts of daily protein. Most research indicates that vegetarians consume enough foods to meet their energy needs and also their protein requirements. A pure vegetarian diet that meets all nutritional needs, however, is generally fairly high in bulk, and sometimes this makes it difficult to take in enough food to meet the energy needs required for rigorous physical activity.

A common problem for those on a vegetarian diet is the selection of foods with a high concentration of iron. Iron is important for the production of hemo-globin and the red blood cells that carry oxygen. Individuals with low hemoglobin and a low red cell count may find it difficult to engage in very rigorous exercise and may fatigue easily. Vegetarians must also be cautious in their selection of iron- and zinc-rich foods or alternative foods because iron and zinc are not well absorbed from vegetable foods.

Fasting

The main source of energy for your exercise comes from your diet. In essence, when you eat, you refuel. When you don't eat, or fast, your body is forced to find other sources of energy and draws upon stored reserves of carbohydrates and fats and eventually upon muscle tissue. Glucose in the blood is quickly used up. The body then draws upon glycogen in the muscles. When the glycogen is burned up, the body depends on fatty acids as an energy source. The problem here is that brain cells cannot depend upon fatty acids for fuel—they need glucose since glucose is the only nutrient that can get through their membranes. When glucose is not available, brain cells find another source of glucose in the form of amino acids that can be converted to glucose. These amino acids are found only in complete protein that is stored in the muscle tissue. Thus, the muscle tissue is broken down to provide energy. As a fast continues, the energy output of the body is sharply reduced and the muscles shrink in mass and have less energy to work.

Fasting also causes the body to produce ketones, which are a combination of fatty acids that normally are found only in small amounts in the body. During fasting, however, very large numbers of ketones are produced and may spill over into the urine, resulting in a serious health condition known as ketosis.

With a balanced perspective on foods and a sense of what's important in diet planning and what's not, you can evaluate various diets by asking yourself the questions that appear in table 9.10.

Carbohydrate Loading

Carbohydrate loading involves increasing the amount of glycogen stored by the skeletal muscles through special diets and exercise. The average individual stores approximately fifteen grams of glycogen for each kilogram of muscle weight.

There are three different methods of carbohydrate loading. In the first, you consume a high-carbohydrate diet for three or four days, after several days of a normal, mixed diet. This technique can increase the amount of stored glycogen by 30 percent.

A second procedure for carbohydrate loading combines exercise and diet. The muscles that you want to load with carbohydrates are first exhausted of their glycogen storage through rigorous exercise. Then, you follow a high-carbohydrate diet for several days. This routine has been shown to double glycogen storage.

The third method of carbohydrate loading involves exercise and two special diets. Once again, exercise is used to induce glycogen depletion. This is followed by a three-day diet that is very low in carbohydrates and high in fats and protein. After this, you consume a diet high in carbohydrates for three additional days. Exhausting exercise may be performed during the days of the high-fat and high-protein diet but not during the high-carbohydrate diet. This last procedure has been shown to increase glycogen storage as much as four times the amount normally stored in the muscle.

Carbohydrate loading is not without its side effects, however, especially when a high-protein, low-carbohydrate diet is combined with exercise. For example, carbohydrate loading can result in a feeling of stiffness and heaviness from the additional glycogen that has been loaded in the muscle. Also, evidence indicates that carbohydrate loading may cause kidney malfunctioning that results

---

TABLE 9.10 Diet Evaluation

---

1. Does the diet provide a reasonable number of kilocalories (enough to maintain weight; not too many; and if a reduction diet, not fewer than 1200 kilocalories for the average-size person)?
2. Does it provide enough, but not too much, protein (at least the recommended intake or RDA, but not more than twice as much)?
3. Does it provide enough fat for satiety, but not so much fat as to go against current recommendations (between 20 and 35 percent of the kilocalories from fat)?
4. Does it provide enough carbohydrate to spare protein and prevent ketosis (100 grams of carbohydrate for the average-size person)? Is it mostly complex carbohydrate (not more than 20 percent of the kilocalories as concentrated sugar)?
5. Does it offer a balanced assortment of vitamins and minerals from whole food sources in all four food groups? The four food groups are milk/milk products; meat/fish/poultry/eggs/legumes; fruits/vegetables; and grains.
6. Does it offer variety in the sense that different foods can be selected each day?
7. Does it consist of ordinary foods that are available locally, and have prices people normally pay?

Source: Reprinted by permission from *Understanding Nutrition,* 4/e by Eleanor Whitney and Eva May Hamilton; p. 274–5. Copyright © 1987 by West Publishing Company. All rights reserved.

in myoglobin in the urine. In addition, athletes who persist in carbohydrate loading may experience chest pain and some electrocardiographic changes similar to those observed in patients with heart disease. These side effects could be very serious and require immediate medical attention.

Most experts now suggest that the best way to insure optimal levels of glycogen is by maintaining a well-balanced diet that draws at least 60 to 65 perent of its calories from complex carbohydrates (preferably complex carbohydrates from foods such as pasta, cereals, bread, legumes, and vegetables), no more than 12 to 15 percent of calories from proteins, and less than 30 percent from fat. On a daily basis, these recommended carbohydrate levels will maintain suffcient muscle glycogen for excercise because most individuals tend to underconsume carbohydrates. Emphasis, therefore, should be on carbohydrate maintenance rather than carbohydrate loading. By sustaining a carbohydrate rich diet, and thereby keeping the muscles continually loaded with glycogen between workouts, you will be able to sustain prolonged and vigorous exercise without suffering from early onset of fatigue. Table 9.11 offers an example of a high carbohydrate diet.

Dietary Guidelines

The content of the daily diet can be closely related to several major risk factors for heart attack and stroke. Elevated blood cholesterol, obesity, and high blood pressure have strong dietary determinants. Reductions in blood cholesterol and

---

TABLE 9.11 Example of a High-Carbohydrate Diet to Support Daily
Vigorous Activity

4000 kcalories:

623 grams of carbohydrates	(61% of kcalories)*
139 grams of protein	(14% of kcalories)*
118 grams of fat	(26% of kcalories)*

Menu	Carbohydrate (Grams)
Breakfast	
Orange	14
Oatmeal, 2 cups	50
Skim milk, 1 cup	12
Bran muffins, 2	48
Snack	
Dates, chopped, 3/4 cup	98
Lunch	
Lettuce salad:	
Romaine lettuce, 1 cup	2
Garbanzo beans, 1 cup	45
Alfalfa sprouts, 1/2 cup	5.5
French dressing, 2 Tbsp	2
Macaroni and cheese, 3 cups	80
Apple juice, 1 cup	28
Snack	
Whole-wheat toast, 2 slices	26
Margarine, 1 tsp	—
Jam, 2 Tbsp	14
Dinner	
Turkey breast (no skin), 2 oz	—
Potatoes, mashed, 2 cups	74
Peas and onions, 1 cup	23
Banana	27
Skim milk, 1 cup	12
Snack	
Pasta, 1 cup, with	33
margarine, 2 tsp. and	—
parmesan cheese, 2 tbsp	—
Cranberry juice, 1 cup	36
Total	628 grams

A carbohydrate:protein:fat ratio of 60:15:25 is a good general goal when planning a diet to aid athletic performance.
Source: From Contemporary Nutrition, Issues and Insides. Wardlaw, G., Insel P. Marolas. Mosby-Yearbook Inc., 11820 Westline Drive, St. Louis, Missouri.

blood pressure have been shown to decrease the incidence of cardiovascular disease in previously healthy adults, therefore, added emphasis is placed on dietary modifications that may minimize these risk factors.

In an effort to prevent heart and vascular diseases, the following dietary guidelines are offered as safe and prudent by the American Heart Association:

1. Total fat intake should be less than 30 percent of calories.
2. Saturated fat intake should be less than 10 percent of calories.
3. Polyunsaturated fat intake should not exceed 10 percent of calories.
4. Cholesterol intake should not exceed 300 mg/day.
5. Carbohydrate intake should constitute 50 percent or more of calories, with emphasis on complex carbohydrates.
6. Protein intake should provide the remainder of the calories.
7. Sodium intake should not exceed 3 g/day.
8. Alcoholic consumption should not exceed one to two ounces of ethanol per day. Two ounces of 100 proof whiskey, eight ounces of wine, or twenty-four ounces of beer each contain one ounce of ethanol.
9. Total calories should be sufficent to maintain the individual's recommended body weight.
10. A wide variety of foods should be consumed.

A number of consumer studies conducted by FDA, as well as outside groups, enabled FDA and the Food Safety and Inspection Service of the U.S. Department of Agriculture to agree on a new nutrition label. The new label is seen as offering the best opportunity to help consumers make informed food choices and to understand how a particular food fits into the total daily diet. Tables 9.12 and 9.13 describe the new labels.

The United States Dietary Association (USDA) revised the Hassle-Free Daily Food Guide to represent a total diet, rather than a foundation for a diet, as was the intention of earlier guides. This latest plan is called the USDA's Food Guide Pyramid. (See figure 9.1.)

Liquid Meals

Some individuals prefer liquid meals before exercise or competition because they empty from the stomach more quickly than solid foods. You might want to experiment with liquified meals to determine whether they are of benefit to you. (See table 9.14.)

TABLE 9.12 Nutrition Label

New heading signals a new label.

More consistent serving sizes, in both household and metric measures, replace those that used to be set by manufacturers.

Nutrients required on nutrition panel are those most important to the health of today's consumers, most of whom need to worry about getting too much of certain items (fat, for example), rather than too few vitamins or minerals, as in the past.

Conversion guide helps consumers learn caloric value of the energy-producing nutrients.

Nutrition Facts

Serving Size 1 cup (228g)
Servings Per Container 2

Amount Per Serving

Calories 260
 Calories from Fat 120

	% Daily Value*
Total Fat 13g	20%
Saturated Fat 5g	25%
Cholesterol 30mg	10%
Sodium 660mg	28%
Total Carbohydrate 31g	10%
Dietary Fiber 0g	0%
Sugars 5g	
Protein 5g	

Vitamin A 4% • Vitamin C	2%
Calcium 15% • Iron	4%

*Percent Daily Values are based on a 2,000 calorie diet. Your daily values may be higher or lower depending on your calorie needs:

		Calories:	2,000	2,500
Total Fat	Less than		65g	80g
Sat Fat	Less than		20g	25g
Cholesterol	Less than		300mg	300mg
Sodium	Less than		2400mg	2400mg
Total Carbohydrate			300g	375g
Dietary Fiber			25g	30g

Calories per gram:
Fat 9 • Carbohydrate 4 • Protein 4

New mandatory component helps consumers meet dietary guidelines recommending no more than 30 percent of calories from fat.

% Daily Value shows how a food fits into the overall daily diet.

Reference values help consumers learn good diet basics. They can be adjusted, depending on a person's calorie needs.

Source: Food and Drug Administration.

TABLE 9.13 Terms on Food Labels

Cholesterol terms:

☐ cholesterol-free: containing fewer than 2 mg of cholesterol per serving.

☐ low-cholesterol: containing fewer than 20 mg of cholesterol per serving.

☐ reduced cholesterol: processed ro reduce the cholesterol by at least 75% compared with the original.

Energy terms:

☐ diet, dietetic: terms used to indicate that a food is either a *low-calorie* or a *reduced-calorie* food.

☐ light, lite: for alcoholic beverages, containing 20 percent fewer calories than regular products; for meat products, 33 percent fewer. For other foods the terms have no definition but can mean light in color, texture, taste, or weight, or it can mean reduced in some component.[a]

☐ low-calorie: containing no more than 40 calories per serving or 0.4 cal/g.

☐ reduced-calorie: containing at least a third fewer calories than the most similar food of the same type.

Fat terms (these apply only to meat and poultry products):

☐ extra lean: containing not more than 5% fat by weight.

☐ lean or low-fat[b]: containing not more than 10% fat by weight.

☐ leaner, lower-fat: reduced in fat by 25% when compared to the company's regular product.

Sodium terms:

☐ low-sodium: containing 140 mg or less sodium per serving.

☐ reduced-sodium: processed to reduce the usual level of sodium by 75%.

☐ sodium-free: containing less than 5 mg sodium per serving.

☐ unsalted, no added salt, salt-free: having no salt added during processing, but not necessarily low in sodium.

☐ very-low-sodium: containing 35 mg or less sodium per serving.

Sugar terms:

☐ sugar-free, sugarless, no added sugar: free of sucrose (table sugar), but possibly containing other energy-providing sweeteners.

---

[a]For example, a ''Light French'' frozen cheesecake may be light in texture but may have more calories than an original frozen cream cheesecake, a fast food ''light'' taco is ''light'' only because it is made with a fried flour tortilla instead of a tougher, but lower-calorie, corn tortilla.
[b]The word *lean* as part of the brand name (as in ''Lean Supreme'') indicates that the product is 25 percent lower in fat than the regular variety. Lean ground beef can be up to 22.5 percent fat by weight.
Source: Food and Drug Administration.

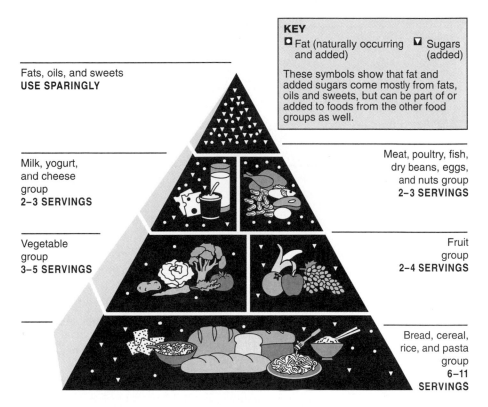

KEY
◻ Fat (naturally occurring ▼ Sugars
and added)   (added)

These symbols show that fat and added sugars come mostly from fats, oils and sweets, but can be part of or added to foods from the other food groups as well.

Fats, oils, and sweets
USE SPARINGLY

Milk, yogurt,
and cheese
group
2–3 SERVINGS

Meat, poultry, fish,
dry beans, eggs,
and nuts group
2–3 SERVINGS

Vegetable
group
3–5 SERVINGS

Fruit
group
2–4 SERVINGS

Bread, cereal,
rice, and pasta
group
**6–11
SERVINGS**

Breads, cereals, rice, and pasta
1 slice of bread
$1/2$ cup of cooked rice or pasta
$1/2$ cup of cooked cereal
1 ounce of ready-to-eat cereal

Vegetables
$1/2$ cup of chopped, raw, or cooked
vegetables
1 cup of leafy raw vegetables

Fruits
1 piece of fruit or melon wedge
$3/4$ cup of juice
$1/2$ cup of canned fruit
$1/4$ cup of dried fruit

Milk, yogurt, and cheese
1 cup of milk or yogurt
$1 1/2$ to 2 ounces of cheese

**Meat, poultry, fish, dry beans, eggs,
and nuts**
$2 1/2$ to 3 ounces of cooked lean meat,
poultry or fish
Count $1/2$ cup of cooked beans, or 1 egg,
or 2 tablespoons of peanut butter as
1 ounce of lean meat (about $1/3$ serving)

Fats, oils, and sweets
Limit calories from these, especially if
you need to lose weight

Figure 9.1 Food Guide Pyramid: A guide to
daily food choices. Source: FDA
Consumer, June 1993

The amount you eat may be more than one serving. For example, a dinner portion of spaghetti would count as two or three servings of pasta.

TABLE 9.14 Liquid Diet	
2 cups lowfat milk	450 calories
1 banana	60% carbohydrates
1 cup dry cereal	20% protein
	15–20% fat
1 cup lowfat yogurt	470 calories
1 apple	75% carbohydrates
1 banana	15% protein
4 graham cracker squares	10% fat

Age and Diet

For each subsequent decade after the age of twenty-five, the body's ability to metabolize food slows down about 4 percent. Thus, if your diet remains unchanged as you get older, you are likely to gain weight because you are not burning up your food as efficiently. One way to counteract this problem is to increase your daily exercise to burn up the extra calories. Another, of course, is to decrease the amount of food that you consume.

As you get older, it also is likely that even if you maintain the same body weight, your percentage of body fat may increase. Over the years, lean muscle tissue can be replaced by increased fat deposits. Again, daily exercise can help to prevent this.

The quantity of essential nutrients in your diet also should be carefully regulated as you age. Protein should constitute about 12 percent of the calories in your diet. No more than 20 percent of your calories should come from fats, with the remainder coming from carbohydrates. While the need for protein is the same for adults as it is for young people, adults have to get their protein from less food to avoid gaining weight. Limiting your fat intake should help you to cut calories and to stop the development of atherosclerosis. Also, excessive fats interfere with calcium absorption and promote osteoporosis. Your vitamins and minerals can be obtained from protein sources and foods high in complex carbohydrates, such as fruits, vegetables, and grains, rather than from fats. Such minerals as calcium and iron are very important in your diet as you age to maintain your hemoglobin since low levels of hemoglobin can result in fatigue and apathy.

Table 9.15 presents basic nutritional guidelines from the U.S. Department of Health and Human Services, while table 9.16 offers three example menus for different levels of calorie intake.

TABLE 9.15	Basic Nutritional Guidelines

1. Eat a variety of foods.
2. Maintain healthy weight.
3. Choose a diet low in fat, saturated fat, and cholesterol.
4. Use sugar only in moderation.
5. Use salt and sodium in moderation.
6. Choose a diet with plenty of vegetables, fruits, and grain products.
7. If you drink alcoholic beverages, do so in moderation.

Source: *Nutrition and your heart: Dieting guidelines for Americans.* U.S. Department of Health and Human Services.

Fiber

As you get older, a high-fiber diet becomes increasingly important and can be obtained through the increased consumption of fruits and vegetables. Essentially, **fiber** is the indigestible substance in plant food. A high-fiber diet is especially important for maintaining the efficiency of your intestinal tract. If there is not regular bulk in your intestines to make the intestinal muscles work, your intestines become ''lazy,'' and you may find yourself needing to rely more on laxatives. Fiber has been found to promote the excretion of bile and to speed up the transit time of materials through the colon. The increased transit time may provide some protection against cancer by reducing the exposure time of cells in the colon to cancer-causing substances.

Cholesterol

Cholesterol is another substance that needs to be monitored closely as you get older. **Cholesterol** is a fatty alcohol manufactured in the body and is associated with heart disease. The amount of saturated fat you consume strongly correlates with your cholesterol levels. If you consume reduced amounts of saturated fat, you have a much better chance of reducing the cholesterol level in your blood. Saturated fat is found mostly in animal fat—in foods such as steaks and chops—and in animal by-products, such as whipped cream, cheese, and milk. Saturated fat is also fairly high in kidneys, shrimp, and lobsters.

The American Heart Association recommends that you limit your diet to about 250 milligrams of cholesterol a day, which is equivalent to approximately one egg. If the amount of cholesterol that is produced by your body is over 150 milligrams, you should try to reduce your saturated fat intake. The American Heart Association also recommends that you reduce the amount of fat in your

TABLE 9.16	Calorie Countdown Menus	
1,200 Calories	**1,800 Calories**	**2,400 Calories**
Breakfast		
Orange juice, ½ cup	Orange juice, ¾ cup	Orange juice, 1 cup
Bran flakes with raisins, ½ cup	Bran flakes with raisins, ½ cup	Bran flakes with raisins, ½ cup
Milk, whole, ½ cup	Milk, whole, ½ cup	Milk, whole, ½ cup
Whole-wheat toast, 1 slice	Whole-wheat toast, 1 slice	Whole-wheat toast, 1 slice
Coffee/tea	Jelly, 2 teaspoons	Jelly, 1 tablespoon
	Coffee/tea	Coffee/tea
Lunch		
Sandwich:	Sandwich:	Sandwich:
Ham, 2 ounces	Ham, 2 ounces	Ham, 2 ounces
Cheese, 1 slice (1 ounce)	Cheese, 1 slice (1 ounce)	Cheese, 1 slice (1 ounce)
Lettuce	Lettuce	Lettuce
Tomato, ½ medium	Tomato, ½ medium	Tomato, ½ medium
Enriched bread, 2 slices	Enriched bread, 2 slices	Enriched bread, 2 slices
Apple, 1 medium	Salad dressing, 2 teaspoons	Salad dressing, 2 teaspoons
Coffee/tea	Apple, 1 medium	Apple, 1 medium
	Coffee/tea	Plain cookies, 4
		Coffee/tea
Dinner		
Beef roast, 3 ounces	Beef roast, 4 ounces	Beef roast, 5 ounces
Baked potato, 1 medium	Baked potato, 1 medium	Baked potato, 1 medium
Broccoli, ½ cup	Broccoli, ½ cup	Broccoli, ½ cup
Milk, skim, 1 cup	Roll, 1	Roll, 1
	Margarine, 1 teaspoon	Margarine, 2 teaspoons
	Milk, lowfat (1%), 1 cup	Milk, lowfat (2%), 1 cup
	Angel food cake (1/16), with strawberries, ½ cup	Angel food cake (1/12), with strawberries, ½ cup, and ice milk, ⅓ cup
Snacks		
Cucumber slices, 1 small cucumber	Peach, fresh, 1 medium	Peach, fresh, 1 medium
Carrot sticks, 3 or 4 strips (2½ to 3 inches long)		Fruit-flavored yogurt, 1 cup
		Banana, 1 small

Source: *Food,* Home and Garden Bulletin Number 228; United States Department of Agriculture.

TABLE 9.17 Cholesterol Content of Some Foods

Food	Serving size	Cholesterol (mg)
Milk		
Skim milk	1 cup	7
Whole milk	1 cup	25
Ice cream	¼ cup	50
Meat		
Beef, lean, cooked	3 oz	110
Chicken, flesh only, cooked	3 oz	90
Egg, whole (50 g)	1	255
Egg white (33 g)	1	0
Egg yolk (17 g)	1	255
Fish fillet, cooked	3 oz	60
Heart, cooked	3 oz	130
Kidney, cooked	3 oz	320
Lamb, lean, cooked	3 oz	110
Liver, cooked	3 oz	260
Lobster, cooked	3 oz	170
Mutton, lean, cooked	3 oz	130
Oysters, raw	3 oz (15)	165
Pork, lean, cooked	3 oz	140
Shrimp, flesh only, cooked	3 oz	105
Veal, lean, cooked	3 oz	180
Caviar	1 oz	85
Cheddar cheese	1 oz	30
Creamed cottage cheese	¼ cup	9
Cream cheese	1 oz	35
Fat		
Butter	1 tsp	12
Margarine, all vegetable	1 tsp	0
Margarine, ⅔ animal fat, ⅓ vegetable fat	1 tsp	3
Lard or other animal fat	1 tsp	5

Chapter 9

TABLE 9.18 Defensive Dining

   Appreciate airline meals for the fresh, wholesome foods you can get from them. Eat selectively. You don't have to eat everything they serve.
   Enjoy frozen meals and "lite" meals for the wholesome ingredients they offer. Supplement with items they do not supply (such as additional vegetables, nonfat milk, fresh fruits).
   In fast-food places, cut kilocalories by ordering diet soft drinks and smaller hamburgers. To cut fat, take the hamburger without the mayonnaise. Cut sodium by having them hold the pickle, ketchup, and mustard. Ask them not to salt your fries. Choose healthier choices such as fish, chicken sandwiches, and lean beef.
   Whenever possible, go to the salad bar. Then choose wisely. Salad bar meals can be high in fat and salt too. Ask for nutrition information on the menu items.
   Don't be fooled by "soda with (selected) vitamins." Drink soda, if you like, but get your vitamins from foods where they are all present, and where minerals and fiber are present too.
   Remember, it's not the item itself that is harmful, but the dose and frequency of consumption. Enjoy treats and convenience foods at intervals—and make the intervals reasonable.
   Eat fresh or minimally processed foods as much as possible, since they usually have few additives. Avoid junk foods (such as cookies, candy, and soda), which are not only chock-full of artificial colors and other additives, but are also of little nutritional value—high in calories, sugar, fats, and/or sodium.
   Read food labels. Remember, additives aren't always listed; more than 300 standardized foods don't have to list ingredients. Ice cream, for example, can contain some 25 specified additives without having to list any of them.
   Limit your intake of foods listing "artificial colors." Products colored by real fruit juice are healthy substitutes. Still, an occasional maraschino cherry won't harm you.
   Eat a variety of foods. This limits your exposure to any one additive, should it turn out to have long-term risks.
   Eat nonfat dairy products.
   Don't fry foods; roast, boil, or bake them.
   Trim all fat and skin from meat and poultry.

---

diet to about 30 percent of your total daily dietary intake and try to keep the amount of saturated fats to about 10 percent. A 20 to 25 percent fat intake is an even better target.

   Table 9.17 shows the cholesterol content of some foods. Refer to table 9.18 to learn how to eat defensively.

204

Key Terms

Antioxidants
A compound that can donate electrons to electron-seeking compounds. Reduces destructive nature of oxidizing compounds

Carbohydrate Loading
A method by which the amount of glycogen stored by the skeletal muscles is increased through special diets and exercise

Carbohydrates
Chemical compounds containing carbon, hydrogen, and oxygen; examples are sugars and starches; major sources of energy

Cholesterol
A fatty alcohol produced by the body and by eating certain foods; elevated levels are associated with an increased risk of heart disease

Fats
Food stuffs containing glycerol and fatty acids

Fiber
The indigestible substance in plant food

Glycogen
The storage form of carbohydrates in the body

Kilocalorie
The amount of energy required to raise one kilogram of water one degree Celsius

Metabolism
The chemical process of the body that allows cells to function

Minerals
Inorganic compounds, some of which are nutrients vital to body function; examples include phosphorus, calcium, potassium, sodium, iron, and iodine

Polyunsaturated Fat
A fatty acid that lacks four or more hydrogen atoms and has two or more double bonds between carbons

Preeclampsia
A toxic condition of pregnancy resulting in increased blood pressure and kidney damage

Protein
Organic material that regulates body processes and builds and repairs body tissue

Saturated Fat
A fatty acid carrying the maximum possible number of hydrogen ions; usually, saturated fats remain solid at room temperature

Toxemia
A serious disease of pregnancy; poisoning the blood, poor kidney function, and high blood pressure

Vitamins
Organic compounds that regulate a number of body processes that are used in the metabolism of carbohydrates and fats

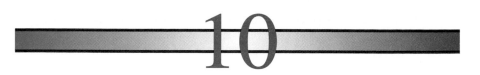

Weight Control

Chapter Concepts

After you have studied this chapter you should be able to

1. discuss the theories for the causes of obesity;
2. calculate desired weight loss;
3. describe daily caloric needs;
4. describe the energy requirements to lose weight through exercise;
5. describe techniques for losing and gaining weight;
6. explain the problems associated with fad diets;
7. describe the effect of using drugs to lose weight;
8. discuss weight- and fat-reduction myths;
9. define anorexia nervosa and bulimia; and
10. discuss behavior modification for changing eating habits.

Weight Control

A major component of physical fitness is body composition. Considerable evidence indicates that **obesity** (a male who has over 20 percent body fat and a female who has over 30 percent body fat) is associated with a number of diseases, such as coronary artery disease, high blood pressure, certain cancers, and diabetes, as well as feelings of insecurity and a lack of self-esteem. Obesity is one of the major health problems in the United States. Fourteen percent of men and 24 percent of women between the ages of twenty and seventy-four, and 10 to 25 percent of all teenagers, are more than 20 percent overweight, the most commonly used definition of obesity. Defined by the National Institutes of Health, obesity is an excessive storage of energy in the form of fat.

Entrepreneurs make millions from Americans desiring to be thin by writing books on how to lose weight. In any given time, about 27 percent of men, 46 percent of women, and 75 percent of teenaged girls, are trying to lose weight.

207

Most diets are usually ineffective and monotonous, and worse, diets can be dangerous if followed for a long period of time by the wrong people, especially young children, teenagers, and pregnant women. The National Institutes of Health's Nutrition Coordinating Committee concluded that none of the conventional approaches to losing weight is effective. In other words most diets don't work; only 3 percent of those who take off weight keep it off for at least five years.

Obesity is an extremely difficult problem to solve. It takes realistic goal setting, patience, counseling, and positive reinforcement. Factors such as the duration of obesity, maturation, motivation, mental state, eating patterns, and socialization must all be considered when treating obesity. Activities such as caloric calculation, nutritional planning, examination of food labels, and maintaining food records may be effective tools in that they provide a sense of responsibility and accomplishment, important components of any weight-loss program. Individual control over food intake is essential, with as much outside assistance as possible.

There are three important principles that need to be understood for any kind of weight-loss program. First, the body resists weight loss. Thyroid hormone levels and consequently basal metabolism drop during weight loss, along with an increase in enzymes that are responsible for storing fat. Second, prevention should be emphasized since curing the disease is extremely difficult. Success in a weight-loss program is only achieved if the person remains at the low weight for three to five years. Third, weight that is lost should be from stored fat and not from lean muscle tissue. Early weight loss may be due to fluid loss and loss of glycogen from the liver and muscle.

Persons who not only want to lose weight but are serious about keeping it off, face a very difficult challenge. Although it can be done, the level of commitment must be high, but unfortunately the probability of long-term reduction is low.

One of the inherent problems with dieting for weight loss is that often the weight is regained. People may end up heavier after their diets than when they began. It appears that dieting itself can promote obesity.

Approximately 60 to 75 percent of the calories you burn are devoted to resting metabolism, basic life support processes of maintaining body heat, and involuntary functions, such as breathing and heartbeat. Another 15 to 30 percent may be burned up through physical activity and the remaining 10 percent used for the digestion and absorption of food.

The problem of losing weight through dieting is that your body responds as it would to starvation—that is, your body burns fewer calories. For example, reducing your caloric intake from 2,000 calories a day to 1,200 calories will reduce resting metabolism by 5 to 10 percent. A more severe reduction to 800 calories a day will lower it by 10 to 20 percent. This protective slowdown in resting metabolism will last as long as you are on the diet. Metabolic rate may remain low even after you start eating normally again.

Much of the weight you lose on a low-calorie diet will come from muscle tissue. The less muscle tissue you have, the lower your metabolic rate will be. The outcome of losing weight through dieting alone is that the more weight you lose, the more your metabolic rate will decline, and you will more likely regain the weight you lost. Dieting should not be undertaken without considerable thought to the problems involved. If a person is not highly motivated and does not have the needed social support, dieting for weight loss should be delayed until a more appropriate time. Repeated weight gain and loss carries with it its own set of problems including difficulty in subsequent attempts at weight loss and an increased risk for a number of diseases.

To date the best results in weight-loss programs are due to some sort of behavior modification. A variety of methods may produce weight loss, but sustained loss requires changes in eating behavior.

Comprehensive Change in Behavior

Research dealing with success in weight-loss programs has centered on a comprehensive change in behavior.[1]

Contrary to popular belief, this research has shown that it is easier for individuals to make a comprehensive change in diet and lifestyle than to make only a moderate change. If you make a moderate change, such as reducing fat intake from 40 percent of calories to the recommended guidelines of 30 percent fat, then you have the worst of two worlds. You feel deprived, hungry, and anxious because you are not eating everything you want and are used to, and you are not making changes substantial enough to significantly affect your weight or to feel better. In other words, you are aware of what you are giving up, but recognize no changes that could reenforce your change in lifestyle. In addition, most diets are too complex to follow for very long, the food doesn't taste good, and you feel hungry and deprived. Making a comprehensive change in diet and lifestyle can be stressful at first because it disrupts old patterns and habits. However, in the long term it is easier to maintain adherence to big changes because they take you out of your old habits and help you form new ones.

This comprehensive approach emphasizes that the type of food you eat is more important than the amount. It recommends reducing fat intake to 10 percent of your total daily calories. By eliminating fat intake, you can eat one-third more

1. Ornish, Dean. *Eat More, Weigh Less*. New York: Harper, Perennial, HarperCollins Publishers, 1994.

food but take in less calories. When you try to lose weight by reducing the amount of food you eat instead of changing the type of food you eat your body responds by increasing the amount and the sensitivity of the body to insulin and lipoprotecylipase. Both act together to increase the body's uptake of fat. Also, increased insulin levels cause your liver to make more of an enzyme called mg-CoA reductase, which causes your body to increase the amount of cholesterol. This program recommends a diet including beans, legumes, fruits, grains, and vegetables, which should be eaten whenever you feel hungry. Avoid the following foods as much as possible: Meats, including chicken and fish; all oils; avocados; olives; nuts, seeds; high fat or "low fat" dairy products; and simple sugar derivatives.

Causes of Obesity

Obesity can be the result of any one or a combination of many factors. Obesity has been linked to both physiological and psychological trauma, hormonal imbalance, and alterations in homeostatic balance. Environmental factors such as cultural habits, inadequate physical activity, and improper diets all contribute to excessive weight gain. Studies have shown a direct genetic influence on height, weight, and Body Mass index.[2] Also, studies on identical twins have provided strong evidence of a significant genetic component.[3] Also, a gene has been discovered that may be linked to certain types of obesity.

In addition, a number of theories have been proposed. Two theories that appear to have some merit are the fat cell theory and the set point theory.

The **fat cell theory** holds that many individuals consume more food than they need during childhood and, as a result, they produce more fat cells (hyperplasia). By the time they reach adolescence, they may have 40 to 50 percent more fat cells than an individual who has not been overeating. The increased number of fat cells makes it much more difficult for them to lose weight as adults and to maintain a proper weight balance. Diet and exercise can reduce the size of the fat cells, but the same number of fat cells is carried for life. According to the fat cell theory, children should not be allowed to routinely take in additional food, and they should be encouraged to develop good psychological eating habits and to participate daily in rigorous exercise.

Some critics argue that fat cells are extremely difficult to count and that empty fat cells may be recruited to store fat, thus showing up as an increase

2. Stunkard, A. J., Jennifer R. Harris, Nancy L. Pedersen, and Gerald E. McClearn. "The Body Mass Index of Twins Who Have Been Reared Apart," *New England Journal of Medicine* 322 (1990):1483–87.

3. Bouchard, C., Angelo Tremblay, Jean-Pierre Després, André Nadeau, Paul J. Lupien, Germain Thériault, Jean Dussault, Sital Moerjani, Sylvie Pinault, and Guy Fournier. "The Response To Long Term Over-Feeding in Identical Twins," *New England Journal of Medicine* 322 (1990):1477–82.

in total fat cells. However, there is agreement that during certain periods of life, such as early infancy (0–1 year), preadolescence, and the third trimester of pregnancy, fat cells increase more rapidly than lean tissue. Therefore, it is important to maintain reasonable caloric intake during these times.

The **set point theory** suggests that the body has a "set point," or a mechanism for stabilizing weight. Within a narrow range, the set point may be affected by such factors as exercise, which lowers the set point, and too many sweets, which raises it. Raising the set point creates a "need" for additional food, resulting in increased body fat. According to this theory, when you attempt to lose weight by dieting, the body tends to view the diet as a threat to the stability of the set point and therefore can make you feel that you need more to eat and also lower the rate at which you burn food.

Other factors indirectly related to these two theories also may play an important part in weight gain. For example, the loss of fat from an obese person may trigger a mechanism designed to put the fat back, making it more difficult to lose weight. Evidence also indicates that obesity may be related to depression levels and that eating is a way of compensating for a personality problem. The brown fat theory holds that some individuals have malfunctioning brown fat, which is less receptive to chemical breakdown than white fat. Because the brown fat resists breakdown, these people lack the ability to lose kilocalories in the form of heat. A more recent theory is that obese individuals' fat cells produce abnormally low levels of a protein adipsin, which may play a role in regulating appetite and metabolism. The low-level production of adipsin may be genetically linked.

Determining Desired Weight Loss

One difficulty that many people have, once they have determined the percentage of body fat that they would like to lose, is how to convert this percentage into pounds. Table 10.1 provides a simple determination method and an example. Use record sheet B-7 in appendix B at the back of the book if you want to determine your desired weight loss.

Daily Caloric Needs

A **kilocalorie** (often referred to simply as a "calorie") is the amount of energy required to raise one kilogram of water one degree Celsius. Your overall caloric intake depends on your degree of activity, sex, age, and weight. Of your total daily caloric intake, approximately 58 percent should be in the form of carbohydrates, 30 percent in fats, and about 12 percent in protein. If you engage in very rigorous activity (running or playing tennis four or five times a week), you need more calories to meet the demands of the exercise. If you lead a sedentary life, you need fewer calories. If you are putting on weight, you probably are

211

Chapter 10

TABLE 10.1 Converting Desired Percentage of Body Fat Loss into Pounds

For an example, let us assume you weigh 180 pounds, have 25 percent body fat, and would like to reduce your body fat by 10 percent. What is the equivalent in pounds of a loss of 10 percent body fat?

Calculation

DBW (desired body weight) = ?

WLR (weight loss required) = ?

PBW (present body weight) = 180 lbs

% Fat (present % of fat) = 25%

FBW (fat body weight) = PBW × % fat = 180 × .25 = 45 lbs

LBW (lean body weight) = PBW − FBW = 180 − 45 = 135 lbs

$$DBW = \frac{LBW}{1 - \text{desired \% fat}}$$

$$DBW = \frac{135}{1.0 - .15} = \frac{135}{.85} = 159 \text{ lbs at 15\% fat}$$

WLR (weight loss required) = PBW − DBW = 180 − 159 = 21 lbs

TABLE 10.2 Daily Caloric Needs (Determined by Multiplying Body Weight in Pounds with the Appropriate Number Relating to Activity Level)

Physical activity	Women	Men
Sedentary	14	16
Moderately active	18	21
Active	22	26

taking in too many calories. If you are losing weight, you are not taking in a sufficient number of calories.

Table 10.2 presents a general idea of daily caloric needs for men and women. Choose your present level of physical activity and multiply the appropriate value by your present weight in pounds to determine your daily caloric needs. Table 10.3 contains more exacting measures of your daily caloric needs.

Tables C-1 and C-2 in appendix C at the back of the book present detailed listings of the caloric content of a variety of foods in the different food groups. Use record sheets B-8 and B-9 in appendix B to record your daily caloric intake.

Goal Setting Weight-Control Guidelines

1. Evaluate your body composition.
2. Set a target body weight (see table 10.1).

212

TABLE 10.3	Mean Heights and Weights and Recommended Energy Intake					
Category	**Age (years)**	**Weight (kg)**	**(lb)**	**Height (cm)**	**(in)**	**Energy needs (kcal) (with range)**
Infants	0.0–0.5	6	13	60	24	kg × 115 (95–145)
	0.5–1	9	20	71	28	kg × 105 (80–135)
Children	1–3	13	29	90	35	1,300 (900–1,800)
	4–6	20	44	112	44	1,700 (1,300–2,300)
	7–10	28	62	132	52	2,400 (1,650–3,300)
Males	11–14	45	99	157	62	2,700 (2,000–3,700)
	15–18	66	145	176	69	2,800 (2,100–3,900)
	19–22	70	154	177	70	2,900 (2,500–3,300)
	23–50	70	154	178	70	2,700 (2,300–3,100)
	51–75	70	154	178	70	2,400 (2,000–2,800)
	76+	70	154	178	70	2,050 (1,650–2,450)
Females	11–14	46	101	157	62	2,200 (1,500–3,000)
	15–18	55	120	163	64	2,100 (1,200–3,000)
	19–22	55	120	163	64	2,100 (1,700–2,500)
	23–50	55	120	163	64	2,000 (1,600–2,400)
	51–75	55	120	163	64	1,800 (1,400–2,200)
	76+	55	120	163	64	1,600 (1,200–2,000)
Pregnancy	—	—	—	—	—	+300
Lactation	—	—	—	—	—	+500

Source: From *Recommended Dietary Allowances,* revised 1980, reprinted with permission of the National Academy Press, Washington, D.C.

3. Set short-term and long-term goals. A short-term goal might be to lose one or two pounds a week. A long-term goal might be a 5 percent fat loss in one year.
4. Use guidelines in tables 10.4 and 10.5 to regulate your eating behavior.

Losing Weight Through Exercise

The belief that the best way to lose weight is to go on a diet is a misconception. Fad and crash diets can result in very serious health consequences. Even normal dieting can cause anxiety and depression. Also, repeated weight gains and losses can cause serious problems, such as an increased percentage of fat. An alternative to dieting is losing weight through exercise.

Calories Burned Through Physical Activity

Exercise is an integral part of any weight-loss program. However, losing weight through exercise takes time. After all, it has taken many years to put on the extra weight, and you cannot expect to lose it in a matter of several days.

TABLE 10.4 Behavior Modification Suggestions for Changing Eating Habits

Cue elimination and physical environment		Manner of eating	Food choice	Alternative activities
Eat only in designated place	Store foods out of sight	Slow rate of eating—chew slowly	Portion control—cut snacks in half	Exercise—walking or jogging, other aerobic activities, recreational activities
Eat only when sitting in designated place	Avoid "problem" places and people	Swallow each bite before taking a second one	Measure foods until portions can be estimated	Relaxation
Set regular eating times	Serve buffets	Put utensils down between bites	Serve only amounts planned	Meditation
Plan snacks and meals ahead	Remove plate from eating place after meal	Count mouthfuls	Preplan eating when guest or entertaining; set aside portions	Imagery (visualize food to be in an inedible form or think of being in another place)
Determine degree of hunger before eating	Clean plates directly into garbage	Pause in the middle of a meal for a few minutes	Share dessert	Do necessary tasks, errands, yard work, or housework
Dissociate eating from other activities (e.g., reading, watching television)	Change route of travel to bypass a tempting eating place	Relax 60 seconds before eating	Include favorite foods	Write a letter
Plan and order restaurant meals ahead	Write notes as reminders or use pictures; put on mirrors or refrigerator	Savor foods; enjoy each bite	Eat a variety of foods	Call someone
Store all foods; use opaque containers or store in inaccessible places		Eat only until reaching a "satisfied" hunger level (*not* until "stuffed")	Have appropriate snacks planned and "ready to go"	Do problem solving
Use small plates and bowls		Allow at least 20 minutes for eating a meal	Serve "on-the-side" dressings and sauces	Reevaluate goals and priorities
Let others get their snacks		Leave 5% to 20% of meal uneaten	Use spices instead of high-calorie condiments	Practice assertiveness
Record food intake		Push food aside ahead of time	Use garnishes (attractive and take up space on the plate)	Make charts for progress
Shop when *not* hungry, and use a list		Cover plate with napkin when finished eating	Use low-calorie ingredient substitutes	Take up a reward for following plans
				Brush teeth
				Take a bath or shower
				Go for a drive

Source: Reproduced by permission. *Health Promotion in the Workplace* By Michael P. O'Donnell & Thomas H. Ainsworth Delmar Publishers Inc., Albany, New York, Copyright 1984

TABLE 10.5 Basic Guidelines

1. Limit your weight loss to two pounds a week.
2. Do not go below 1,200 kilocalories daily for women and 1,500 kilocalories for men. More drastic plans should only be undertaken with a doctor's supervision.
3. Eat a variety of foods from all food groups (see table 9.3), including dark green and yellow vegetables.
4. The diet should contain easily obtainable foods.
5. The diet should meet nutritional needs except for kilocalories.
6. The diet should minimize hunger and fatigue.
7. The diet should help reshape eating habits.
8. The diet should improve overall health.
9. Aerobic exercise should be a vital part of any weight-loss program.

Approximately 3,500 calories must be burned to use up one pound of stored fat. If, for example, your food intake in one day is equivalent to 2,400 calories and you burn up 2,400 calories in your everyday activities, you will be in **caloric balance**—you will not gain or lose weight. If, however, you burn up an additional 100 calories a day (for a total of 2,500 calories) by jogging or walking a mile, in thirty-five days you probably would lose one pound of fat. If this loss of 100 extra calories a day was extended for one year, you could lose approximately twelve to thirteen pounds of fat, assuming that you haven't increased your food intake. By increasing your exercise to burn up 200 calories a day, you could lose almost twenty-four pounds in a year. Combining increased exercise with a decrease in food intake usually increases weight loss. Maximum weight loss a week, however, should not exceed two pounds, or a one thousand calories per day deficit.

At rest and during light exercise (up to 50 percent of maximum oxygen uptake) the predominant fuel is fat. When maximum oxygen uptake exceeds 50 percent, carbohydrates are the predominant fuel. At exercise levels of 85 to 90 percent of maximum oxygen uptake, nearly all energy is derived from carbohydrates.

The more rigorous or exhausting the physical activity, the greater the number of calories burned per minute. For example, activities like running and cross-country skiing probably burn up the highest number of calories—up to twenty calories per minute! Swimming also rates very high in caloric expenditure.

You can approximate the number of calories you are burning per minute during rigorous activity by monitoring your pulse. Generally, if your pulse rate is about 120 or below, you probably are burning about five calories per minute. If your pulse rate is 120 to 150 beats per minute, you are burning five to ten calories per minute. If your pulse rate is about 150, you probably are burning ten or more calories per minute. For example, if you jog thirty minutes with a pulse rate that averages between 130 and 140, you might burn up to three hundred calories (10 cal × 30 min) in a half hour.

The speed at which you run is another important factor in caloric expenditure. If you run at 5 miles per hour, your caloric expenditure will be about ten calories per minute. If you speed up to about 7.5 miles per hour, you burn about fifteen calories per minute. At ten miles per hour, you might burn as many as twenty calories per minute, while at twelve miles per hour, you have the potential of using up twenty-five calories per minute.

Tables 10.6 and 10.7 give you a general idea of the number of kilocalories expended per minute during exercise. Tables 10.8–10.11 indicate how much walking, jogging, bicycling, and swimming you must do to burn enough calories to lose weight. Use record sheets B-8 and B-9 in appendix B to keep track of your daily caloric intake and expenditure.

Weight loss without exercising can have a negative effect on body composition. Frequent, intermittent dieting, alternating with weight gain, in the absence of exercise will result in a loss of lean body tissue and an increase in body fat content. To avoid lean body losses it is essential to include rigorous exercise along with a sensible diet program.

Losing Fat

Exercise affects your body's ability to use fat in a number of ways. For example, the amount of fat lost due to exercise generally is proportional to the intensity and duration of the exercise. The body tends to shift from burning fat during moderate activities to burning stored carbohydrates (glycogen) during very rigorous activities. Therefore, at very high levels of exercise, when the amount of oxygen is limited, carbohydrates are burned in preference to fat. During moderate physical activity, such as jogging, which can be continued for a much longer period of time, fat is the main source of energy. Even though you burn fewer calories per unit of time during moderate exercise as compared to rigorous exercise, you are able to continue exercising for a much longer period, thus producing a greater overall caloric expenditure.

As mentioned before, while the number of fat cells does not decrease as a result of exercise, their size can be substantially reduced through diet and exercise. Also, blood flow through stored fat increases during exercise, which aids in the transport of fat to working muscles. An interesting corollary is that research indicates that high levels of lactic acid can interfere with fat breakdown. Thus, individuals in good physical condition, who do not usually accumulate as high a level of lactic acid as those who are not as physically fit, can continue exercising

216

TABLE 10.6 Approximate Energy Cost (in Kilocalories) of Various Physical Activities

Sport or activity	Kilocalories expended per minute (kcal/min) of activity
Climbing	10.7–13.2
Cycling 5.5 MPH	4.5
9.4 MPH	7.0
13.1 MPH	11.1
Dancing	3.3–7.7
Football	8.9
Golf	5.0
Gymnastics	
Balancing	2.5
Abdominal exercises	3.0
Trunk bending	3.5
Arm swinging, hopping	6.5
Rowing 51 str/min	4.1
87 str/min	7.0
97 str/min	11.2
Running	
Short distance	13.3–16.6
Cross-country	10.6
Tennis	7.1
Skating (fast)	11.5
Skiing, moderate speed	10.8–15.9
Uphill, maximum speed	18.6
Squash	10.2
Swimming	
Breaststroke	11.0
Backstroke	11.5
Crawl (55 yd/min)	14.0
Wrestling	14.2

Source: Reprinted by permission of the American Alliance for Health, Physical Education, Recreation and Dance, 1900 Association Drive, Reston, Virginia 22091.

for much longer periods of time before lactic acid accumulates and interferes with fat breakdown.

Abdominal Fat

Fat around the abdomen may represent a greater risk to health than fat elsewhere in the body. Abdominal fat, unlike fat in other parts of the body, goes directly to the liver when it is metabolized. While in the liver it may be made into

Chapter 10

TABLE 10.7 Typical Criteria for the Classification of Exercise Intensity

Exercise intensity classification	Criteria heart rate	Energy expenditure (kcal/hr)	Perceived exertion
Very light	<110	<110	Very, very easy
Light	110–120	111–270	Easy, no pain or discomfort
Moderate	121–150	270–400	Somewhat difficult and slight discomfort
Heavy	151–160	401–550	Difficult, uncomfortable, and some pain
Very heavy	161–180	550–669	Very difficult and painful
Exhaustive	>180	>700	Extremely difficult and painful

Source: From Hage, Phillip, "Perceived Exertion: One Measure of Exercise Intensity," in *The Physician and Sports Medicine*, September 1981, pp. 136–46. © 1981 McGraw-Hill Healthcare Group. Reprinted by permission.

TABLE 10.8 Days Required to Lose Five to Twenty-Five Pounds by Walking* and Lowering Daily Calorie Intake

Minutes of walking +	Reduction of calories per day (in kcal)	Days to lose 5 pounds	Days to lose 10 pounds	Days to lose 15 pounds	Days to lose 20 pounds	Days to lose 25 pounds
30	400	27	54	81	108	135
30	600	20	40	60	80	100
30	800	16	32	48	64	80
30	1,000	13	26	39	52	65
45	400	23	46	69	92	115
45	600	18	36	54	72	90
45	800	14	28	42	56	70
45	1,000	12	24	36	48	60
60	400	21	42	63	84	105
60	600	16	32	48	64	80
60	800	13	26	39	52	65
60	1,000	11	22	33	44	55

Source: From *Exercise Equivalents of Foods: A Practical Guide for the Overweight*, by Frank Konishi. Copyright © 1983 by Southern Illinois University Press. Reprinted with permission of the publisher.
*Walking briskly (3.5 to 4 MPH), calculated at 5.2 cal/min.

218

TABLE 10.9	Days Required to Lose Five to Twenty-Five Pounds by Jogging* and Lowering Daily Calorie Intake						
Minutes of jogging	+	Reduction of calories per day (in kcal)	Days to lose 5 pounds	Days to lose 10 pounds	Days to lose 15 pounds	Days to lose 20 pounds	Days to lose 25 pounds
30		400	21	42	63	84	105
30		600	17	34	51	68	85
30		800	14	28	42	56	70
30		1,000	12	24	36	48	60
45		400	18	36	54	72	90
45		600	14	28	42	56	70
45		800	12	24	36	48	60
45		1,000	10	20	30	40	50
60		400	15	30	45	60	75
60		600	12	24	36	48	60
60		800	11	22	33	44	55
60		1,000	9	18	27	36	45

Source: From *Exercise Equivalents of Foods: A Practical Guide for the Overweight,* by Frank Konishi. Copyright © 1983 by Southern Illinois University Press. Reprinted with permission of the publisher.
*Alternate jogging and walking, calculated at 10 cal/min.

cholesterol-carrying LDL (low-density lipoproteins), which are associated with a higher incidence of diabetes and coronary heart disease.

Increased Caloric Expenditure After Exercise

The increased **metabolism** brought about by rigorous physical exercise can persist for a number of hours after the exercise has ceased and may even enable you to burn up more fat. For example, while jogging a half hour, you may burn around ten calories a minute for a total of 300 calories. After you stop jogging, instead of returning to preexercise levels, your metabolism is stimulated to about 25 percent above resting rate for as long as three hours after an intensive bout of exercise and may remain elevated at approximately 10 percent above resting rate for another two days.

"Diet Foods"

A common food myth is that certain kinds of foods burn up stored fat and play a part in weight reduction. All foods contain calories; therefore, no foods can serve as weight reducers. Grapefruit and the other substances around which this myth flourishes, such as safflower oil, vinegar, vitamin B6, and lecithin, have no effect whatsoever on fat loss. Substances that are referred to as ''diet foods,''

TABLE 10.10	Days Required to Lose Five to Twenty-Five Pounds by Bicycling* and Lowering Daily Calorie Intake						

Minutes of bicycling	+	Reduction of calories per day (in kcal)	Days to lose 5 pounds	Days to lose 10 pounds	Days to lose 15 pounds	Days to lose 20 pounds	Days to lose 25 pounds
30		400	25	50	75	100	125
30		600	19	38	57	76	95
30		800	17	34	51	68	85
30		1,000	13	26	39	52	65
45		400	22	44	66	88	110
45		600	17	34	51	68	85
45		800	14	28	42	56	70
45		1,000	12	24	36	48	60
60		400	19	38	57	76	95
60		600	15	30	45	60	75
60		800	13	26	39	52	65
60		1,000	11	22	33	44	55

Source: From *Exercise Equivalents of Foods: A Practical Guide for the Overweight,* by Frank Konishi. Copyright © 1983 by Southern Illinois University Press. Reprinted with permission of the publisher.
*Bicycling at approximately 7 MPH, calculated at 6.5 cal/min.

such as diet bread, diet cookies, and diet beer, all contain calories, and if you consume enough of them, you will gain weight.

Using Drugs to Lose Weight

A number of prescription drugs, such as amphetamines and barbiturates, have been used as diet aids to reduce appetite. These drugs, however, have many dangerous side effects and really don't get at the overweight individual's major problem—changing his or her eating pattern. No over-the-counter drugs are effective in reducing fat or appetite. The so-called bulk reducers, such as glucomanan, have little effect on the appetite; neither do other so-called appetite depressants, such as propradine.

Commercial Weight Loss Programs

Despite their sales pitches, there is no evidence that commercial weight loss programs help most people achieve significant permanent weight loss. Your best bet is to place less emphasis on cutting calories and more emphasis on exercising and eating a healthy diet. Everyone will not respond the same to the same program used to lose weight. Those trying to lose weight should understand this so that they will not be easily discouraged.

| **TABLE 10.11** | Days Required to Lose Five to Twenty-Five Pounds by Swimming* and Lowering Daily Calorie Intake | | | | | |

Minutes of swimming	+	Reduction of calories per day (in kcal)	Days to lose 5 pounds	Days to lose 10 pounds	Days to lose 15 pounds	Days to lose 20 pounds	Days to lose 25 pounds
30		400	23	46	69	92	115
30		600	18	36	52	72	90
30		800	14	28	42	56	70
30		1,000	12	24	36	48	60
45		400	19	38	57	76	95
45		600	15	30	45	60	75
45		800	13	26	39	52	65
45		1,000	11	22	33	44	55
60		400	16	32	48	64	80
60		600	14	28	42	56	70
60		800	11	22	33	44	55
60		1,000	10	20	30	40	50

Source: From *Exercise Equivalents of Foods: A Practical Guide for the Overweight,* by Frank Konishi. Copyright © 1983 by Southern Illinois University Press. Reprinted with permission of the publisher.
*Swimming at about thirty yards per minute, calculated at 8.5 cal/min.

How to Gain Weight

If you want to gain weight in a hurry and it does not matter to you if the additional weight is in muscle or fat, you can add any kind of calories to achieve the desired gain. Fatty foods have more calories than protein or carbohydrates per weight; therefore, you can gain weight more quickly and easily with a high-fat diet. Eating fat to gain weight, however, can increase the possibility of nutrition-related diseases, such as coronary heart disease.

The best way to gain weight is to build yourself up through very careful and consistent physical training. Weight training is an effective technique to build muscle mass, which weighs more than an equal volume of fat. Eat a well-balanced nutritious diet with enough calories in the form of complex carbohydrates to support a weight gain. Table 10.12 presents an example of a high-calorie diet.

Weight and Fat Reduction Myths

Weight and fat reduction myths that need to be dispelled include cellulite, saunas and steam baths, and spot reducing.

TABLE 10.12 High-Calorie Diet—Six Thousand Calories in Six Meals

Breakfast	Snack	Dinner	Snack
1/2 cup orange juice	1 peanut butter sandwich	1 cup cream of mushroom soup	1 cup cashew nuts
1 cup oatmeal	1 banana	2 pieces oven-baked chicken	1 cup cocoa
1 cup lowfat milk	1 cup grape juice	1 candied sweet potato	Total calories: 1,045
1 scrambled egg	Total calories: 485	1 dinner roll and margarine	
1 slice whole-wheat toast		1 cup carrots and peas	
1½ teaspoons margarine		1/2 cup coleslaw	
1 tablespoon jam		1 piece cherry pie	
Total calories: 665		1 beverage	
		Total calories: 1,615	

Lunch	Snack		
5 fish sticks with tartar sauce	1 cup mixed dried fruit		
1 large serving, French fries	1½ cups malted milk		
1 green salad with avocado and French dressing	Total calories: 660		Daily total calories: 5,975
1 cup lemon sherbet			
2 granola cookies			
1 cup lowfat milk			
Total calories: 1,505			

Source: High-Calorie Diet Table, *Food for Sport,* by N. J. Smith, Copyright 1976, Bull Publishing. Palo Alto, CA.

Cellulite and Health Spas

For some time there has been a popular myth that there are two kinds of body fat—regular fat and cellulite—and that cellulite is a sort of lumpy, hard fat that can be broken and burned up only through the vigorous massages provided by massage machines found in health spas. The reality, however, is that cellulite is just another word for fat.

The American Medical Association evaluated the evidence on cellulite and concluded that cellulite is a hoax. Also, the health spa techniques, such as rolling, vibrating, and thumping the body through passive exercise, are completely ineffective in weight reduction. For the body to lose fat, the muscles have to contract and perform work, and the body has to go into **negative caloric balance** (the amount of energy burning up calories is greater than the number of calories consumed), which results in stored fat being used.

Saunas and Steam Baths

Saunas and steam baths do not increase your metabolic rate and do not melt off fat, as some claim. They can, however, cause dramatic dehydration from the large water losses that occur because of increased body temperature. Although this rapid water loss may be interpreted by some as a weight loss, this ''weight loss'' will be regained as soon as normal body fluid levels are restored through drinking and eating.

The increased body temperature that results from saunas and steam baths also can dangerously stress the kidneys, heart, and blood vessels. Middle-aged and older individuals and anyone with heart and circulatory problems should be particularly cautious of saunas and steam baths, especially when such methods are accompanied by wrapping in hot towels.

Spot Reducing

Spot reducing (exercising specific areas of the body to reduce stored fat in those areas) is widely accepted, even though there is no evidence that it works. Generally, overall exercise, such as jogging, swimming, and bicycling, is the most efficient way to burn a large number of calories. If the result of such exercise is a negative caloric balance, there is a reduction of fat in the areas of greatest fat concentration, regardless of which part of the body the exercise focused on.

Another thing to keep in mind is that muscle tissue is much more compact than fat tissue. Therefore, a pound of fat takes up a great deal more room than a pound of muscle. Through aerobic exercise, you can burn up fat and at the same time increase your lean body mass, which reduces inches from your girth.

Eating Disorders

Two eating disorders that are especially prevalent in adolescent females are anorexia nervosa and bulimia.

Anorexia Nervosa

Anorexia nervosa is a state of emaciation brought on by voluntary starvation. Estimates indicate that possibly one out of every 200 adolescent girls has this disease. Unless it is recognized in its earliest stages, anorexia nervosa is very difficult to treat since the individual simply refuses to eat. Most cases have a psychological basis and represent a form of malnutrition far more serious than that resulting from a lack of food.

Anorexic adolescent females usually experience cessation of menstruation (amenorrhea) and sometimes a fatal electrolyte imbalance. They deny that they are emaciated in spite of a skeletonlike appearance and usually continue to pursue thinness by refusing to eat and maintaining a hyperactive exercise program. Treatment consists of psychiatric as well as nutritional management.

Characteristics of anorexia nervosa include:

1. Avoidance of food, with a loss of at least 25 percent (and sometimes as much as 50 percent) of preillness body weight
2. Onset before twenty-five years of age
3. Distorted attitudes toward food, eating, or weight, including denial of illness, enjoyment of extreme weight loss, and unusual hoarding or handling of food
4. No other medical or psychiatric illness that could account for the weight loss
5. At least two of the following:
   a. Cessation of menstrual periods
   b. Lanugo (fine coat of hair over the body)
   c. Slow heartbeat
   d. Periods of overactivity
   e. Episodes of bulimia

Bulimia

A related phenomenon to anorexia nervosa—known as binge and purge, or **bulimia**—also is seen among adolescents, especially girls. Individuals with bulimia consume unrealistic quantities of food and then induce vomiting or take laxatives to purge themselves of food. This disease has primarily a psychological origin.

Characteristics of bulimia include:

1. Recurrent episodes of binge eating (rapid consumption of a large amount of food in a short period of time, usually less than two hours)
2. At least three of the following:
   a. Consumption of high-calorie, easily ingested food during a binge
   b. Secrecy during a binge

c. Termination of a binge because of abdominal pain, sleep, or self-induced vomiting

d. Repeated attempts to lose weight by severely restrictive diets, self-induced vomiting, or use of laxatives

e. Frequent weight fluctuations greater than ten pounds due to alternating binges and fasts

3. Awareness that eating pattern is abnormal and fear of not being able to stop eating voluntarily

4. Depressed mood and self-deprecating thoughts following binges

Key Terms

Anorexia Nervosa
An eating disorder characterized by voluntary starvation and a state of emaciation

Bulimia
An eating disorder characterized by alternating binging and purging

Caloric Balance
The total calories ingested are equivalent to the total calories burned

Fat Cell Theory
Excessive fat cells are produced resulting from overeating during childhood

Kilocalorie
The amount of energy required to raise one kilogram of water one degree Celsius

Metabolism
The chemical process of the body that allows cells to function

Negative Caloric Balance
The amount of calories coming in are less than the amount of calories expended

Obesity
Excessive body fat (a male who has over 20 percent body fat and a female who has over 30 percent body fat)

Set Point Theory
Body has an automatic mechanism for stabilizing weight

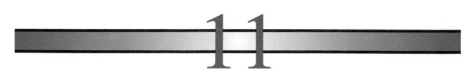

c h a p t e r

Drugs

After you have studied this chapter you should be able to

1. describe the effects of psychoactive drugs;
2. describe motives for using drugs;
3. discuss some danger signals of drug abuse;
4. discuss the problem of drug interaction;
5. describe the effects of alcohol and cigarettes;
6. describe the symptoms of alcohol abuse;
7. describe some tips for quitting smoking;
8. discuss some reasons for alcohol abuse;
9. describe the effects of smokeless tobacco;
10. describe the effects of anabolic steroids; and
11. describe the effects of amphetamines, cocaine, and caffeine.

Psychoactive Drugs

More than one-fourth of legal drugs sold in the United States and virtually all illegal drugs are psychoactive. That is, they alter your feelings, thoughts, perceptions, and moods. Legal and illegal psychoactive drugs are used by millions of individuals to cope with mental and emotional problems as well as to alter moods and behavior.

Psychoactive drugs include tranquilizers that function to reduce anxiety; stimulants that are used in an attempt to increase energy and physical activity; **narcotics** that depress the central nervous system, thus preventing pain and inducing sleep; **sedatives** that slow down the nervous system and also induce sleep; **analgesics** that block pain; and **hallucinogens** that alter mood and perception (see table 11.1 for a complete list of psychoactive drugs).

227

TABLE 11.1 Classifications of Drugs That Affect the Central Nervous System (Psychoactive Drugs)

Drug classification	Common and trade names	Medical uses	Effects of average dose	Physical dependence	Tolerance develops
Narcotics	Codeine Demerol Heroin Methadone Morphine Opium Percodan	Analgesic (pain relief)	Blocks or eases pain; may cause drowsiness and euphoria; some users experience nausea or itching sensations	Marked	Yes
Analgesics	Darvon Talwin	Pain relief	May produce anxiety and hallucinations	Marked	Yes
Sedatives	Amytal Nembutal Phenobarbital Seconal Doriden Quaalude	Sedation, tension relief	Relaxation, sleep; decreases alertness and muscle coordination	Marked	Yes
Minor tranquilizers	Dalmane Equanil/Miltown Librium Valium	Anxiety relief, muscle tension	Mild sedation; increased sense of well-being; may cause drowsiness and dizziness	Marked	No
Major tranquilizers (phenothiazines)	Mellaril Thorazine Prolixin	Control psychosis	Heavy sedation, anxiety relief; may cause confusion, muscle rigidity, convulsions	None	No
Alcohol	Beer Wine Liquor	None	Relaxation; loss of inhibition; mood swings; decreased alertness and coordination	Marked	Yes

TABLE 11.1 Classifications of Drugs That Affect the Central Nervous System (Psychoactive Drugs) (*Continued*)

Drug classification	Common and trade names	Medical uses	Effects of average dose	Physical dependence	Tolerance develops
Inhalants	Amyl nitrite Butyl nitrite Nitrous oxide	Muscle relaxant, anesthetic	Relaxation, euphoria; causes dizziness, headache, drowsiness	None	?
Stimulants	Benzedrine Biphetamine Desoxyn Dexedrine Methedrine Preludin Ritalin	Weight control, narcolepsy; fatigue and hyperactivity in children	Increased alertness and mood elevation; less fatigue and increased concentration; may cause insomnia, anxiety, headache, chills, and rise in blood pressure; organic brain damage after prolonged use	Mild to none	Yes
Cocaine	Cocaine hydrochloride	Local anesthetic, pain relief	Effects similar to stimulants	None	No
Cannabis	Marijuana Hashish	Relief of glaucoma, asthma, nausea accompanying chemotherapy	Relaxation, euphoria, altered perception; may cause confusion, panic, hallucinations	None	No
Hallucinogens	LSD PCP Mescaline Peyote Psilocybin	None	Altered perceptions, visual and sensory distortion; mood swings	None	Yes
Nicotine	(In tobacco)	None	Altered heart rate; tremors, excitation	Yes	Yes

---

TABLE 11.2   Danger Signals of Drug Misuse

Many persons are prescribed drugs that affect their moods. Using these drugs wisely can be important for physical and emotional health. But sometimes it is difficult to decide when using drugs to handle stress becomes inappropriate. It is important that adaptive use of drugs does not result in maladaptation. Here are some "danger signals" that can help you evaluate your own way of using drugs.

1. Do those close to you often ask about your drug use? Have they noticed any changes in your moods or behavior?
2. Are you defensive if a friend or relative mentions your drug or alcohol use?
3. Are you sometimes embarrassed or frightened by your behavior under the influence of drugs or alcohol?
4. Have you ever gone to see a new doctor because your regular physician would not prescribe the drug you wanted?
5. When you are under pressure or feel anxious, do you automatically take a tranquilizer or drink or both?
6. Do you take drugs more often or for purposes other than those recommended by your doctor?
7. Do you mix drugs and alcohol?
8. Do you drink or take drugs regularly to help you sleep?
9. Do you have to take a pill to get going in the morning?
10. Do you think you have a drug problem?

If you have answered yes to a number of these questions, you may be misusing drugs or alcohol. There are places to go for help at the local level. One such place might be a drug abuse program in your community, listed in the Yellow Pages under Drug Abuse. Other resources include community crisis centers, telephone hotlines, and the Mental Health Association.

Source: National Institute on Drug Abuse

As a result of the media explosion, today's young adults have a much broader appreciation for perceptive experiences, sensory awareness, and altered consciousness than past generations. These factors may provide a fertile environment for the experimentation and use of various drugs. People's motives for taking drugs vary enormously and include curiosity, thrill seeking, relaxation, increased sense of well-being, peer acceptance, and religious experience. Others use drugs to escape from the present reality of their lives or to achieve happiness and provide meaning to their existence. They are eager to change their state of consciousness and ingest substances that promote mental and emotional changes, particularly if those changes are perceived as pleasurable. However, problems inevitably arise when drugs become a substitute for a sense of purpose or meaning in life. (See table 11.2.)

It is essential to help individuals to resist drugs before they develop dependency and abuse. Continuing support and direction to young individuals who are

TABLE 11.3 Drug Interactions

Listed below are some of the more dangerous combinations that can result when psychoactive drugs are taken together with other types of drugs or medication. These drugs should never be combined without the consent and supervision of a physician.

Barbiturates in combination with tranquilizers, alcohol, drugs for high blood pressure, stimulants, cortisone, painkillers, diuretics, anticonvulsants, or birth control pills.

Tranquilizers in combination with barbiturates, antihistamines, alcohol, drugs for high blood pressure, stimulants, antidepressants, or painkillers.

Stimulants in combination with barbiturates, tranquilizers, beer, drugs for high blood pressure, antidepressants, anticonvulsants, drugs for diabetes, or digitalis.

Antidepressants in combination with tranquilizers, alcohol, drugs for high blood pressure, stimulants, diuretics, anticoagulants, or asthma spray.

Source: National Clearinghouse for Alcohol Information, as modified

uncertain, have a sense of not belonging, and are in need of help and sensitive understanding are key ingredients in prevention.

The persistent use of drugs by healthy individuals can result in impairment of health status and functional ability. The danger of continuing use of a particular drug is often associated with the drug's ability to cause addiction or physical dependence. Many legal drugs, including barbiturates, tranquilizers, analgesics, opiates, alcohol, and tobacco, are addictive and can cause physical dependence. Unfortunately a number of psychoactive drugs, such as beer, coffee, tea, wine, cola, cigarettes, and sleep-enhancing and alertness-promoting preparations, are integrated into everyday lifestyles. Interactions of some of these drugs can result in serious problems. (See table 11.3.)

Cocaine

Cocaine is a central nervous system stimulant producing similar effects as caffeine. Cocaine enhances alertness and relieves fatigue. It produces a state of excitement, restlessness, and talkativeness. Euphoria, heightened self-confidence, temporary relief from depression, and a suppressed appetite all result from cocaine use. As these effects wear off, the user will experience a period of depression, confusion, and dizziness. Small doses slow the heart, but larger amounts stimulate the heart. Blood pressure increases as a result of constricted blood vessels and respiration becomes shallow and rapid. Repeated use of large doses will lead to weight loss, insomnia, anxiety, and paranoid delusion. Inhaling and snorting may also result in ulceration of the nasal tissue and accidental death due to respiratory failure.

Amphetamines

Amphetamines are a group of drugs that stimulate the central nervous system of the body. They generally cause a rise in blood pressure, cardiac output, blood sugar, breathing rate, and metabolism. Athletes take amphetamines in hopes that the increased arousal level, which depresses the sensation of muscle fatigue, will enable them to maintain high-performance levels for longer periods of time. There is very little scientific evidence, however, that amphetamines improve performance or increase endurance. In fact, most of the studies report that the drugs have very little effect on performance level. Some athletes use amphetamines to ''get them up'' for competition or psychologically ready to compete. This practice may require the athlete to resort to the use of barbiturates to bring them down from the amphetamine high in order to sleep. The result is a dangerous stimulant-to-depressant combination. Another danger of taking amphetamines during exercise is that the individual may overstress the body with possible damage to the heart. Other risks include psychological dependence with the possibility of circulatory collapse.

Caffeine

There is some recent evidence that caffeine can, in some circumstances, increase endurance in moderately strenuous activity. Caffeine facilitates the use of fat as fuel and increases the permeability of the muscle cell to calcium, resulting in a more efficient contraction of the muscle and sparing the glycogen in the muscles. Caffeine may also have a psychostimulating effect causing the athlete to feel that the exercise was easier. The adverse effects of using caffeine are that in some individuals it may produce an allergic response, cardiac arrhythmia, headache, insomnia, irritability, or a diuretic effect.

Alcohol

The consumption of alcohol and beverages is a relatively permanent feature in our society. Alcohol abuse has become the principal drug abuse problem in the United States. Twelve million Americans of all religions, races, educational, and socioeconomic levels have problems with alcohol, including over three million American teenagers between the ages of fourteen and seventeen.

Alcoholism is generally described as long-term, repeated, uncontrolled, compulsive, and excessive use of alcoholic beverages that significantly impairs the drinker's health and interpersonal relationships. The chief characteristic of the disease is the drinker's inability to control when he or she begins and/or stops drinking. (See table 11.4, What Kind of Drinker Are You?)

Unfortunately our society not only allows but encourages tension reduction and escape by drinking alcohol. In addition, we seem to give status to the person

---

TABLE 11.4 What Kind of Drinker Are You?

Directions: Check the appropriate box to the left of each question.

Yes	No	
☐	☐	1. Do you think about drinking often?
☐	☐	2. Do you drink more now than you used to?
☐	☐	3. Do you sometimes gulp your drinks?
☐	☐	4. Do you often take a drink to help you relax?
☐	☐	5. Do you drink often when you are alone?
☐	☐	6. Do you sometimes forget what happened while you were drinking?
☐	☐	7. Do you keep a bottle hidden somewhere—at home or at work—for a quick pick-me-up?
☐	☐	8. Do you need a drink to have fun?
☐	☐	9. Do you ever just start drinking without really thinking about it?
☐	☐	10. Do you drink in the morning to relieve a hangover?

If you had four or more yes answers, you may be one of the ten million Americans with a drinking problem.

Source: National Institute on Alcohol Abuse and Alcoholism

who can drink large amounts of alcohol, and we laugh at those who get drunk. These attitudes in combination with heavy consumption of alcoholic beverages, reinforced by the popular media, are underlying factors of alcohol abuse.

Many young people begin drinking as a normal process of assuming adult roles in society. The use of alcohol is such an integral part of our culture that its use is often accepted without question. The decision to drink is determined by various social, cultural, and personal factors that are difficult to identify and control. It is important for young people to be prepared to meet the needs and challenges regarding the use of alcohol and to be equipped with the knowledge to enable them to handle situations involving alcohol.

Alcohol acts as a general depressant on the central nervous system. Problems occur when alcohol is consumed in quantities that exceed the body's capability to metabolize it. Unlike most substances, alcohol is absorbed directly from the stomach. An adult can metabolize about one-half to three-fourths of an ounce of pure alcohol per hour. (Two ounces of a 100-proof bourbon, for example, equals one ounce of pure alcohol.) One ounce of pure alcohol produces a blood alcohol level of 0.05 percent in a large adult. Four ounces of pure alcohol produce a blood alcohol level of 0.20 percent, resulting in severe intoxication. A blood alcohol level over 2.0 percent produces coma and sometimes death.

Alcohol interferes with coordination, vision, and judgment. It also slows reaction time and can produce severe motor disturbances, such as staggering, and impaired sensory perception. Long-term damage to the brain and liver may also result from use of alcohol. In addition, alcohol negatively affects the controlling impulses to the heart. Thus, individuals who exercise after drinking alcohol run the risk of irregular heartbeats. Increased heart rate also is common because of alcohol's depressant effect upon the central nervous system, which is unable to regulate and control the heart properly. Finally, evidence indicates that alcohol taken prior to rigorous physical activity can result in a reduced blood supply to the heart tissue. For all of these reasons, alcohol obviously has no place in physical exercise.

Cigarettes

People have turned to cigarettes for some of the same reasons others use psychoactive drugs: to reduce tension and anxiety, enhance pleasure of the moment, promote stimulation, and counteract boredom. Specifically, cigarettes are popular because they provide the users with certain personal gratifications unobtainable in other tobacco forms. Cigarettes provide the smoker with an oral activity, an occupation for idle hands, a sensation of relaxation due to the deep rhythmical breathing of inhaling the smoke, and an immediate stimulatory effect. They are also readily available, socially acceptable, and relatively inexpensive. Unfortunately smoking cigarettes carries a very high price tag physiologically in the forms of drug dependency and predisposition to serious, sometimes fatal diseases.

The United States Public Health Service estimates that 54 million Americans smoke 615 billion cigarettes a year. Of those smokers, 37 percent are men, 28 percent are women, and 35 percent are teenagers. Twelve percent of the teenagers between twelve and eighteen years of age smoke at least weekly. Among teenagers, more females than males smoke. The influence of peers and parents who smoke continues to attract new teenaged smokers (approximately one million a year), despite the serious health hazards.

Cigarette smoking is now characterized as one of the most serious and yet preventable health problems. The greater number of cigarettes smoked, the greater the health risk and the more days of disability and workdays lost. Cigarette smoking is directly linked to bronchitis; emphysema; coronary heart disease; cirrhoses of the liver; accidents; peripheral vascular disease; bladder cancer; peptic ulcer; lung cancer; larynx cancer; lip, tongue, gum cancers; tobacco amblyopia; and adverse drug reactions. In addition, 14 percent of all premature deliveries may be due to maternal smoking.

Cigarette smoking reduces the oxygen-carrying capacity of the blood, reduces the efficiency of the lungs to take in oxygen, increases heart rate and blood pressure, and decreases motor performance. The negative effects that smoking has on individuals prevent them from attaining a high level of fitness. For additional information about smoking, see page 36.

Current cigarette smokers have about a 70 percent greater chance of dying from disease than nonsmokers. In excess of 350,000 deaths a year are attributed to cigarette smoking, with 13 billion dollars in direct medical costs. One-third, or 125,000, of all cancer deaths are attributable to cigarette smoking. The American Cancer Society's findings indicate that only 5 percent of lifetime smokers are still alive by the age of eighty-five, while 37 percent of those who never smoked are still alive at that age. In addition, smokers at age thirty can expect to live to an average age of 64.8 years if they continue to smoke, while nonsmoking thirty-year-olds can expect to reach the age of eighty-two.

Quitting

Whatever the specific method people use to stop smoking, a major factor is the personal resolve of the smoker to want to quit. Become aware of your personal motives for smoking. It is necessary to eliminate those thoughts and behaviors that lead to smoking. Integrate positive and rewarding activities, thoughts, and feelings in place of those that lead to smoking. For some tips on how to quit see table 11.5.

Smokeless Tobaccos

An alternative to smoking cigarettes that has gained popularity among young people in recent years is the use of smokeless tobacco, such as snuff and chewing tobacco. The chemicals from this tobacco can mix with saliva and find ready access to the bloodstream. Smokeless tobacco has been found to cause cancer of the mouth and throat and is associated with a number of other cancers in the body.

Drugs Used to Improve Athletic Performance

The use of drugs by professional and amateur athletes to improve performance has become common these days at all competitive levels. Athletes have always looked for that "extra edge" that will give them the advantage over their opponent. With only hundredths of seconds or a few inches separating the winner from the losers, it is not surprising that drugs thought to increase performance are finding wide acceptance among athletes. Both male and female competitive athletes are presently using a wide range of pharmacological agents in hopes that it will increase their strength, endurance, speed, power, and skill. One of the most unfortunate aspects of drug use to increase performance is that many athletes appear to be willing to court major health risks just to be competitive.

Such drugs as anabolic steroids, growth hormones, and amphetamines are used in an attempt to increase muscle strength and endurance and delay the onset of fatigue, while in fact, these drugs can adversely affect performance and lead

TABLE 11.5 Tips for Smokers Who Want to Quit

When Thinking About Quitting . . .

1. List all the reasons you want to stop smoking.

2. Keep a diary of the times of the day and the circumstances of your smoking behavior. Be particularly mindful of your feelings that lead you to light up.

3. Tell your family and friends you are going to quit and ask for their support.

4. Switch to a brand of cigarettes you dislike. Try not to smoke two packs of the same brand in a row.

Cut Down the Number of Cigarettes You Smoke

1. Smoke only half of each cigarette.

2. Don't smoke when you first experience a craving. Wait several minutes. During this time change your activity or talk to someone.

3. Do not buy cigarettes by the carton. Wait until one pack is empty before buying another.

4. Make cigarettes difficult to get. Don't carry them with you.

5. Don't smoke automatically. Smoke only when you really *want* to.

6. Reward yourself in some way other than smoking.

7. Reach for a glass of juice instead of a cigarette for a pick-me-up.

Immediately After Quitting

1. Whenever you feel uncomfortable sensations from having stopped smoking, remind yourself that they are signs of your body's return to health and that they will soon pass.

2. If you miss the sensation of having a cigarette in your hand, play with something else—a pencil, a paper clip, a marble.

3. Instead of smoking after meals, get up from the table and brush your teeth or go for a walk.

4. Temporarily avoid situations you strongly associate with the pleasurable acts of smoking.

5. Develop a clean, fresh nonsmoking environment around yourself—at work and at home.

6. Until you are confident of your ability to stay off cigarettes, limit your socializing to healthful, outdoor activities or to situations in which smoking is prohibited.

7. Look at cigarette ads more critically. Remind yourself that cigarette companies are making money at the expense of your health and well-being.

Find New Habits

1. Change your habits to make smoking difficult and unnecessary.

2. Keep a clean-tasting mouth.

3. Substitute relaxation and deep breathing for stressful situations.

4. Absorb yourself in activities that are meaningful to you.

5. Never allow yourself to think that "one won't hurt"—it will!

Based on *Calling It Quits,* U.S. Department of Health, Education, and Welfare Publication No. (NIH) 79–1824.

to long-term health problems. Alcohol, cigarettes, and cocaine also can pose a serious threat if used prior to and during physical exercise.

Anabolic Steroids

Anabolic steroids are synthetic hormones and close relatives of the male hormone testosterone. Anabolic steroids have had their chemical structure altered so that the androgenic, or masculinizing, effect has been reduced and their anabolic protein-producing characteristics have been enhanced in order to promote muscle growth. There is also speculation that small residual androgenic effects increase performance by making the athletes more aggressive and competitive, resulting in increased intensity of training motivation. Steroids have been used frequently in medical practice in cases of replacement therapy, malnutrition, infection, skeletal disorders, and some cancers and growth problems. Anabolic steroids promote anabolism by increasing nitrogen retention. They may convert a mildly negative nitrogen balance to a positive one, dependent on adequate protein and caloric intake. They may build lean body mass and provide strength only in individuals intensively training in heavy resistance activities, such as weight lifting. They do not directly improve performance in aerobic activities such as long-distance running, skiing, or swimming. The real possibility of harmful side effects greatly outweighs the still questionable increases in performance. Because of the irreversible side effects in women and children, they should never be used in this population. Anabolic-androgenic steroids have been associated with adverse effects on the liver, cardiovascular system, reproductive function, and psychological status. Steroids that are alkalated at the 17-carbon position (most all oral forms) are especially dangerous because of the strong link between this chemical structure and liver dysfunction.

The adverse side effects associated with anabolic steroid use are liver tumors and blood-filled cysts on the liver, decreased HDLs, elevated blood pressure, hyperinsulinism, altered glucose tolerance, reduced sperm count, reduction in testosterone, and reduced estrogen and progesterone in females. Both males and females experience mood swings, aggressive behavior, and decreased libido.

The American College of Sports Medicine Position Statement on Anabolic-Androgenic Steroids in Sports

It is the position of the American College of Sports Medicine that:

1. Anabolic-androgenic steroids in the presence of an adequate diet can contribute to increases in body weight, often in the lean mass compartment.

2. The gains in muscular strength achieved through high-intensity exercise and proper diet can occur by the increased use of anabolic-androgenic steroids in some individuals.

3. Anabolic-androgenic steroids do not increase aerobic power or capacity for muscular exercise.

4. Anabolic-androgenic steroids have been associated with adverse effects on the liver, cardiovascular system, and psychological status in therapeutic trials and in limited research on athletes. Until further research is completed, the potential hazards of the use of the anabolic-androgenic steroids in athletes must include those found in therapeutic trials.

5. The use of anabolic-androgenic steroids by athletes is contrary to the rules and ethical principles of athletic competition as set forth by many of the sports governing bodies. The American College of Sports Medicine supports these ethical principles and deplores the use of anabolic-androgenic steroids by athletes.

Growth Hormones

There is a major concern that growth hormones (somatotrophic hormones) will replace anabolic steroids as the new high-tech drug. Growth hormone is produced by the pituitary gland located in the brain. Its main function is to stimulate and control the tissue-building process associated with normal growth and development. It has been used medically to treat children with retarded growth. With the advancement of bioengineering it will soon be possible to produce large amounts of this hormone inexpensively. Athletes are attracted to the drug because it increases protein synthesis and fat breakdown and decreases the amount of carbohydrates used by the body. Its use in adults, however, could lead to symptoms similar to those of acromegaly, enlarged bones of the face, hands, and feet, overgrowth of soft tissue, and a most dangerous abnormal enlargement of cardiac tissue. This hormone is most difficult to detect in screening tests because it occurs naturally in the body. Unfortunately, with the new techniques of producing the hormone synthetically through recombinant DNA techniques, the price will fall sharply, thus making it more available.

Key Terms

Amphetamines
A group of drugs that stimulate the central nervous system

Anabolic steroids
Synthetic hormones that are similar to the male hormone testosterone

Analgesics
Drugs that block pain

Hallucinogens
Drugs that alter mood and perception

Narcotics
Drugs that depress the central nervous system

Psychoactive drugs
Drugs that alter feelings, insights, perception, and moods

Sedatives
Drugs that slow down the nervous system and induce sleep

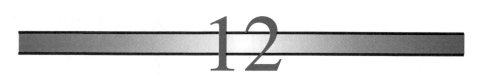

12

c h a p t e r

Exercise and Stress Reduction

C h a p t e r   C o n c e p t s

After you have studied this chapter you should be able to

1. describe the relationship between physical exercise and stress response;
2. describe the three stages of stress response;
3. differentiate between type A, type B, and type C personalities;
4. describe the Coping Lifestyle Inventory (table 12.4);
5. describe techniques useful in managing stress response;
6. describe the purpose and method of relaxation techniques;
7. describe the seven-step relaxation program; and
8. describe the progressive relaxation exercise.

S tudents bring to campus a variety of needs, expectations, and experiences that influence the way they react and adjust to their new environment. Factors such as their academic strengths and weaknesses, social insecurity, fear of failure, lack of challenge, autonomy and responsibility, and role strain all play a vital part in this adjustment. Unfortunately, many young people are unable to adjust to the demands of their new environment and fall victim to the effects of stress response.

A fundamental assumption of one approach to stress is that mind, body, and behavior are closely intertwined. The interconnectiveness of these three factors occur all day and every day as one continually adjusts to the demands of daily living. Also, physical wear and tear on the body may result in chronic mental strain associated with coping with the demands of college life. Destructive distress often develops in precisely this way as mind, body, and behavior affect each other in an accelerating cycle of stress buildup.

There are, however, positive aspects of stress. To many, involvement with a variety of stimuli and stressors provides a number of interesting and stimulating aspects to a full life. Learning, developing, and striving for optimal potential all require an encounter with stress. Many of our most memorable peak moments in our lives involve stressful events.

We all have our unique zone of positive stress, the zone in which we feel healthy, productive, and satisfied. It is important for us to be able to recognize the limits of this zone. We must be able to distinguish warning signs that bring us close to the borders of this zone and live within them.

Exercise Benefits

A vital step in controlling stress and preventing illness is to maintain a periodic exercise program. Exercise can be a very effective means of managing the physical and psychological effects of stress response. Physical activity can prevent stress-induced illnesses such as ulcers, back pain, migraine headaches, and high blood pressure. In addition, physical activity can play a major part in reducing the destructive coping behavior in our society as evidenced by the abuse of alcohol and other drugs, smoking, overeating, and violence. There is substantial evidence that exercise can positively affect a wide variety of physical and psychological stress-related responses. A sound program of physical exercise may increase body awareness, reduce muscle tension, burn up stress-produced adrenalin, quiet the sympathetic nervous system, lower base line tension levels, and produce faster recovery time of stress response. Psychological benefits of rigorous exercise are the release of emotional tension, feelings of well-being and calmness, less anxiety, less depression, and enhanced self-esteem.

The Stress Response

When you experience stress, which can be loosely defined as anything that you experience as a threat to your stability or equilibrium, a portion of your nervous system comes into play to ready the body to meet the demands brought on by this emotional upset. Your heart rate speeds up, your breathing is faster, your pupils dilate, and your muscles become more tense, resulting in an overall heightened mental and physical awareness. This phenomenon is referred to as the **stress response.** Also, personality is related to stress in that a person's perception of a stimulus or situation determines to a large extent how stressful the situation is.

Whether you suffer from stress or thrive on it, your system must be prepared to withstand it. The stress response readies your body to deal with threats efficiently and effectively. It gives your body the stimulus to perform amazing feats, both mental and physical; yet, at the same time, it also can wreak havoc on your health. If the stress is prolonged, it can weaken your body defenses, accelerate the aging process, and lead to chronic disease.

Table 12.1 shows important life events and the degree of stress associated with each measured on a point scale.

TABLE 12.1 SUGGESTED LAB ACTIVITY: Life Change Scale for Youth

The following scale, developed by Martin B. Marx, ranks life changes in order of the amount of stress they cause college-age youths. For each time one of the events listed below has happened in your life in the past year, write the point value on each line as many times as each of these events occurred. A score below 600 suggests a low life change and a small possibility of illness in the coming year; 600 to 1,000 points represents a medium change; anything exceeding 1,000 is high. A high score does not mean you will necessarily get sick, but it does mean that in a large sample of people like you, a substantial percentage will get sick.

Life event	Stress rating	Your score
Death of spouse	100	
Divorce (of yourself or parents)	73	
Pregnancy (or causing pregnancy)	68	
Marital separation	65	
Jail term	63	
Death of close family member	63	
Broken engagement	60	
Engagement	55	
Personal injury or illness	53	
Marriage	50	
Entering college	50	
Varying independence or responsibility	50	
Conflict or change in values	50	
Drug use	49	
Fired at work	47	
Change in alcohol use	47	
Reconciliation with mate	45	
Trouble with school administration	45	
Change of health in family member	44	
Working while attending school	42	
Changing course of study	40	
Sex difficulty	39	
Changing dating habits	39	
Gaining a new family member	39	
Business readjustments	39	
Change in financial state	38	
Changing participation in courses, seminars	38	

TABLE 12.1	Life Change Scale for Youth (*Continued*)	
Death of close friend	37	_____
Change to different line of work	36	_____
Change in number of arguments with mate	35	_____
Trouble with in-laws	29	_____
Outstanding personal achievement	28	_____
Mate begins or stops work	26	_____
Begin or end school	26	_____
Change in living conditions	25	_____
Revision of personal habits	24	_____
Trouble with boss	23	_____
Change in work hours or conditions	20	_____
Change in residence	20	_____
Change in schools	20	_____
Change in recreation	19	_____
Change in church activities	19	_____
Change in social activities	18	_____
Going into debt	17	_____
Change in sleeping habits	16	_____
Change in frequency of family gatherings	15	_____
Change in eating habits	15	_____
Vacation	13	_____
Christmas	12	_____
Minor violation of the law	11	_____
Your Total		_____

Reprinted with permission from M. B. Marx, T. F. Garrity, and F. R. Bowers, "The Influence of Recent Life Experiences on the Health of College Freshmen," *Journal of Psychosomatic Research, 19:* 1975. Pergamon Journals, Ltd.

Generally, the stress response can be broken down into the three stages defined by Hans Seyle, a pioneer in stress research: (1) the alarm reaction stage, (2) the resistance stage, and (3) the exhaustion stage.

The **alarm reaction stage,** or fight or flight response, is the initial reaction of your body to stress. This response mobilizes the body's resources for immediate physical activity. Increased activity of the sympathetic nervous system and suprarenal glands brings about a wide range of physical changes that are necessary to prepare the body to deal with the impending threat. These changes include increased heart rate and stroke volume and decreased digestion.

During the **resistance stage,** the body increases its capacity to deal with stress. However, if the stressor continues for a prolonged period of time, the heightened physiological adjustment that is maintained may have a detrimental effect on the body.

When the body can no longer deal effectively with stress, the **exhaustion stage,** or distress, is evident. The exhaustion stage may manifest itself in high blood pressure, extra heartbeats, and emotional problems.

Determine your behavioral and physiological reactions to stress from tables 12.2 and 12.3. Table 12.4 measures your style of coping with stress. This self-evaluation may help to give you some perspective on developing techniques for stress reduction.

Your Personality—Type A, Type B, or Type C?

Research over the past ten years has focused on what is perhaps one of the most critical personal influences on stress. This characteristic was first introduced by Friedman and Rosenman and is called type A personality (as opposed to type B and C personalities). Type A personality is characterized by impatience, restlessness, aggressiveness, competitiveness, and intolerance to frustration. Type A individuals tend to invest long hours on the job to meet pressing and recurring deadlines. Type B and C people, on the other hand, experience no pressing deadlines or conflicts and are relatively free of any sense of time, urgency, or hostility.

Research indicates that type A individuals are more prone to heart disease and more prone to second heart attacks than type B and C individuals. However, a number of other variables are associated with heart disease in addition to your physiological response to stress. Most importantly, keep in mind that it is possible to modify your personality type and subsequent response to stress.

Use table 12.5 to determine your personality type.

The type A pattern exists to the degree that the person is hard-driving, maintains excessively high expectations towards self and/or others, is chronically overloaded and in a hurry, and, most important of all, tends to be easily aggravated, irritated, and angered.

Type B behavior is the absence of type A. While the person who exhibits type B behavior may be ambitious and successful, he or she is generally calmer, more patient, and less hurried. Of course there are gradations within each behavior type. Most of us go back and forth between type A and type B as our activities and pressures vary from one day or week to the next. Type A personalities experience a higher continuous stress level than type Bs because they are more likely to be stress-seekers, and thereby expose themselves to more challenges than type Bs. The response to these challenges turns on the sympathetic nervous system and increases secretions of hormones such as norepinephrine, which combine to produce elevated heart rates.

TABLE 12.2 SUGGESTED LAB ACTIVITY: Behavioral Reactions to Stress

Circle the number that best represents frequency of occurrence of the following behavioral symptoms and add up the total number of points.

	Never	Infrequently (more than once in six months)	Occasionally (more than once per month)	Very often (more than once per week)	Constantly
1. Difficulty relaxing	1	2	3	4	5
2. Generalized anxiety (no known cause)	1	2	3	4	5
3. Easily angered	1	2	3	4	5
4. Short attention span	1	2	3	4	5
5. Bored	1	2	3	4	5
6. Sexual difficulties or problems	1	2	3	4	5
7. Accident prone	1	2	3	4	5
8. Overeating	1	2	3	4	5
9. Drug usage	1	2	3	4	5
10. Alcohol usage	1	2	3	4	5
11. Inability to control emotions	1	2	3	4	5
12. Inability to concentrate	1	2	3	4	5
13. Distortions in memory	1	2	3	4	5
14. Difficulty in making decisions	1	2	3	4	5
15. Racing thoughts	1	2	3	4	5
16. Pessimistic	1	2	3	4	5
17. Sleeping difficulties	1	2	3	4	5
18. Urge to cry	1	2	3	4	5
19. Blaming others for your anxiety	1	2	3	4	5
20. Frustration	1	2	3	4	5
21. Hostility	1	2	3	4	5
22. Irritability	1	2	3	4	5
23. Impatience	1	2	3	4	5
24. Inflexibility	1	2	3	4	5
25. Powerless	1	2	3	4	5
26. Agitated	1	2	3	4	5
27. Out of control	1	2	3	4	5

Interpretation

40—Low psychological symptoms of stress response
41–60—Moderate psychological symptoms of stress response
61–80—High psychological symptoms of stress response
Over 80—Excessive psychological symptoms of stress response

Source: From *Presidential Sports Award Fitness Manual,* edited by H. Ebel, N. Sol, D. Bailey, and S. Schecter. Copyright © 1983 FitCom Corporation, Havertown, PA.

TABLE 12.3 SUGGESTED LAB ACTIVITY: Physiological Reactions to Stress

Circle the number that best represents the frequency of occurrence of the following physical symptoms and add up the total number of points.

	Never	Infrequently (more than once in six months)	Occasionally (more than once per month)	Very often (more than once per week)	Constantly
1. Tension headaches	1	2	3	4	5
2. Migraine (vascular) headaches	1	2	3	4	5
3. Stomachaches	1	2	3	4	5
4. Increase in blood pressure	1	2	3	4	5
5. Cold hands	1	2	3	4	5
6. Acidy stomach	1	2	3	4	5
7. Shallow, rapid breathing	1	2	3	4	5
8. Diarrhea	1	2	3	4	5
9. Palpitations	1	2	3	4	5
10. Shaky hands	1	2	3	4	5
11. Burping	1	2	3	4	5
12. Gassiness	1	2	3	4	5
13. Increased urge to urinate	1	2	3	4	5
14. Sweaty feet/hands	1	2	3	4	5
15. Oily skin	1	2	3	4	5
16. Fatigue/exhausted feeling	1	2	3	4	5
17. Panting	1	2	3	4	5
18. Dry mouth	1	2	3	4	5
19. Hand tremor	1	2	3	4	5
20. Backache	1	2	3	4	5
21. Neck stiffness	1	2	3	4	5
22. Gum chewing	1	2	3	4	5
23. Grinding teeth	1	2	3	4	5
24. Constipation	1	2	3	4	5
25. Tightness in chest or heart	1	2	3	4	5
26. Dizziness	1	2	3	4	5
27. Nausea/vomiting	1	2	3	4	5
28. Menstrual distress	1	2	3	4	5
29. Skin blemishes	1	2	3	4	5
30. Heart pounding	1	2	3	4	5

TABLE 12.3 SUGGESTED LAB ACTIVITY: Physiological Reactions to Stress (*Continued*)

	Never	Infrequently (more than once in six months)	Occasionally (more than once per month)	Very often (more than once per week)	Constantly
31. Colitis	1	2	3	4	5
32. Asthma	1	2	3	4	5
33. Indigestion	1	2	3	4	5
34. High blood pressure	1	2	3	4	5
35. Hyperventilation	1	2	3	4	5
36. Arthritis	1	2	3	4	5
37. Skin rash	1	2	3	4	5
38. Bruxism/jaw pain	1	2	3	4	5
39. Allergy	1	2	3	4	5

Interpretation

40–75 Low physiological symptoms of stress response
76–100 Moderate physiological symptoms of stress response
101–150 High physiological symptoms of stress response
Over 150 Excessive physiological symptoms of stress response

Source: From *Presidential Sports Award Fitness Manual,* edited by H. Ebel, N. Sol, D. Bailey, and S. Schecter. Copyright © 1983 FitCom Corporation, Havertown, PA.

TABLE 12.4 SUGGESTED LAB ACTIVITY: Coping Lifestyle Inventory

For each of the items listed, circle the number that best represents what you do when you feel stressed.

	Never	Infrequently (more than once in six months)	Occasionally (more than once per month)	Very often (more than once per week)	Constantly
1. Lose control (e.g., excessive crying)	1	2	3	4	5
2. React on emotions and not intellect	1	2	3	4	5
3. Freeze—controlled by physical symptoms (e.g., shaking)	1	2	3	4	5
4. Use drugs	1	2	3	4	5
5. Use alcohol	1	2	3	4	5

TABLE 12.4 SUGGESTED LAB ACTIVITY: Coping Lifestyle Inventory (*Continued*)

	Never	Infrequently (more than once in six months)	Occasionally (more than once per month)	Very often (more than once per week)	Constantly
6. Avoid stressor as best I can	1	2	3	4	5
7. Ignore or run from stressor	1	2	3	4	5
8. Internalize feelings (keep inside)	1	2	3	4	5
9. Allow people to take advantage of me	1	2	3	4	5
10. Remain passive because of fear of hurting others	1	2	3	4	5
11. Put off stressful situations until they "come to a head"	1	2	3	4	5
12. Watch television	1	2	3	4	5
13. Read nonprofessional material	1	2	3	4	5
14. Spend time working on hobbies	1	2	3	4	5
15. Binge eat	1	2	3	4	5
16. Listen to music	1	2	3	4	5
17. Face situation head-on	1	2	3	4	5
18. Do something physical (i.e., exercise related)	1	2	3	4	5
19. Ask friends for advice	1	2	3	4	5
20. Get involved with formal relaxation activity	1	2	3	4	5
21. Do yoga, t'ai chi, or meditate	1	2	3	4	5
22. Use positive self-talk (e.g., "Things will work out—I just know it")	1	2	3	4	5

TABLE 12.4 SUGGESTED LAB ACTIVITY: Coping Lifestyle Inventory (*Continued*)

	Never	Infrequently (more than once in six months)	Occasionally (more than once per month)	Very often (more than once per week)	Constantly
23. Do imagery or fantasy activities	1	2	3	4	5
24. Engage in self-hypnosis	1	2	3	4	5
25. Do nothing (let it be)	1	2	3	4	5
26. Feel the stressor is out of your control	1	2	3	4	5
27. Expect the worst to happen	1	2	3	4	5
28. Try to face or attack your fears head-on	1	2	3	4	5
29. Say it's stupid or illogical to get upset	1	2	3	4	5
30. Work out a plan to control stressor	1	2	3	4	5
31. Take out time from daily activities to improve your mental state or well-being	1	2	3	4	5
32. Put off tasks when they aren't important to immediate or future goals	1	2	3	4	5
33. Seek medical help when stress becomes excessive	1	2	3	4	5

Your Style?

This inventory is not intended to judge your coping lifestyle as good or bad, but rather to make you more aware of what your present style is, so that you can make any adjustments that might be necessary.

TABLE 12.4	SUGGESTED LAB ACTIVITY: Coping Lifestyle Inventory (*Continued*)

Coping Styles

A study of many stress intervention techniques identified the following ten most commonly used styles of coping. Try to identify any that you often use.

1. Lose Control—You freeze, cry excessively, engage in binge eating, or hyperventilate. In other words, your symptoms control you instead of you controlling them. (numbers 1, 2, 3, and 9 on the "Coping Lifestyle Inventory")

2. No Active Involvement (Negative)—You feel that stress is out of control and think the worst will probably happen to you. You tell yourself that things won't work out and that there is no reason to try and do anything about it. You are simply pessimistic. (numbers 26, 27)

3. No Active Involvement (Positive)—You don't do anything at all because of your belief that things will work out for the best or that *someone* is watching out for you. You are simply optimistic. (numbers 22 and 25)

4. Divert—You try to distract your mind away from stressful thoughts and emotions. To accomplish this, you might watch television, read books, clean, exercise, work, listen to music, cook, or involve yourself in a hobby. (numbers 12, 13, 14, 15, and 16)

5. Escape—You try to disassociate and run from stressful thoughts and emotions. You might go on vacation, sleep, drink enough alcohol to forget, work long hours, use drugs, and even engage in sexual activity as a means of escaping. (numbers 4, 5, 6, and 7)

6. Suppress—You avoid, deny, rationalize, and use any other mental device ("defense mechanism") to protect you from directly facing the stress of daily living. Passive individuals often use suppression as their primary means of coping. (numbers 8 and 11)

7. Active Involvement—This is when you really enter into and attack your problems realistically. Examples of active involvement are when you assert yourself and engage in direct problem solving. In addition, you should set up a schedule of exercise and relaxation. (numbers 17, 18, 19, and 20)

8. Altered State of Confusion—This is when you try to change your frame of mind by getting into activities like imagery, sensory deprivation (isolation tanks), meditation, and self-hypnosis. (numbers 21, 23, and 24)

9. Prevent Stress Reactions—This is really not a coping method. Its objective is to prevent you from experiencing excessive stress by making changes in your lifestyle and interactions. Examples of preventive coping techniques include time management, cognitive restructuring, fear control training, and taking an occasional day off for "mental health." (numbers 28, 29, 30, 31, and 32)

10. Seek Medical Help—Sometimes, all of the books and self-training programs are not helpful enough, and there is a need to seek additional medical or psychological assistance. This may be a most important coping method under certain circumstances. (number 33)

Source: From *Presidential Sports Award Fitness Manual,* edited by H. Ebel, N. Sol, D. Bailey, and S. Schecter. Copyright © 1983 FitCom Corporation, Havertown, PA.

TABLE 12.5 Determining Your Degree of Type A Behavior

If you find a majority of the following statements describe you, you probably possess some degree of type A behavior.

1. Rush your speech
2. Hurry other people's speech
3. Hurry when you eat
4. Hate to wait in line
5. Never seem to catch up
6. Schedule more activities than time available
7. Detest "wasting time"
8. Drive too fast most of the time
9. Often try to do several things at once
10. Become impatient if others are too slow
11. Have little time for relaxation, intimacy, or enjoying your environment.

Type C Behavior and Hardiness

Research has also turned attention to those individuals who tend to thrive and stay well during challenge and difficulty. They are able to interpret change and difficulty as positive challenges or opportunities rather than as threats. They tend to be committed rather than detached or alienated. They feel in control of events and their reactions to those events, withstanding everyday stressors. Maddi and Kobasa of the University of Chicago have identified "a distress resistance pattern."[1] They call it "hardiness," consisting of three Cs, relating to attitude or perception: challenge, commitment, and control. Type C people tend to engage in regular exercise and are involved in a number of social support groups. Kriegel and Kriegel have also identified a type C behavior, or what they call a "C zone," similar to hardiness, which consists of two of Kobasa and Maddi's three Cs, challenge and control, but replaces commitment with confidence.[2]

The Type C person perceives situations in regard to:

Challenge—Interprets a difficult task or change as a challenge rather than as a threat.

Confidence—Believes in one's ability to master a difficult problem or challenge, rather than approaching it with self-doubt.

1. Maddi, Salvador, and Suzanne Kobasa. *The Hardy Executive*. Homewood Princeton, N.J.: Dow Jones, 1984.
2. Kriegel, Robert, and Marilyn Kriegel. *The C Zone: Peak Performance under Pressure.* New York: Anchor-Double Day, 1984.

Commitment—Positively engages with one's job, family, and friends, rather than feeling alienated.

Control—Believes in one's ability to control events and reactions to events, rather than feeling helpless.

Stress Management

In this section, we discuss ten useful ways to turn off stress and also a variety of relaxation techniques that are helpful in stress management. The recommendations that follow are not a panacea for stress but may give you some insight into dealing with it effectively. In the final analysis, however, the best recommendation for dealing with stress is: Know your limits. You must know when your various frustrations, conflicts, and stresses are getting to you and take appropriate action to limit or modify these stresses.

Turning Off Stress

Ten ways to turn off stress are:

1. **Try to Change How You Perceive Specific Stress-Inducing Events.** For example, the next time a person in another car does something foolish, try not to perceive him or her as the enemy who is out to run you off the road, but as a friend who has simply made a driving mistake.

2. **Try to Understand and Deal with Your Anger.** Acknowledge your anger to yourself. Learn to differentiate between levels of anger. Try to diagnose the threat that is causing you to be angry— it may be the result of a difference in values or in style and be no real threat to you at all. Finally, try letting go of anger through forgiveness and by canceling the charges against the other person.

3. **Take Time to Relax or Meditate.** Try to manage your time more effectively so that you don't court stress through disorganized scheduling.

4. **Expand Your Social Support System.** Contact and try to establish relationships with new individuals or groups who may be able to give you emotional support.

5. **Regular Exercise Is an Essential Ingredient in Reducing Stress.** Considerable evidence indicates that individuals who regularly exercise have a lower arousal to stress than individuals who are less fit. Exercise aids in balancing and stabilizing the physiological consequences of emotional stress. Exercise also

maintains your body systems in a fit state so that they are able to effectively handle any additional stress. Exercise also ensures normal fatigue and relaxation.

6. **Good Nutrition Is Vital.** Eat regular, well-balanced meals, and avoid alcohol and cigarettes.

7. **Slow Down.** Learn to slow your pace of talking, walking, and eating.

8. **Don't Take on Too Many Responsibilities.** Measure success by quality rather than quantity.

9. **Don't Set Unrealistic Deadlines.** Learn to live with unfinished tasks.

10. **Practice Effective Listening.** Avoid interrupting out of impatience.

Relaxation Techniques

There probably are times during the day when you just want to unwind, relax, take time out, and turn off anxiety-producing stimuli. Both psychologically and physiologically, there is a need to relax the tension that is an ever-present companion in all of us. Tension manifests itself in muscle contractions, shallow breathing, clenched jaws, and a variety of other involuntary responses. With a little practice and patience, you can begin to free yourself of tension with such simple relaxation and meditation techniques as the seven-step relaxation program, hatha-yoga, the progressive relaxation exercise, and autogenic training. It is important to relieve the tension in both your body and your brain so that they both relax as one.

Keep in mind, however, that even though relaxation can reduce arousal and be just as effective as exercise in reducing the stress response, it does not bring with it the physiological advantages of rigorous exercise.

The Seven-Step Relaxation Program

1. **Establish a Quiet Environment.** Arrange for things to be as quiet as possible. Avoid having to answer the phone or door or respond to other distracting stimuli.

2. **Find a Comfortable Position.** Sit in a comfortable chair or lie on the floor. The main thing is that you have full body support.

3. **Close Your Eyes.** Now use your imagination. Place yourself in a relaxing environment, such as a beach or another enjoyable place.

4. **Maintain a Passive Attitude.** Focus your attention on your bodily sensations. Diffuse your concentration by letting thoughts pass out of your awareness.

5. **Take a Deep Breath.** Tighten your muscles for a few seconds.

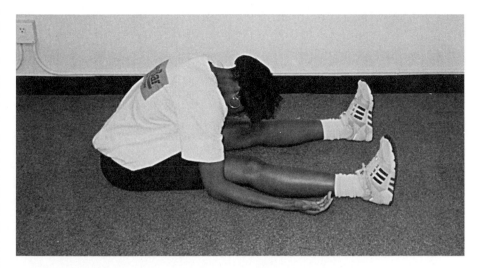

Figure 12.1 Child's pose (darnikasava). Sit on a mat, with your feet slightly apart. Bend forward at the groin and stretch your trunk until your forehead rests on the mat. Tuck in your chin slightly to lengthen your neck. Place your hands by your feet, palms up. Relax your entire body. You may place a small pillow under your head if your head does not touch the floor. Remain in this position for five to ten minutes.

6. **Exhale and Relax.** Feel the release in tension and the heaviness of your muscles as you exhale and fall into the comfortable position.
7. **Repeat Steps 1–6 Two or Three Times or Until You Are Relaxed.** Take fifteen to twenty minutes to achieve complete relaxation, with about thirty seconds between each phase.

Hatha-Yoga Rest Procedures

The hatha-yoga rest procedures illustrated in figures 12.1 and 12.2 also may be valuable in achieving relaxation and in releasing tension.

The Progressive Relaxation Exercise

The **progressive relaxation exercise** that follows constitutes a more comprehensive muscle relaxation program.

General Instructions

1. The progressive relaxation exercise follows a systematic pattern: right hand (or dominant hand), left hand, right bicep, left bicep, forehead, eyes, facial area, chest, abdomen, and both legs and feet.

255

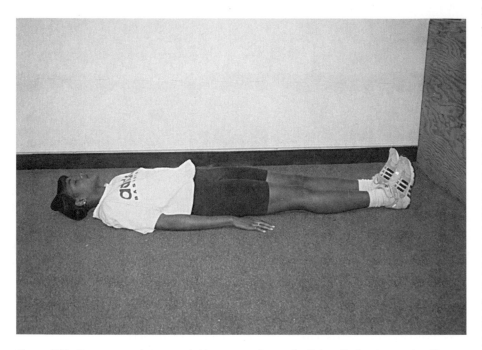

Figure 12.2 Corpse pose (savasana). Lie on your back with your legs straight and your feet about eighteen inches apart, toes falling out. Your hands should be about a foot away from your thighs. Close your eyes, breathe, and relax with each exhalation. Let your entire body sink toward the earth. Relax all of your muscles. Keep your jaw loose so that your teeth are not touching. Remain in this position for five to twenty minutes. You also may try placing your hands, palms down, across your chest, and bending your knees with your feet on the floor near your buttocks.

At the start, repeat the exercise for each group twice before going to the next group. After completing each muscle group, refrain from moving that area so that it remains relaxed.

2. If you are doing the relaxation exercise for the first time, have someone else read the instructions aloud for you to follow.

3. Whoever reads the instructions should do so in a normal voice, pacing the speed by doing the tension exercises. The aim is to tense the muscle group long enough to be noticeable but not long enough to be painful or to lead to cramps or fatigue.

4. Some muscle groups (for example, the eyes, the jaws, and the feet) should be tensed for a shorter span—about three seconds—to avoid pain or cramping.

5. After you have done the exercise once under the direction of someone else, you can practice the exercise alone by simply tensing and relaxing each muscle group in sequence.

6. After three or four practice sessions, omit the muscle-tensing exercises and concentrate simply on having each muscle group become relaxed or limp, again in sequence. With training, you should be able to develop a state of relaxation within five minutes; with more practice, you may be able to establish relaxation control within one minute. Some individuals are able to achieve relaxation while sitting in chairs or riding in vehicles, and can practice it prior to competition. Control in relaxing specific muscle groups is possible with repetition.

7. Repetition of the deep-breath technique (described in the exercise directions that follow) can establish this as a signal for the initiation of relaxation on a quick-reflex basis.

8. Although the relaxation exercise can be used for other forms of training, the directions here are aimed at teaching you how to control muscle groups to achieve relaxation. As with other physical exercise, your success will depend upon how often you practice and your adherence to the exercise steps. Practice the exercise once a day, five times a week. More frequent practice speeds up training.

Directions for the Progressive Relaxation Exercise Before beginning the progressive relaxation exercise, get into a comfortable position, preferably lying down on your back. You may use a small pillow for your head. Choose a time of day when you will not be disturbed for an hour. Many people practice in the evening since the relaxation achieved is an especially good way of going to sleep at night. The read-aloud directions for the progressive relaxation exercise follow.*

> **Hands** Close your eyes so as not to be distracted by your surroundings. Now tense your right hand into a fist, as tight as you can get it so that you feel the tension . . . really tight, the tighter the better, so that you can really feel the tension. . . . Now relax the hand, let the tension remove itself . . . feel the muscles become loose . . . and notice the contrast between the tension a moment ago and the relaxation, the absence of tension. . . . Allowing the fingers to relax . . . and then the entire right hand.

*Reprinted with permission of Macmillan Publishing Company from *Psychology in Sports: Method and Application,* by Richard M. Suinn. Copyright © 1980 by Macmillan Publishing Co.

(Repeat the exercise for the right hand once.)

Now we'll leave the right hand relaxed and focus on the left hand. Tense the left hand by making it into a fist . . . very tight . . . and again notice how that tension feels . . . focus your attention on the muscles as they are tense. . . . All right, now relax the hand, and notice the contrast between the tension of a moment ago and the relaxation. . . . Continue to be aware of the relaxation of the muscles . . . in the fingers . . . and throughout the entire hand.

(Repeat the exercise for the left hand once.)

Arms (Biceps)   We'll leave the hands and the fingers relaxed and move to the biceps. In order to tense the biceps, you will be bending the arm at the elbow and tightening the biceps by moving your hand toward your shoulder. Let's start with the right arm.

Bend your right arm at the elbow so that your hand moves toward your shoulder . . . tight. . . . Keep tightening the biceps as hard as you can . . . focusing your attention on the muscle tension. . . . Really notice how that feels. . . . Now relax . . . letting the arm and hand drop back down . . . and noticing the relaxation, the absence of tension. . . . Feel the relaxation as it takes over the upper arm. . . . Notice the feeling of relaxation in the lower arm, the hand, and the fingers.

(Repeat the exercise for the right arm once.)

Now leave the right arm relaxed and move to the left arm. Tense up the left arm by bending it at the elbow . . . really tense, as tense as you can get it . . . and focus your attention on the feelings of tension. . . . Now relax, letting your arm drop back down. . . . Notice the difference in feeling between the tension and relaxation. . . . Permit the relaxation to take over the entire left arm . . . the upper arm . . . the forearm . . . the hands . . . and fingers.

(Repeat the exercise for the left arm once.)

Forehead   We'll leave the hands and the arms comfortably relaxed and move to the forehead. In order to tense up the forehead, you will frown.

All right, I want you to tense the forehead by frowning. . . . Wrinkle up the forehead area . . . very tight . . . and notice how the tension feels. . . . Now relax. . . . Let the wrinkles smooth themselves out. . . . Allow the relaxation to proceed on its own . . . making the forehead smooth and tension free, as though you were passing your hand over a sheet to smooth it out.

(Repeat the exercise for the forehead once.)

Eyes   We'll leave the forehead relaxed and move to the eyes. What I want you to do is close your eyes tighter than they are . . . tighter . . . feeling the tension. . . . (Use less time for tension here so as to avoid afterimages). . . . Now relax . . . keeping the eyes comfortably closed . . . noticing the contrast between the tension and the relaxation now.

(Repeat the exercise for the eyes once.)

Facial Area   We'll leave the eyes relaxed and go on to the facial area. To tense up the facial area, I want you to clench your jaws. . . . Bite down on your teeth hard now. . . . Really pay attention to the tension in the facial area and jaws. . . . (Use less time for tension here). . . . Now relax. . . . Let the muscles of the jaws become relaxed. . . . Notice the feeling of relaxation across the lips, the jaws, the entire facial area. . . . Just allow the relaxation to take over.

(Repeat the exercise for the facial area once.)

All right, notice the relaxation in the right hand and the fingers . . . and the feeling of relaxation in the forearm and the upper arms. . . . Notice the relaxation that is present in the left hand and the fingers . . . in the forearm. . . . Let the relaxation take over and include the forehead . . . smooth and without tension . . . the eyes . . . the facial area . . . and the lips and the jaws.

Chest   All right, we'll now proceed to help the relaxation across the chest. I want you to tense up the chest muscles by taking a deep breath and holding it for a moment. . . . Notice the tension. . . . Now slowly exhale, breathing normally again . . . and notice the chest muscles as they become more and more relaxed.

(Repeat the exercise for the chest once.)

Abdomen   Now we'll move to the stomach. I want you to tense your stomach right now . . . very tight. . . . Pay attention to the tension. . . . Now relax . . . letting the feeling of relaxation take over. . . . Notice the difference in the feeling of tension a moment before and the relaxation.

(Repeat the exercise for the abdomen once.)

Legs and Feet   Now we'll proceed with the relaxation. To tense your legs and feet, I want you to point your toes downward until you can feel the muscles of your leg tense. . . . Notice the tension. . . . (Maintain the tension for only about three seconds to avoid cramping of the toes or feet). . . . Now relax. . . . Let the relaxation take over. . . . Feel the comfort.

(Repeat the exercise for the legs and feet once.)

All right, simply enjoy the sense of relaxation and comfort across your body . . . feeling loose and relaxed in the hands and fingers . . . comfortable in the forearms and upper arms . . . noticing the relaxed feeling as it includes the forehead . . . the eyes . . . the facial area . . . the lips and the jaws . . . letting the relaxation include the chest . . . the abdomen . . . and both feet.

Now, to further increase the relaxation, I want you to take a deep breath and slowly exhale . . . using your rhythmical deep breathing to deepen the relaxation and to permit you to become as relaxed as you want . . . breathing slowly in and out . . . using your rhythm to achieve whatever level of relaxation you want . . . and in the future you can use this deep-breathing technique to initiate or to deepen the relaxation whenever you want.

All right, that's fine. . . . Now let your breathing continue normally.

Termination of Exercise In a moment, I'll count backward from three to one. When I get to one, you'll feel alert and refreshed . . . no aches or pains. . . . You can retain the relaxed feeling as long as you wish. . . . All right, three . . . more and more alert . . . two . . . no aches or pains . . . and one . . . you can open your eyes.

Autogenic Training

Autogenic training also has been useful in modifying the stress response. Autogenic training emphasizes concentrating on your muscular and involuntary functions, as well as on your mental state, to regulate yourself perceptually, physiologically, mentally, and muscularly. Through autogenic training, for example, you can regulate your heart rate, respiration, and muscle tension. In addition, self-regulation of your mental state allows you to imagine various states of feeling, to visualize concrete and abstract objects, and to experience colors.

Autogenic training involves three phases: (1) the preparation phase, (2) the relaxation phase, and (3) the activation phase.

Preparation Phase

1. Find a comfortable position—lying on your back is the most common.
2. Breathe deeply and concentrate on your depth of breathing.
3. Tighten all of the muscles in your body as hard as you can for a brief second and then relax as completely as possible. Repeat this procedure three times.

Relaxation Phase

4. Think about making one of your arms as heavy as possible—so heavy that it cannot be lifted.
5. Repeat this with the other arm and then with each of your legs, one at a time, and then with your chest muscles and abdominal muscles.

6. Repeat this procedure several times until you feel totally relaxed.

7. Ignore your environment and concentrate on yourself, particularly your body parts.

8. After a few minutes of relaxation, imagine that first one limb and then another are becoming warm. Repeat this several times with all of the muscle groups until you experience a feeling of warmth.

Activation Phase

9. At the end of the relaxation exercise, you will feel relaxed and refreshed. If you fall asleep during the procedure, don't worry about it. Don't be in a hurry to activate yourself. Stay under the ''spell'' for a while, enjoying the feeling of relaxation. Let the feeling of relaxation reinforce you for the events to come.

10. After several minutes of relaxation or when you desire to become activated, gradually tighten your muscles in the same order that you relaxed them. Imagine a level of activation that you would like to assume while you are tightening the muscles. Once you have achieved a satisfactory level of activation, reintroduce yourself to your daily activities.

Key Terms

Alarm Reaction Stage
The first stage of the stress response, during which your body initially reacts to stress

Autogenic Training
A stress management technique that emphasizes concentrating on your muscular and involuntary functions, as well as on your mental state, to regulate yourself perceptually, physiologically, mentally, and muscularly

Exhaustion Stage
The third stage of the stress response, during which your body can no longer deal effectively with stress

Progressive Relaxation Exercise
A stress management technique involving progressive muscle relaxation

Resistance Stage
The second stage of the stress response, during which your body increases its capacity to deal with stress

Stress Response
A physiological response to stress that results in heightened mental and physical awareness

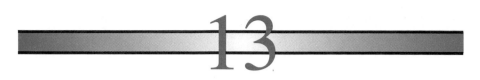

Other Risks to Health and Fitness

After you have studied this chapter you should be able to

1. differentiate between a sprain and a strain;

2. describe injury to the growth plate of the long bones;

3. describe the causes of leg cramps and the purpose of muscle massage;

4. describe tennis elbow;

5. describe shinsplints;

6. describe stress fractures;

7. describe Achilles tendon problems;

8. discuss the important criteria in selecting a running shoe;

9. describe the problems associated with exercising in hot weather;

10. describe the problems associated with exercising in cold weather;

11. describe altitude sickness;

12. describe the risk factors associated with sexually transmitted diseases; and

13. discuss preventive measures against sexually transmitted diseases.

Risk Factors in Exercise

A variety of problems and risks to your general health and fitness can be associated with rigorous physical exercise. These risks and problems are divided into three major areas: common injuries, environmental problems, and sexually transmitted diseases. The section on common injuries deals with injuries to the ligaments, tendons, muscles, and bones and offers tips on prevention and treatment. The next section concerns exercise and environmental problems such as altitude and warm and cold weather. Special precautions and clothing requirements also are discussed. The final section in the chapter deals with sexually transmitted diseases and includes information on risk factors and prevention.

Common Injuries

Many of the injuries that occur during exercise are avoidable (see table 13.1). Some athletes are injured because they push themselves too hard and too long, or they take unnecessary risks, such as running over rough and uneven terrain, where injuries are more likely to occur. Also, many individuals are unaware of how easily they can injure themselves. They launch into such activities as tennis and racquetball, which require a lot of repetitions, without a proper warm-up. As a result, the continuous hitting and running movements required in these sports greatly stress muscles, tendons, and ligaments, causing breakdowns, inflammation, and pain. Even well-conditioned individuals who have played tennis for a long time can be afflicted with an inflamed elbow from overuse. Individuals who do a lot of rope jumping or jogging on hard surfaces run the risk of tendon injuries and stress fractures.

Probably the most common injury to the average exerciser, however, is tendinitis. Tendinitis occurs when the tendon is overstressed during exercise. The resulting inflammation and pain may make the area tender and sore for a long time. A good example is jumper's knee, which is an inflammation of the tendon where it attaches to the patella or the kneecap. Jumper's knee usually is the result of small tears in the tendon that have not healed properly. This condition is most common in basketball players and high jumpers, but also can occur in individuals who do a lot of running, jogging, or jumping.

In any exercise or sport in which you participate, make sure that you (1) warm up properly, (2) don't overstress the muscles and joints at the beginning of an activity, and (3) use moderation in repetitive activity. If you don't, you may find yourself suffering from one or more of the common injuries discussed here.

Sprains and Strains

A **sprain** is an injury to a ligament, a fibrous tissue that holds bones together and stabilizes them to form a joint. A ligament has very little elasticity, and if it is stretched beyond its elastic limit, the result may be a permanent injury. In some cases, the ligament may even rupture and break.

Ligament sprains are very common injuries in sports, occurring frequently in the knees and ankles. Many times, a ligament sprain results in immediate pain, but the degree of pain is not always related to the severity of the injury. Less severe ligament injuries may be very painful, while more severe ligament injuries, particularly around the knee, may become painless in a few minutes. If a

TABLE 13.1	Factors That Lead to Injuries

- Overdoing it and pushing too hard
- Inadequate footwear and equipment
- Poor conditioning
- Weak, tight muscles
- Improper training technique

- No warm-up or stretching
- Ignoring aches and pains
- Repetitive activities
- Exercising too soon after injury

ligament is completely torn, there may be an absence of pain but abnormal motion when the joint is moved.

The treatment for a ligament sprain generally involves protecting the ligament until it has the opportunity to grow together. A unique characteristic of the new growth after injury is that it does not consist of more ligament tissue, but rather heals with a scar. Sometimes, surgeons suture the torn ligament together so that the scar that connects the two ends will be shorter. Excessive scar tissue can predispose the joint to further injury.

A **strain** is an injury to a muscle or tendon and results when the muscle or tendon is pulled excessively or torn. A tendon is the end of the muscle that attaches to the bone. A tendon is elastic, but in some cases its elasticity is limited, and it can be overstretched and pulled away from the bone. Often, a strain is accompanied by the swelling and bleeding of soft tissue, and this may increase the severity of the pain. As with a ligament sprain, the degree of pain associated with muscle or tendon strain may not be related to the severity of the injury.

There is some debate as to how a strain should be treated. One method involves actively stretching the muscle and tendon throughout the healing process so that the muscle or tendon does not heal shortened, which could lead to subsequent injuries. Another treatment prohibits all activity until the muscle and tendon heal. Then the muscle is gradually stretched to its normal length.

Bone Growth and Injury

The long bones in the body, before reaching maximum length between the ages of sixteen and eighteen, are divided into three separate parts—two ends and a shaft. The ends are connected to the bone shaft by cartilage (semielastic hard tissue covering bones) at a location called the growth plate. The cells of the growth plate eventually mature and fuse the ends of the bones to the shaft to form one solid bone. An injury to the growth plate can damage these cell layers and prevent them from growing properly. As a result, the bone may be deformed or not grow as long as it should have. It is therefore vital that anytime a child injures a bone or joint in an arm or leg that the injury be carefully examined by a physician to determine if the growth plate has been damaged.

Leg Cramps

Cramps are sustained muscle contractions and usually occur in the calf muscle and the lower leg. Early research indicated that cramps resulted from the salt loss that occurred because of excessive sweating. Research now, however, indicates that cramps may result from a reduction in fluid volume. Therefore, an individual who has frequent cramps in hot weather should try to drink as much fluid as possible (hydrate) before and during rigorous activity.

When a muscle goes into a cramp, it squeezes against the artery and partially cuts off the flow of blood. A reduced flow of blood to the muscle (ischemia) results in pain. Generally, when the muscle goes into **muscle tetanus** (sustained contraction), the best treatment is to stretch the muscle by extending the joint or to press gradually on the body of the muscle, forcing it to stretch. This allows blood to flow to the muscle again, thereby reducing the spasm and pain.

A muscle that has gone into tetanus or that has been injured should not be vigorously massaged. In these situations, massage actuates the stretch reflex, which increases the muscle spasm and leads to further pain and swelling. Generally, massage should be used for body relaxation. During massage, small skin receptors set off a reflex activity, which relaxes the body. Massage also results in the dilation of blood vessels close to the skin surface, which may aid in the return of blood flow to the limb.

Tennis Elbow

Tennis elbow is pain in the upper arm near the elbow and is caused by injury to the muscles that extend the wrist. This affliction gets its name because of the constant hand and wrist flexing and extension of the forearm during tennis that can lead to injury and produce severe pain. In some cases, tennis elbow can be disabling to the point where the person no longer can shake hands or move the hand in a rotating motion.

Generally, X rays of tennis elbow show no sign of change in the bone. In some cases, there may be swelling and inflammation of the tendon (tendinitis). Aspirin is sometimes effective in reducing the pain, and avoiding tennis for two weeks may be the best remedy. In some cases, cortisone is injected into the area of pain; this results in immediate relief, but the pain, unfortunately, returns in a few hours. In very severe cases, surgery is a possibility since the muscle attachment may have pulled away from the bone.

Shinsplints

Shinsplints is a term given to a number of injuries that produce pain in the lower leg. The symptoms are pain on the inner side of the shinbone (tibia) in the front part of the leg. The pain usually is associated with running or jogging. Sometimes, it comes on very slowly and eventually may become quite severe. In some cases, the muscle may even pull away from the bone, or there may be small tears in the muscle where it attaches to the shinbone. In other cases, the pain may be due to a stress fracture, blocked circulation, lowered arch, or damage to nerves in the leg. The condition generally does not result in permanent disability.

The best cure for shinsplints is rest. Wearing good shoes with a firm heel support, avoiding running on hard surfaces, and proper warm-up before running sometimes can prevent or reduce the severity of this kind of injury. Running in a reversed direction (clockwise) on a curved track along with concentrating on a heel-to-toe foot stride also have been found to be preventive measures.

Stress Fractures

Stress fractures are very small, minute cracks appearing in any bone that has been stressed repeatedly in such activities as jogging on hard surfaces or jumping for long periods of time. Although a stress fracture becomes painful and during activity is very tender to the touch, this condition cannot be detected in an X ray until two or three weeks after the injury. For this reason, it is important that you don't ignore the pain and continue with your activity, since then an actual break can occur in the bone.

Achilles Tendon Problems

A common running injury occurs in the Achilles tendon, the tendon that connects your calf muscle with your heel. Under the normal stress of running, small tears may occur in the Achilles tendon, but they normally heal in a short time. Once the tendon has been weakened by small tears, however, stair climbing, running up a hill, or similar activities may cause additional tearing. If the leg is continually stressed by exercise, the tendon may become inflamed.

Treatment for an inflamed Achilles tendon consists of ice massage twice a day. If the tendon is torn, ice massage and a heel lift (a small piece of material placed under the heel in the shoe to slightly elevate the heel), along with a four- to six-week layoff from exercise, are recommended. If the tear requires surgery, it is important to consult an orthopedic expert who knows something about the problems of runners.

Preventing Injuries Through Proper Shoe Selection

Jogging or running with improperly fitting or poor-quality shoes can result in a variety of back, knee, ankle, and foot problems. When selecting a shoe, keep some basic principles in mind:

1. Purchase a quality shoe. A number of good brands are on the market. Be wary of so-called low-priced running shoes. Proper footwear is important in any physical activity. Remember—you are going to spend many hours in them in all kinds of conditions. So don't be afraid to invest a few extra dollars.

2. Solicit advice about what shoe to purchase from some of your running friends, and check a few specialty stores.

3. If you run on a grass or dirt surface, you need less cushion in the shoe but good traction and stability. If you run on pavement, you need adequate cushioning. Be careful, however, because too much cushion leads to reduced stability.

4. Do you have a rigid foot or a floppy foot? If you have a rigid foot, the wear spots will be on the outside of your shoe. You probably should select a cushioned shoe that is slip-lasted. If you have a floppy foot, your shoe will wear in various spots on the sole where your foot pushes against the ground. You need a more stable shoe with a little less cushion and a broad last (wider form).

5. Do you have a straight foot or a curved foot? If you have a straight foot and wear a curved shoe, you will feel pressure on the outside of each foot. If you have a curved foot and wear a straight shoe, you will feel pressure on your toes. The shape of your shoe should correspond to the shape of your foot. Be sure there are no areas of pressure or pain or a feeling of binding.

6. The ball of the foot of the shoe should be flexible, the heel should be flared for greater stability, and the tread should be grooved for enhanced gripping.

Environmental Problems

Hundreds of thousands of individuals who live in a variety of extreme climatic conditions in the United States actively participate in year-round sports. Few cross-country and downhill skiers, hikers, and mountaineers, however, understand the environmental problems associated with high altitudes and cold; few marathon runners and tennis players understand the environmental problems associated with extremely hot climates. Exercise in cold and hot climates without taking the proper precautions may not only lead to slight discomfort but also to serious injury and death.

Exercise in Hot Weather

Exercise in hot environments increases the need for an excess amount of blood flow to the working muscles and also to the skin to maintain body temperature. If the amount of blood necessary to meet the demands exceeds the amount the heart can pump out, a type of circulatory shock or overload occurs. This overload can result in problems with temperature regulation, accompanied by symptoms of dizziness and fainting. In some cases, there may be serious medical consequences.

In temperatures above ninety to ninety-five degrees Fahrenheit exercise should be prohibited. With high humidity, 40 to 50 percent, and temperatures between seventy-five and ninety degrees Fahrenheit exercise intensity should be reduced. Any sudden feeling of being chilled, signaling a failure in the sweating mechanism, may lead to a high body temperature and heat stroke. Acclimatization to heat generally takes from one to two weeks. See table 13.2 for other heat-related problems.

To avoid problems when exercising in hot weather, begin with moderate exercise and gradually increase to the desired intensity over a period of days. This gives the body time to physiologically acclimate itself to the demands made by high temperatures. For example, the heart rate generally decreases, and the amount of blood that flows through the skin decreases, which allows more blood to flow through the deep muscles, where it is needed for the exercise. Also, blood pressure is more adequately maintained, sweating is more efficient, and the sweat that is produced evaporates more effectively. You also lose less salt. In addition to those physiological changes, you are more resistant to dizziness, fainting, and nausea, which are common problems for individuals who exercise in hot weather.

Also important when exercising in hot weather is the frequent ingestion of water and the wearing of clothing that allows for a large skin surface and sweat evaporation. Wear light, porous, short-sleeved shirts and shorts and avoid long socks and warm-up suits. It also is important to protect the top of your head from overheating. In severe heat, a wet cloth, handkerchief, or sock on the top of your head underneath your hat will prove invaluable in keeping the top of your head cool.

Other hot-weather exercise topics include water substitutes, salt needs in hot weather, water loss from exercise in a hot environment, sweating, and long-distance running under very warm conditions.

TABLE 13.2 Heat-Related Problems

Heat illness	Signs and symptoms	Immediate care
Heat syncope	Headache, Nausea	Normal intake of fluids
Heat cramps	Muscle cramping (calf is very common)	Isolated cramps: Direct pressure to cramp and release, stretch muscle slowly and gently, gentle massage, ice
	Multiple cramping (very serious)	Multiple cramps: Danger of heat stroke, *treat as heat exhaustion*
Heat exhaustion	Profuse sweating	Move individual out of sun to a well-ventilated area
	Cold, clammy skin	
	Normal temperature or slightly elevated	Place in shock position (feet elevated 12–18 in); prevent heat loss or gain
	Pale	Gentle massage of extremities
	Dizzy	Gentle range of motion of the extremities
	Weak, rapid pulse	Force fluids
	Shallow breathing	Reassure
	Nausea	Monitor body temperature and other vital signs
	Headache	Refer to physician
	Loss of consciousness	
Heat stroke	Generally, no perspiration	This is an *extreme medical emergency*
	Dry skin	Transport to hospital quickly
	Very hot	Remove as much clothing as possible without exposing the individual
	Temperature as high as 106° F	
	Skin color bright red or flushed (blacks—ashen)	Cool quickly starting at the head and continuing down the body; use any means possible (fan, hose down, pack in ice)
	Rapid and strong pulse	
	Labored breathing—semi-reclining position	Wrap in cold, wet sheets for transport
		Treat for shock; if breathing is labored, place in a semi-reclining position

---

From ''Injury Prevention & Treatment'' by Sue Carver. In Health Fitness Instructor's Handbook, 2nd Edition (pp. 300) by E. T. Howly & B. D. Franks (Eds.). Champaign, IL: Human Kinetics Publishers. Copyright 1992 by Edward T. Howley and B. Don Franks. Reprinted by permission.

Water Substitutes

Water substitutes—or as they are more commonly called, sweat replacers—are used frequently by athletes who exercise in hot weather. Gatorade thirst quencher is one example. These water substitutes are mixtures of glucose, sodium, chloride, potassium, magnesium, calcium, and water—all substances that the body loses through sweat during exercise in intense heat. Sweat replacers put these important substances back into the system more efficiently than water. Even though these mixtures resemble the composition of sweat (except for the glucose), they probably are absorbed less rapidly than water because of the glucose, which tends to slow down absorption. In fact, it takes an hour for the stomach to absorb one liter of water; it takes even longer for it to absorb a liter of sweat replacer. A good replenishing drink aside from plain water should consist of approximately 2.5 grams of sugar per 100 milliliters of water, forty to fifty-five degrees, and consumed in a volume ranging from three to ten ounces.

Salt Needs in Hot Weather

The normal daily intake of salt is about ten to twelve grams. Even under very severe conditions, you do not lose more than thirteen to seventeen grams of salt a day. Normally, the amount of salt needed can be supplied to the body through a normal diet; therefore, the use of salt tablets is unnecessary. Also keep in mind that more water than salt is lost during exercise. Therefore, taking salt tablets without an adequate amount of water is far worse than taking no salt tablets at all. Modest salting of food should be followed for athletic events exceeding fifty to sixty minutes.

Water Loss

In hot weather, the weight lost from exercising over short periods of time is primarily due to water loss, not a breakdown of fatty tissue. This weight quickly returns when you eat and drink. More important, however, is that a large water loss can be very dangerous.

The best way to determine your water loss is to weigh yourself before and after exercise. Water loss of 3 percent or less of total body weight is fairly safe, 5 percent or less is borderline, but anything over 7 percent can severely affect the functioning of the heart and circulatory system. It is possible to lose six to seventeen pounds of water within twenty-four hours, and this amount of water lost through exercise must be replaced. If it isn't, the body stops producing sweat, body temperature increases sharply, and an imbalance in electrolytes occurs. (Sodium, potassium, and chloride collectively are referred to as **electrolytes.** They are present in the body in the form of electrically charged particles called ions. Electrolytes' main function is to control fluid exchange in various body tissues.)

It is not uncommon for a person exercising in hot weather to lose considerable amounts of water and not feel thirsty. You should not depend on your natural feeling of thirst to satisfy your body's needs for water replacement.

Sweating

During rigorous exercise, efficient sweating indicates that the body is responding well to the increase in body temperature. Sweating provides water to the surface area of the skin; there the water evaporates into the air, which cools the body and regulates body temperature. Evaporation of sweat depends upon three fac-tors: the skin surface area exposed to the environment, temperature and relative humidity of the air, and convective air currents around the body. High levels of relative humidity (ratio of water to air) reduce evaporation of sweat, which then rolls off the skin instead of drying and cooling it. Also, toweling off frequently prevents sweat from evaporating and cooling the body.

Large areas of the skin should be exposed for efficient sweating because the skin surface is important for sweat evaporation. Approximately 50 percent of all sweat is lost from the trunk area of the body, 25 percent is lost from the head and the upper limbs, and 25 percent is lost from the lower limbs. When exercising in hot weather, wear light, loose-fitting clothing, such as shorts and a shirt made of light-weight material or a cotton/polyester blend with large holes. Avoid hoods, towels around your head and neck, rubber belts, and sweat suits, which increase body temperature and cause fluid loss.

Long-Distance Running in Hot Weather

Competitive races covering distances over ten miles should not be conducted when the temperature exceeds twenty-eight degrees Celsius or eighty-eight de-grees Fahrenheit (wet bulb). During periods of the year when the daylight tem-perature exceeds these limits, races should be conducted before 9:00 A.M. or after 4:00 P.M. Race sponsors should provide fluids that contain small amounts of sugar (less than 2.5 grams glucose per 100 milliliters of water) and electrolytes, such as sodium and potassium. Frequent ingestion of fluids during competition is im-portant, as is consuming thirteen to twenty ounces of fluid thirty minutes before the race and 3.6 to 5 ounces during the activity. There should be water stations at every 2- to 2.5-mile interval for all races ten miles and longer. Unless these simple precautions are taken, endurance running in hot climates can result in serious physical disability and sometimes death.

Exercise in Cold Weather

Exercise in cold weather is generally less stressful on the circulatory system because there is less body heat production. Running or cycling in cold weather, however, can reduce body temperature because of the chill factor, especially if there is a wind. In these cases and also when the temperature drops below forty degrees Fahrenheit, you need some protection. Make sure that your head and hands are covered. Materials made from wool or polypropylene are excellent. Wind or rain suits made from Goretex or PTFE-film keep you dry and also allow heat to escape. When it is extremely cold, dress in layers, so that when you exercise, you can take off clothing as your body temperature goes up.

Keep in mind that retention of heat causes excessive sweating, even in freezing weather. If your skin surface is covered by heavy clothing, sweat cannot evaporate efficiently and cool the body. As a result, body temperature rises further, and large amounts of sweat permeate socks and underclothing. When you stop exercising, the sweat-soaked clothing may freeze, which could result in some very severe consequences.

Downhill Running

Running downhill, contrary to popular belief, is much riskier for the joints and muscles in your feet and legs than running uphill. As you go downhill you speed up, your stride lengthens, and your impact with the ground increases. These factors cause you to run with a distorted gait that can leave you with muscle soreness and pain behind the kneecap (runner's knee). To avoid injury, never run straight down a steep hill; walk or run in a zigzag pattern, leaning slightly forward and keeping your knees bent.

Altitude Sickness

Many individuals experience headaches, feelings of drowsiness, insomnia, and a lack of appetite at altitudes as low as 2,600 meters. This is called **altitude sickness.** In serious cases of altitude sickness, fluid accumulates in the lungs, which sometimes is erroneously diagnosed as pneumonia. If individuals in this condition are given antibiotics without being taken to lower altitudes, they may die. Altitude sickness also produces an intolerance to fatty foods that may result in nausea and vomiting. In some cases, the symptoms of altitude sickness are paradoxically euphoric, rather than disabling, and the individual may experience feelings of well-being, especially during the first night. Most people are affected to some degree by altitude sickness at altitudes over 4,300 meters.

The most effective remedy for altitude sickness is gradual descent to lower altitudes to minimize the symptoms. A diet high in carbohydrates and low in fat and the avoidance of strenuous exercise at high altitudes also can reduce the severity of altitude sickness.

Air Pollution and Exercise

In some parts of the United States, the atmosphere contains many pollutants, such as nitrogen oxide, sulfur oxide, carbon dioxide, and particulate matter such as dust and solid particles. Also, ozone, which results from the sun's action on nitrogen dioxide, and hydrocarbon from automobile exhaust are major pollutants. Some evidence indicates that ozone can reduce an individual's ability to bring in oxygen and thus interferes with such aerobic activities as long-distance running and jogging. Also, particulate matter and fumes can increase resistance to air flow to the lungs and result in less efficiency. Pollutants not only affect physical

---

TABLE 13.3 Risk Factors for STDs

1. If you do not have sex, you have virtually no chance of getting an STD.
2. If you only have sex with a single partner who does not have sex with other partners and both of you do not have an STD, you have practically no risk of being infected.
3. If you have sex with a few people you know well, your risk increases.
4. If your partner has sex with others, you are more at risk because you have no control over your partner's partner.
5. If you have sex with many partners, you are at high risk, particularly with people you do not know well.

The use of condoms, along with spermicidals (containing nonoxynol-9), is the most effective preventative measure against STDs. Other important measures include washing and urinating after sex. While these measures do not provide infallible protection, they can weigh the odds significantly in your favor.

---

performance—their long-term toxic effects on the lungs and circulatory system are well documented. If air is particularly smoggy, exercise indoors; otherwise, exercise outdoors after morning rush hour, in open windy areas. In the afternoon the wind is stronger and helps disperse pollutants.

STDs and Wellness

STDs may be a new term for you. It stands for sexually transmitted diseases. Over ten million people from all walks of life get STDs every year. Most STDs are easily treatable, yet many people suffer guilt, embarrassment, anger, and fear when notified that they have an STD. The force of their reaction, the hostility, guilt, and fear, is a reflection of our society's attitude towards sexuality. In one society, many people—out of their own fear of illness—judge the sick and handicapped as responsible for their own illness and consequently treat them with indifference and disdain. To avoid identifying with the afflicted people, many may ignore STD symptoms, avoid screening tests, feel embarrassed to seek care, and continue to engage sexually with others, in spite of the possibilities of transmitting the infection.

Risk Factors

If you are sexually active, whatever your age, race, occupation, or sexual preference, you are at risk, and your risk is increasing because more and more people are getting STDs (see table 13.3 for risk factors). Furthermore, new STDs are being identified. The key to reducing your risks is to be informed. If you think you have an STD, go to a doctor or clinic right away. While some STDs are minor, others may have serious consequences. If you learn to recognize STD symptoms (see appendix D) and get early treatment, most infections can be quickly and painlessly cured.

The following are some tips on dealing with STDs.

Key Factors in Dealing with STDs

Be able to recognize symptoms; they are the body's warning signs of disease.

Be aware that some STDs are symptomless, especially in early stages.

Get early treatment; if treated early, most STDs can be cured, and others can be controlled.

Early treatment reduces complications and keeps you from infecting others.

Tell the doctor everything.

When being treated don't share medication.

Don't take old medication for STDs.

Tell your partner to get treatment.

Take precautions during treatment.

Take all medications prescribed.

Go back for a follow-up.

Practice prevention.

Exercise and Disease Resistance

There is very little evidence to link rigorous exercise with increased susceptibility to disease. It is possible that hormones released by the adrenal glands during stress from overexertion may inhibit certain immune responses, but the facts are not clear as to whether this leads to an increase in the infection process. No evidence at the present time indicates that the physical stress resulting from athletic activity predisposes an individual to susceptibility to infection.

Another related question is whether stress resulting from physical activity can aggravate an already existing infection. Again, there is very little evidence in this regard. If a person has a very high body temperature and an infection, especially a respiratory infection, rigorous physical activity can cause sudden changes in body temperature and can irritate the infected tissue, thereby increasing the infection.

Exercising when you have a virus infection, runny nose, sneezing, aching, and other symptoms of mild upper respiratory infection is not advised. Working off the infection through exercise may even be dangerous since the virus could find its way to your heart muscle, resulting in myocarditis, which inflames and damages the heart muscle. Avoid exercise until your symptoms have disappeared.

Individuals with asthma who overexert themselves through exercise or breathe in too much cold air may induce bronchial spasms. Also, some evidence indicates that a small percentage of the population who do not have classical asthma can bring on asthmatic-like symptoms by rapidly breathing in cool air. This is a common occurrence among runners in cool environments.

Key Terms

Altitude Sickness
A serious disease encountered at levels as low as 2,600 meters that may produce headaches, insomnia, drowsiness, lack of appetite, nausea and vomiting, and lung congestion

Electrolytes
Electrically charged particles, such as sodium, potassium, and chloride

Muscle Tetanus
Sustained muscle contraction

Shinsplints
A number of injuries that produce pain in the anterior portion of the lower leg

Sprain
An injury to a ligament

STDs
Sexually transmitted diseases

Strain
An injury to a muscle or tendon

Stress Fracture
Small, minute cracks in the bone

Tennis Elbow
Pain in the upper arm near the elbow; caused by injury to the muscles that extend the wrist

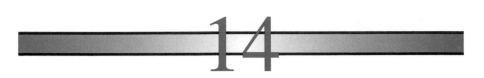

chapter

Special Considerations

Chapter Concepts

After you have studied this chapter you should be able to

1. describe the major differences between male and female athletes in relation to physical performance;
2. describe the effects of rigorous exercise on menstruation, pregnancy, childbirth, and osteoporosis;
3. describe the effects of maintaining fitness with age;
4. discuss the main benefits of competitive sports;
5. describe important factors in preparing for competition;
6. describe the effect that individual differences have on competitive intensity;

7. discuss methods of achieving and maintaining advanced fitness;
8. discuss the physical requirements for long aerobic competition;
9. explain the general guidelines for long-distance running;
10. describe interval training;
11. describe over-distance training; and
12. describe other aerobic and anaerobic options for advanced fitness.

Females and Exercise

F emale athletic competition and participation in physical activities has increased markedly, as antiquated social mores regarding women's involvement in sports and exercise have fallen away. Research on the effects of exercise on the female is scarce. The following sections discuss differences between male and female athletes; how exercise affects menstruation, pregnancy, and childbirth; and the iron and calcium needs of females.

277

Cultural images about women participating in athletics are changing. Male and female collegiate students in one survey[1] describe female athletes as strong, brave, strong willed, healthy, and leaders. The stigma of athletic competition for women is finally on the decline.

In physical performance women are gaining on men. Although the gap in performance and standards between men and women continues, it has narrowed markedly since 1970. In running (100 meter dash and marathon) and swimming (100 meter freestyle and butterfly) women athletes are within 98 percent of the men's records. Also, women's marathon times have dropped by nearly an hour in just fifteen years.

Differences Between Male and Female Athletes

A number of physiological differences between females and males can result in differences in physical performance. For example, women have a lower center of gravity, which means that they are not as top-heavy as men. As a result, women have better stability, which gives them an advantage in such sports as the martial arts and balancing activities. In addition, women have approximately 19 to 24 percent body fat compared to 12 to 17 percent for males. The additional fat gives them better buoyancy in the water. This, combined with their lower center of gravity, enables females to maintain body alignment with less physical effort in the water, which results in more efficient swimming movements. The additional fat also serves as insulation, giving women the advantage of being able to maintain body temperature more efficiently in cold water.

Men, on the other hand, exceed women in maximum oxygen consumption during exercise. This is believed to be due to greater cardiac output, blood volume, and oxygen-carrying capacity of the blood. Also, because men have more lean muscle in relation to total body weight than women, they have about 30 to 40 percent greater absolute strength. Their overall stores of energy-rich compounds, such as ATP, PC, and glycogen, also are greater.

Women's response to physical training in terms of cardiorespiratory endurance, muscle metabolism, and strength, however, is similar to that of men.

Rigorous Exercise and Menstruation

While a variety of misconceptions and taboos have had women believe otherwise, no research indicates that exercise causes serious health problems during menstruation. Many women do have pain with menstruation, called **dysmenorrhea,** with the degree of discomfort varying from one individual to another. Normally,

1. C. Atkin, C. Mores and R. Schweigenhaft. "The Stereotyped and Recognition of Female Athletes." *Journal of Psychology* 100 (1978): 27–31.

however, this discomfort should not prevent women from participating in physical activity. As a matter of fact, evidence indicates that physical activity may in some cases reduce the symptoms of menstrual pain.

Some physicians believe that certain exercises, such as skiing, tennis, gymnastics, and rowing, carry greater incidence of menstrual disorder, and they support reduced competition in these areas when women are menstruating. However, little evidence supports this concept.

Evidence has shown that approximately one-third of competitive female long-distance runners between the ages of twelve and forty-five experience **amenorrhea** (cessation of menstruation) or **oligomenorrhea** (irregular menstruation) for brief periods. The incidence is usually related to the number of miles run: the longer the distance, the higher the incidence of irregularity. These problems also are found in some gymnasts, swimmers, and dancers, and typically are more common in women who have not given birth or who began menstruating late. The cause of exercise amenorrhea is still unknown. Some of the theories include increased testosterone levels, decreased ovarian function, loss of body fat, and altered pituitary functioning. Presently there is a strong indication that a change in hypothalamic functioning may be responsible. Sufficient calcium replacement is essential for individuals encountering amenorrhea.

Exercise During Pregnancy

No scientific evidence supports the old theory that pregnant women who exercise rigorously develop tense abdominal muscles, which result in problems during delivery. On the contrary, some evidence indicates that women who are athletic have easy labor and fewer undesirable side effects during delivery. If a pregnant woman has medical problems, disease, or other complications, she should seek advice from her obstetrician before undertaking or continuing an exercise program. Extremely rigorous activities that require prolonged endurance or produce a large oxygen debt are discouraged since they could result in reduced oxygen in the circulatory system and an increase in the internal body temperature of the mother and the fetus. Rhythmic, moderate activity, however, is well advised and safe for both mother and fetus. A program of thirty minutes of exercise three times a week is recommended. The following are exercise guidelines during pregnancy:

1. Exercise intensity should not go beyond the 70 percent threshold level. The American College of Obstetricians and Gynecologists cautions against heart rates exceeding 140 beats per minute. However, prepregnancy fitness level is probably a better predictor of maximum allowable heart rate than 140 beats per minute.

2. Exercise should be stopped if there is any pain or bleeding.
3. Adequate intakes of iron, calcium, and vitamins should be maintained before and during pregnancy.
4. Avoid rigorous exercise at high altitudes.
5. Avoid bouncing, jarring, and twisting activities that put your abdomen in jeopardy.
6. If you feel very tired, experience discomfort, or unusual symptoms occur stop and rest.
7. You should not exercise so intensely that you are unable to talk.
8. Don't exercise while lying on your back after the fourth month; this can block blood supply to the uterus and depress fetal heart rate. If you need to rest lie on your side.
9. Don't exercise rigorously in hot humid weather. (Core body temperature should not go above 101 degrees Fahrenheit.) Avoid hot tubs and saunas.
10. Always drink plenty of water before, during, and after exercise.
11. Your exercise program should be started well in advance of pregnancy.
12. Research is not confirmed in the area of the detrimental effects of a pregnant mother being inverted as in such activities as gymnastics and yoga.

Exercise After Childbirth

Women who have just given birth should start exercising as soon as possible if there were no complications and if they have received medical clearance from their physician. They should start slowly because their red blood cell count may be a little low, resulting in feelings of fatigue and shortness of breath. Gradually, over four to six weeks, they should be able to work up to the exercise routine they maintained before they became pregnant. If, during exercise, they feel themselves getting overly tired, they shouldn't force themselves to complete the exercise. Moderation is the key until their bodies start responding and they feel as though they can exercise without undue stress.

Female Iron Needs

The average female needs approximately eighteen milligrams of iron a day. (A pregnant woman, however, needs thirty to sixty milligrams.) The average balanced diet offers about six milligrams of iron per one thousand calories; thus, the less you eat, the less likely you are to get enough iron. In particular, women consuming less than 1,500 calories a day will find it hard to get their recommended daily allowance. Long-distance runners tend to have increased iron losses and lower absorption rates. This may lead to a higher incidence of iron depletion, manifested by below-normal iron stores. The physiological significance of these changes is uncertain, and it is not known whether they impair performance in the absence of anemia.

Liver is the best source of iron, with no other food having such a large concentration. Other fairly good sources, however, include meats, cereals, fruits, and vegetables. Eating meat and vegetables at the same meal enhances the absorption of iron. For the same reason, iron supplements should be taken before meals because high-bulk diets reduce iron absorption.

Exercise requires a great deal of oxygen, which is carried by the red blood cells. Red blood cells are composed of iron. Thus, if you are not getting enough iron, your red blood cell count will be low, and your body won't be getting enough oxygen when you exercise, resulting in excessive fatigue. If you are eating a nutritionally balanced diet and taking iron supplements of eighteen milligrams, however, you should have sufficient energy for exercise.

The use of an intrauterine device (IUD) for contraception carries with it the potential loss of more than normal amounts of menstrual blood each period. Thus, a woman who chooses this method of contraception should be certain that her daily iron intake is sufficient to meet this increased need.

Female Calcium Needs and Osteoporosis

Osteoporosis is a disease in which bone tissue degenerates. It ranks closely behind arthritis as a major chronic disease of older people, especially women. Susceptibility to the disease appears to increase with menopause. It may be that the estrogen decreases that accompany menopause hasten the destruction of bone tissue and also decrease the body's absorption rate of calcium, which is vital for the integrity of the bones.

There is a wide variation in bone density among women. Physical activity, calcium intake throughout life, ability to adapt to low-calcium diets, and fluoride intake are all associated with higher bone density. On the other hand a lack of regular menstruation, premature menopause, use of some medications, and prolonged bed rest are associated with low bone density. It is important, therefore, not to focus attention on calcium when a number of factors play a significant part in this disease. Evidence from the National Institutes of Health indicates that taking calcium supplements after menopause has only a marginal effect on bone loss. The NIH recommends that all adults consume 1,000 milligrams of calcium daily, and post-menopausal women considered to be at high risk for development of osteoporosis should consume an additional 500 milligrams.

Women who take in very little calcium in their diet also may be more susceptible to osteoporosis. Before menopause, approximately 800 milligrams of calcium a day is sufficient for normal nutrition. After menopause, however, women need between 1,000 and 1,500 milligrams of calcium to maintain bone tissue. Milk, which is one of the best sources of calcium, contains only about 1,000 milligrams of calcium per quart. Obviously, then, many older women need calcium supplements to their diets.

Estrogen replacement therapy will eliminate risks for significant osteoporosis in some women who begin this therapy right after menopause and take it for the rest of their lives. However, long-term studies are still lacking even though this therapy is thought to be safe. Unfortunately estrogen therapy is not without some risks. Other therapies such as vitamin D hormone, calcitriol or the hormone calcitonin are available and effective.

More than 1.2 million bone fractures of the hip, spine, and wrist in the elderly are associated with osteoporosis. Between 12 and 20 percent of all elderly who suffer hip fractures eventually die from fracture-related complications. About one-third of all women experience osteoporosis-related fractures in their lifetime.

Don't bank on calcium supplements to prevent osteoporosis. Many calcium pills on the market cannot be effectively absorbed by the body much less forestall the disease. You should only purchase tablets that meet United States pharmacopeia standards. Your best bet is to get your calcium from natural sources. One lowfat cup of milk will provide 300 milligrams, and one cup of lowfat yogurt, 415 milligrams. Other good sources of calcium are salmon, sardines, cheese, and green leafy vegetables.

Lack of exercise also seems to be a contributing factor to osteoporosis. Exercise helps to stimulate the production of new bone tissue. Also, the activity of muscles working against gravity is crucial in maintaining strong bones. Exercise such as walking and jogging adequately satisfies this need. Even though there is no hard evidence that regular exercise prevents osteoporosis, there is plenty of evidence that shows a lack of physical activity hastens bone loss. It is also known that drinking beverages high in phosphorus (such as colas) causes the body to excrete more calcium.

Maintaining Fitness with Age

The health of an individual at each stage of the aging process is based upon the foundations that were laid down in previous years. It is necessary to know what those changes are and how they can be affected by our living habits, such as nutrition and exercise. There is interest in what causes the body to prematurely age or run down.

In addition, exercise for the older person is a phenomenon brought about by a change in social mores and a new perception of the role of exercise in life. It is not uncommon to see older people jogging, swimming, and engaging in a variety of activities. The increased number of individuals exercising has generated an increased interest in the effects of exercise on the body. The interest in exercise is not only limited to maintaining physical fitness but also involves its relationship with chronic diseases associated with aging, such as heart disease, diabetes, high blood pressure, and osteoporosis.

Statistics on population trends indicate that we are becoming a nation of older people. As a result, there is an increased need for evaluation of the aging process, its effects on physical performance, and the roles of exercise and nutrition in preserving our health and vitality.

Aging and Performance Levels

In general, an individual's ability to perform physical activities declines with age. This area, however, has not been researched thoroughly because a number of factors make it very difficult to assess. For example, as a person ages, he or she is more susceptible to a number of diseases, which can affect physical performance. Also, because of the sedentary nature of most Americans, it is very difficult to find an old population to compare with a young population at equal levels of physical activity. Very few studies have analyzed individuals from birth to old age within the same population.

Research, however, has been able to establish a number of facts about how aging affects our bodies. First, overall muscle strength decreases slightly with age. An individual generally achieves maximum strength at about thirty years of age, and there is a slight decrease from that time on. Even at the age of sixty, however, a person's loss of maximum muscle strength is only about 10 to 20 percent of that at age thirty. Research also has determined that the muscles' ability to increase in size (muscle hypertrophy) decreases with age. Muscle hypertrophy, however, usually is not responsible for an increase in strength level. Strength increases usually are due to better coordination and skill and to nerve innervation. However, recently it has been shown that individuals in their seventies and eighties who have undergone a weight-resistance program have gained strength along with muscle hypertrophy. An individual's maximum heart rate (220 minus age) also decreases with age—about forty beats per minute from the age of twenty to the age of seventy-five. Cardiac output, the amount of blood pumped out by the heart, decreases after the age of thirty by approximately 1 percent per year. Also, peripheral blood flow to the extremities decreases. An increased resistance to blood flow caused by hardening of the arteries results in higher blood pressure. Research also has established that the amount of air an individual can bring into the lungs decreases with age because of decreased efficiency of the muscle of the chest wall and also of the lung tissue itself. Two final changes with age: body fat tends to increase as individuals get older and reaction time slows down.

The physiological trainability of an older individual is roughly equal to that of a young adult when expressed on a relative basis, taking into account the various physiological factors of aging. In other words, older persons exercising in an individualized program can maintain levels of strength, cardiac output, and oxygen uptake that are as reasonable for them as are comparable programs for younger individuals.

If the exercise program is of adequate intensity, sequence and duration, physical adaptations will most definitely take place in older people. In addition, healthy, fit elderly can acclimatize to changing environmental conditions. Exercise has shown to produce muscle hypertrophy in the elderly with subsequent increases in muscular strength. Exercise also has a mediating effect on high blood pressure, ischemic heart disease, and a slowed decline in bone density.[2]

Types of Exercise for Older Individuals

An exercise program for an older person should consist of flexibility exercises, calisthenics, and a continuous fast walking or jogging program. Stretching exercises and light calisthenics stimulate the muscles and circulation and also maintain good joint flexibility. In addition, they put a slight load upon the heart. However, it also is important to engage in some continuous, rhythmic activity, such as fast walking or jogging, which is of greater benefit to the cardiovascular system. Heart rate should reach levels of about 112 to 120 beats per minute. The flexibility exercises and calisthenics should be done every day, while the jogging or fast walking exercise is important at least three times a week.

The specific level of fitness needed to mitigate cardiac and other health risk factors in older individuals is an important but still unanswered question. Considerable research indicates that the training level necessary for the heart is approximately 70 percent of maximum. This may not be an appropriate standard, however, for individuals over sixty. It has been found that training responses of the heart in individuals over sixty years of age can be elicited at heart rates as low as 90 to 100 beats per minute. Well-conditioned individuals over sixty years of age require heart rates of approximately 103 to 106 beats per minute to produce a training stimulus. The important point to remember is that training response levels are produced at far lower exercise intensities than was first thought. Older individuals should start at very low heart rate levels—under 100 beats per minute—and increase progressively. The intensity level of the exercise, not the type of exercise, is the critical factor, and the pulse rate should be monitored very carefully. While a younger person usually can proceed rapidly with

2. Evans, W. S. "Exercise, Nutrition and Aging." *Journal of Nutrition* 122 (1992): 796–801.

increasing levels of activity, the older person should take care to gradually increase the exercise load and to recheck with a physician every six weeks early in the program.

Finally, it is important for older individuals to avoid sudden, rigorous bursts of exhaustive anaerobic activity, such as sprinting or weight lifting, and to concentrate mainly on endurance activities that are moderate and rhythmic in nature, such as jogging, walking, swimming, and bicycling.

Aging and the Benefits of Exercise

Considerable evidence indicates that the physiological consequences of aging increase if the cardiovascular and respiratory systems are weak. Regular and rhythmic exercise that increases the heart and respiratory rates, then, is an extremely important factor in maintaining health during the older years.

Older individuals derive a number of benefits from physical conditioning. Evidence indicates that the process of aging is delayed. Also, the ability of older individuals to transport oxygen increases, which increases their aerobic capacity to do work for longer periods of time. There also is some indication that physical conditioning can decrease blood pressure, improve breathing capacity, and make the muscles of the respiratory system more efficient. Other research shows that degenerative bone changes, such as osteoporosis, can be reduced through exercise, which prevents the bones from losing organic matter. Older people who engage in exercise programs benefit from improved joint mobility. In addition, such conditions as chronic lung disease, diabetes, coronary artery disease, and angina pain tend to be less severe in older individuals who are physically fit. Finally, some evidence indicates that arteriosclerosis is reduced in individuals who engage in long-term, continuous exercise. All of this adds up to an increase in life expectancy.

Whatever benefit an older person derives from exercise depends upon the type, intensity, and duration of the exercise the person participates in. For example, an older person who has been jogging three to five days a week at a training effect level for many years can expect greater benefits than an individual who plays a round of golf each week.

Nutrition and Aging

Research indicates that the physiological consequences of aging increase if a nutritionally sound diet is not maintained. While the energy needs of older people remain fairly constant, the digestive process slows down, and the amount of nutrients absorbed is reduced. Therefore, the quality of the diet has added importance. More nutrients need to be derived from less food. The decreased energy

285

requirements are due to a decrease in basal metabolism, which is about 10 percent slower for every ten years over sixty.

Older people should observe the following basic principles of nutrition, whether they are exercising or not:

1. Take in fewer overall calories.
2. Increase slightly the amount of protein in the diet.
3. Reduce the amount of fat in the diet.
4. Ensure that sufficient complex carbohydrates are in the diet.
5. Maintain appropriate vitamin and mineral levels, especially vitamin C, iron, and calcium.
6. Include adequate fiber, fruits, vegetables, and whole grains in the diet.
7. Ingest adequate water (six to seven glasses a day).

A Word About Competitive Sports

Once you have achieved an advanced level of cardiorespiratory endurance, you may be tempted to get involved in competitive running, cycling, skiing, swimming, or other competitive sports. This is perfectly understandable and may even increase your motivation. The important point to remember is that you must keep competitive sports in the proper perspective.

Competition is neither inherently good nor bad but simply one type of human behavior. It is good when it stimulates interest and leads to continued participation, gratification, and self-improvement. It is bad when it promotes hostility, anxiety, and dissatisfaction.

It is self-destructive to judge your success in competitive sports solely on your ability to win. Agonizing about losing a match in the local tournament or finishing way back in the pack in the Sunday morning ten-kilometer run leads only to dissatisfaction. Also, all too often we tend to perceive an opponent as an obstacle blocking our goals. In a very real sense, however, an opponent is a fellow competitor who is presenting us with a challenge. Viewed in this context, competition can provide self-fulfillment for both the "loser" and the "winner."

Too many people are concerned only with winning, and they lose sight of many of the important intrinsic benefits that can be derived from competition, such as increases in skill and endurance and the satisfaction derived from meeting new challenges. Set your own standards and create your own criteria for success and failure. Be aware of your uniqueness and the importance of defining the quality of your personal competitive experience. If you emphasize these values instead of focusing only on winning, competition can enrich your life.

Individual differences with regard to skill level, motivation, strength, endurance, and so on can directly affect the degree of fitness benefits derived from participating in sports activities. For example, an individual with low-level swimming skills may find water polo much more exhausting than a highly skilled swimmer. The same is true of a beginning skier as compared to an expert. The beginner is much less efficient in controlling extraneous muscle movement and in pacing the activity and probably will require much more energy expenditure than the highly skilled performer. Even equally skilled individuals display different levels of aggression and intensity, especially while competing, and thus may derive different degrees of fitness benefits.

Preparing for Competition

One of the most common problems facing the highly fit individual who decides to get involved in such competition as running, skiing, swimming, or bicycling is determining the sequence of training leading up to competition. Generally, in the early part of the training season, increases in volume (frequency and duration) are most important. As the competition season approaches, however, the intensity of the exercise should be increased and the volume should be decreased. As the competition date nears, both the volume and the intensity of the exercise should be reduced. This is sometimes referred to as the **tapering period.** Most runners use a tapering period of between one and two weeks. Swimmers generally use about two to four weeks for the tapering period.

Determining the volume and intensity of exercise during the tapering period is difficult since there has been very little research in this area. Evidence does indicate, however, that glycogen storage is maximized in about one week and that minor injuries, discomfort, and soreness generally clear up in about two weeks. Both of these are good arguments for a one- to two-week tapering period.

Most training regimens, however, are based upon the past experiences of individual athletes and coaches. Individualized training is important, since you are the best judge of how you are responding to exercise. Also, keep a log of the volume and intensity of your training, and think of long-term, not short-term, competitive goals.

Achieving Advanced Fitness

Methods of achieving advanced fitness include long-distance running, interval training, over-distance training, and many other aerobic and anaerobic options.

Long-Distance Running

Long-distance aerobic events can be extremely challenging and satisfying, yet they pose a number of problems not encountered in lower levels of aerobic activity. As you increase your exercise intensity, your heart, muscles, bones, and joint structures are subjected to increased levels of stress, thereby increasing the possibility of injury and disability. Peak physical condition is vital before attempting long-distance aerobic activities.

The distance you decide to run should be determined by your current fitness level and not by your psychological motivation. You should not attempt distances of five to ten kilometers unless you score in the "good" to "superior" category on the 1.5-mile run in chapter 4 and also are currently running approximately twenty-five to forty miles a week. You also should be able to cover the competitive distance comfortably during training at a target heart rate level of between 70 and 75 percent. This is important because during actual competition your target heart rate level may go as high as 85 to 95 percent.

A four-hour period of abstinence from food and even fluid containing sugar or carbohydrates should be maintained before running a marathon. Carbohydrates will increase the secretion of insulin in the blood and interfere with the mobilization of fatty acids from adipose tissue, which are the essential fuels in long-distance running.

The following are some general guidelines for long-distance running:

1. Ten to fifteen minutes of warm-up (stretching, slow jogging) should precede a run, and the run should be followed by at least an eight- to ten-minute cooling-down period.

2. Twenty to twenty-five percent of competitive training should be above the 70 percent target heart rate level.

3. Four to five months of training should precede competitive runs of five to ten kilometers.

4. If you are running between thirty-five and fifty-five miles a week (training for a ten-kilometer competition), one run a week should be six to ten miles in length.

5. Do not try to increase drastically the number of miles you run from one week to the next. Keep increases at approximately 8 to 10 percent per week.

6. Every four to five weeks, reduce your total weekly mileage by approximately 8 to 10 percent and then increase it by 10 percent the following week.

7. Vary your running distance each day.

8. Practice running both uphill, downhill, and on the level to ensure proper conditioning of all leg muscles and reduce the chances of soreness and injury.

9. Two days out of the week should include interval speed work: for five-kilometer races, two to three miles of 200 to 300 yard runs at a speed faster than your competitive pace with two minutes rest

recovery between runs; for ten-kilometer races, five to six miles of 200 to 300 yard runs at a speed faster than your competitive pace with two minutes rest recovery between runs.

10. The week before a ten-kilometer race, you should be able to run six to eight miles comfortably with a fast recovery (forty-five minutes to an hour) and no adverse effects the next day.

11. When your body signals that you are overextending yourself or when you experience pain in your muscles or joints, give way to your feelings and don't try to ''run through them.''

12. Set your own goals and limits. Don't let others dictate your pace or push you into an unnecessary risk zone.

Interval Training

Interval training is used primarily in competitive training programs for such sports as swimming, skiing, basketball, sprinting, and middle-distance running. It involves periods of intense training interspersed with rest periods. During the rest periods, the chemicals, fatigue products of exercise, can be paid off and new sources of energy resupplied to the muscles. For example, a 1,500 meter runner might run eight repetitive sixty-second 400 meter runs with three-minute resting periods between each.

One advantage of this regimen over distance running is that the athlete can practice specific pacing and intensity skills involved in running 1,500 meters. Another advantage is that the intensity of training on the cardiorespiratory system is much greater than in distance running. Also, interval training stresses the glycogen system, which results in the production of high levels of lactic acid. High levels of lactic acid produce the feelings of discomfort associated with all intensive exercise. As a result, interval-trained athletes are subject to high levels of physiological stress and thus are familiar with this stress and know how to adjust to it when it confronts them during competition.

Table 14.1 presents an eight-week aerobic interval training program for competitive athletes. During the first two weeks of the program, you need to train four days a week; during the remaining six weeks, you train three days a week. The program consists of grouped exercises (sets), a number of exercises per set (repetitions), and resting times between repetitions (relief intervals). For example, table 14.1 indicates that, on Day 1 of the first week, Set 1 should consist of: 4 × 220 at easy (1:3), where 4 is the number of repetitions, 220 is the training distance in yards, the term *easy* refers to running the 220 at an easy pace, and (1:3) indicates the relief interval (rest three times the amount of time it takes you to run 220 yards before running the next 220). In other words, in the first set,

TABLE 14.1 Aerobic Interval Training Progam for Competitive Athletes

Day		First week		Day		Fifth week	
1	Set 1	4 × 220 at easy	(1:3)	1	Set 1	4 × 660 at 2:05	(4:10)
	Set 2	8 × 110 at easy	(1:3)		Set 2	2 × 440 at 1:30	(2:40)
2	Set 1	2 × 440 at easy	(1:3)	2	Set 1	4 × 220 at 0:37	(1:51)
	Set 2	8 × 110 at easy	(1:3)		Set 2	4 × 220 at 0:37	(1:51)
3	Set 1	2 × 440 at easy	(1:3)		Set 3	4 × 220 at 0:37	(1:51)
	Set 2	6 × 220 at easy	(1:3)		Set 4	4 × 220 at 0:37	(1:51)
4	Set 1	1 × 880 at easy		3	Set 1	2 × 880 at 2:55	(2:55)
	Set 2	6 × 220 at easy	(1:3)		Set 2	2 × 440 at 1:30	(2:40)

		Second week				Sixth week	
1	Set 1	2 × 880 at easy	(1:3)	1	Set 1	4 × 660 at 2:00	(4:00)
	Set 2	2 × 440 at easy	(1:3)		Set 2	2 × 440 at 1:18	(2:36)
2	Set 1	6 × 440 at easy	(1:3)	2	Set 1	4 × 220 at 0:36	(1:48)
3	Set 1	3 × 880 at easy	(1:3)		Set 2	4 × 220 at 0:36	(1:48)
4	Set 1	1 × 2,640 at easy			Set 3	4 × 220 at 0:36	(1:48)
					Set 4	4 × 220 at 0:36	(1:48)
				3	Set 1	2 × 880 at 2:50	(2:50)
					Set 2	2 × 440 at 1:18	(2:36)

		Third week				Seventh week	
1	Set 1	2 × 660 at 2:25	(4:30)	1	Set 1	2 × 880 at 2:45	(2:45)
	Set 2	2 × 440 at 1:20	(2:40)		Set 2	2 × 440 at 1:26	(2:32)
2	Set 1	4 × 220 at 0.38	(1:54)	2	Set 1	4 × 220 at 0:35	(1:45)
	Set 2	4 × 220 at 0.38	(1:54)		Set 2	4 × 220 at 0:35	(1:45)
	Set 3	4 × 220 at 0.38	(1:54)		Set 3	4 × 220 at 0:35	(1:45)
3	Set 1	1 × 880 at 3:00	(3:00)		Set 4	4 × 220 at 0:35	(1:45)
	Set 2	2 × 440 at 1:20	(2:40)	3	Set 1	1 × 1,320 at 4:30	(2:15)
					Set 2	2 × 1,100 at 3:40	(1:50)

		Fourth week				Eighth week	
1	Set 1	3 × 660 at 2:10	(4:20)	1	Set 1	2 × 880 at 2:40	(2:40)
	Set 2	3 × 440 at 1:20	(2:40)		Set 2	2 × 440 at 1:16	(2:32)
2	Set 1	4 × 220 at 0:38	(1:54)	2	Set 1	4 × 220 at 0:34	(1:42)
	Set 2	4 × 220 at 0:38	(1:54)		Set 2	4 × 220 at 0:34	(1:42)
	Set 3	4 × 220 at 0:38	(1:54)		Set 3	4 × 220 at 0:34	(1:42)
	Set 4	4 × 220 at 0:38	(1:54)		Set 4	4 × 220 at 0:34	(1:42)
3	Set 1	2 × 880 at 2:55	(2:55)	3	Set 1	1 × 1,320 at 4:24	(2:12)
	Set 2	2 × 440 at 1:20	(2:40)		Set 2	2 × 1,100 at 3:34	(1:47)

Source: From *Sports Physiology* 2/e by Edward L. Fox. Copyright © 1984 by CBS College Publishing.
Reprinted by permission.

you run 220-yard runs at an easy pace. Between each run, you rest three times the amount of time it takes you to run the 220-yard distance.

Starting with the third week of the interval training program, table 14.1 lists suggested times for running the distances and also for the lengths of the relief intervals. For example, table 14.1 indicates that, on Day 1 of the third week, Set 1 should consist of: 2 × 660 at 2:25 (4:30), which translates into running two 660-yard runs, each in two minutes and twenty-five seconds, and resting four minutes and thirty seconds between each run. These are suggested times. Your best judge is your heart rate response to the exercise.

It is very important that you observe two rules when following the interval training program presented in table 14.1:

1. Do not start the next repetition until the heart rate is down to 150 beats per minute.
2. Do not begin the next set until the heart rate is down to approximately 125 beats per minute.

Over-Distance Training

Over-distance training involves running, skiing, swimming, or bicycling for a longer distance at a slower pace than that intended for competition; for example, a 1,500 meter competitor might run 1,600 meters at a slower time than it takes to run 1,500 meters. Over-distance training is effective for building respiratory capacity, but this training technique violates the principle of specificity. It is difficult to develop a sense of pace because the skill, coordination, and intensity needed, for example, to run 1,500 meters are not the same as in running 1,600 meters.

Other Options for Advanced Fitness

Anaerobic options for advanced fitness include:

1. **Sprint Training** Repeated sprints of fifty to one hundred yards each with complete recovery between each sprint.
2. **Hollow Sprints** Running two sprints with walking or jogging between sprints. For example, sprinting sixty yards, jogging sixty yards, and then walking sixty yards.
3. **Accelerated Sprints** Increasing running speed from a jog to a stride to a run in fifty- to one-hundred-yard segments.

Aerobic options for advanced fitness include:

1. **Continuous, Fast Running** Long-distance running or swimming at a fast pace. For example, an athlete who usually runs one mile might run 1¼ to 1¾ miles.
2. **Continuous, Slow Running** Long-distance running or swimming (two to five times longer than competitive distance) at a slow pace. The training heart rate should be approximately 150 beats per minute.
3. **Jogging** Continuous, slow running over moderate distances.

Options for advanced fitness that are both aerobic and anaerobic include:

1. **Repetition Running** Repeated periods of exercise interspersed with long rest intervals. For example, running half of a race distance at a slower than competitive time.
2. **Speed Play** Alternating fast and slow running over natural terrain. Can include sports skills—for example, dribbling, kicking.

Key Terms

Amenorrhea
An abnormal cessation of menstruation

Dysmenorrhea
Painful menstruation

Interval Training
Periods of intense training interspersed with rest periods

Oligomenorrhea
Irregular menstruation

Osteoporosis
A disease in which the bone tissue degenerates

Over-Distance Training
Training for a longer distance at a slower pace than that intended for competition

Tapering Period
A period of time prior to competition during which the volume and the intensity of the exercise is reduced

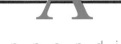

American College of Sports Medicine Position Statement

*The Recommended Quantity
and Quality of Exercise
for Developing and Maintaining
Cardiorespiratory and Muscular
Fitness in Healthy Adults*

With more and more people becoming involved in endurance training and other forms of physical activity, guidelines for exercise prescription have become necessary. Based on the existing evidence concerning exercise prescription for healthy adults and the need for guidelines, the American College of Sports Medicine (ACSM) makes the following recommendations for the quantity and quality of training for developing and maintaining cardiorespiratory fitness, body composition, and muscular strength and endurance in the healthy adult:

1. Frequency of training: three to five days per week.
2. Intensity of training: sixty to ninety percent of maximum heart rate (HRmax), or fifty to eighty-five percent of maximum oxygen uptake ($\dot{V}O_2$ max or HRmax reserve).
3. Duration of training: Twenty to sixty minutes of continuous aerobic activity. Duration is dependent on the intensity of the activity; thus, lower-intensity activity should be conducted over a longer period of time. Because of the importance of the "total fitness" and the fact that it is more readily attained in longer duration programs, and because of the potential hazards and

Source: Reprinted with permission of the American College of Sports Medicine. Copyright 1990 American College of Sports Medicine.

compliance problems associated with high-intensity activity, lower- to moderate-intensity activity of longer duration is recommended for the nonathletic adult.

4. Mode of activity: Any activity that uses large muscle groups, can be maintained continuously, and is rhythmical and aerobic in nature, for example, walking-hiking, running-jogging, cycling-bicycling, cross-country skiing, dancing, rope skipping, rowing, stair climbing, swimming, skating, and various endurance game activities.

5. Resistance training: Strength training of a moderate intensity, sufficient to develop and maintain fat-free weight (FFW), should be an integral part of an adult fitness program. One set of 8–12 repetitions of eight to ten exercises that condition the major muscle groups at least 2 days per week is the recommended minimum.

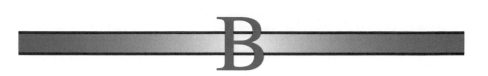

Record Sheets

RECORD SHEET B-1 Daily Exercise Program

Name _____   Date _____

Exercise

Fitness level
_____

Flexibility	Repetitions
Lower-leg stretch	
Back stretch	
Groin stretch	
Quadriceps stretch	
Abdominal stretch	
Lower-back stretch	
Upper-trunk stretch	

Fitness level
_____

Floor Exercise	Repetitions
Modified push-up	
Full push-up	
Head-and-shoulder curl	
Bent-knee sit-up	

Fitness level
_____

Strength	RM	Repetitions	Sets
Zottman curl			
Bent-arm lateral			
Heel raise			
Bent-over rowing			
Lateral arm raise			
Standing overhead press			
Bent-arm pullover			
Bench press			
Biceps curl			

Fitness level
_____

Cardiovascular	Distance	Duration	Heart rate training effect level
Jogging			
Swimming			
Bicycling			
Walking			
Rope jumping			
Other			

RECORD SHEET B-2 Flexibility and Floor Exercise Record

Name _____

Week	Day	Repetition	Lower-leg stretch	Back stretch	Groin stretch	Quadriceps stretch	Abdominal stretch	Upper-trunk stretch	Lower-back stretch	Modified push-up	Full push-up	Head-and-shoulder curl	Bent-knee sit-up

RECORD SHEET B-3 Aerobic Exercise Record

Name _____

Week	Day	Exercise	Heart rate training effect level	Distance	Duration

RECORD SHEET B-4 Weight-Training Record

Exercise	Date					Date				
	RM	Rep.	Set 1	Set 2	Set 3	RM	Rep.	Set 1	Set 2	Set 3

| **RECORD SHEET B-5** | Circuit-Training Record |

Exercise	Date _____ I Repetitions completed	Date _____ II Repetitions completed	Date _____ III Repetitions completed	Date _____ IV Repetitions completed
1				
2				
3				
4				
5				
6				
7				
8				
9				
10				
11				
12				
13				
14				
15				
16				
17				
18				
19				
20				
Target time				
Actual circuit time				
Postcircuit heart rate				

RECORD SHEET B-6 Strength Record

Name _____

Week	Day	RM	Zottman curl	Bent-arm lateral	Bent-over rowing	Lateral arm raise	Standing overhead press	Bent-arm pullover	Bench press	Biceps curl	Heel raise
		Repetition									

RECORD SHEET B-7 Weight-Reducing Record

Name _____ Date _____

1. Determine your individual caloric allowance, see table 10.2.   _____ KCal
2. Determine your percentage of body fat (chapter 4): _____
3. Weight = _____

Percentage of body fat _____ X Body weight _____ = Total fat _____ lbs

Body weight _____ − Total fat _____ = Lean body weight _____

      y= Desired weight   Desired body fat = _____ %

y − (y X Percentage of desired body fat _____) = Body weight _____ −
                                                (Body weight _____ X
                                                Percentage of body fat _____)

      Body weight _____ − y _____ = Weight loss required _____

Source: Preventive Medicine Center, Weight Control, Palo Alto, CA, 1978.

RECORD SHEET B-8 Daily Caloric Intake

Date _____   Weight _____

                                      Percentage of body fat _____

Day	Food	Portion	Calories (from Appendix C)
Breakfast			
Lunch			
Dinner			
Desserts			
Snacks			
Drinks			
Other			

                             Total caloric intake _____

                   Total caloric expenditures _____
                         (from tables 10.8–10.11)
       Caloric difference (positive or negative) _____

RECORD SHEET B-9 Caloric Record

Name _____

Week	Day	Total caloric intake	Exercise	Caloric expenditure	Weight

Appendix B

| RECORD SHEET B-10 | Cardiorespiratory Exercise Contract |

Name _____

Date _____

1. Fitness category _____

2. Goals (specific behavior to be changed) _____

_____

3. Beginning target heart rate _____

Week	Day	Exercise	Intensity	Duration
1				
2				
3				
4				
5				
6				
7				
8				

Signature _____   Sponsor _____

Date _____   Date _____

RECORD SHEET B-11 Muscle Strength Contract

Name _____

Date _____

1. Fitness category _____

   a. Bench press _____

   b. Leg press _____

   c. Biceps curl _____

   d. Shoulder press _____

   e. Push-ups _____

   f. Bent-knee sit-ups _____

2. Strength and Endurance goals _____

Week	Day	Exercise	Repetition max	Sets
1				
2				
3				
4				
5				
6				
7				
8				

Signature _____   Sponsor _____

Date _____   Date _____

Appendix B

Name _____

Date _____

Present weight _____ Weight to be lost _____ Desired weight _____

Week	Day	Exercise	Intensity	Duration	Lbs. to be lost	Desired caloric intake
1						
2						
3						
4						
5						
6						
7						
8						

Signature _____ Sponsor _____

Date _____ Date _____

RECORD SHEET B-13 Flexibility Contract

Name _____

Date _____

1. Fitness category _____

   a. Sit-and-reach test _____

   b. Back hyperextension _____

2. Flexibility goals _____

Week	Day	Stretching exercise
1		
2		
3		
4		
5		
6		
7		
8		

Signature _____   Sponsor _____

Date _____   Date _____

RECORD SHEET B-14 Fitness and Health Diary

Week	Day	Date	Activity	Evaluation special problems positive/ negative outcome	Comments
1					
2					
3					
4					
5					
6					
7					
8					
9					
10					
11					
12					

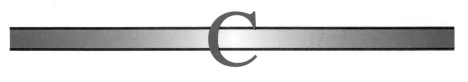

app p e n d i x

Calorie Values,
Vitamins, and Minerals

TABLE C-1	Caloric Content of Food Groups

Milk and milk products

	Amount	Calories
Milk, pasteurized, whole	1 cup	165
Milk, canned, evaporated, unsweetened	½ cup	140
Milk, condensed, sweetened	½ cup	480
Milk, nonfat	1 cup	80
Skim milk	1 cup	86
Goat's milk	½ cup	71
Buttermilk, cultured	1 cup	80
Ice cream	1/6 quart	200
Cream, light	1 teaspoon	30
Cream, heavy or whipping	1 teaspoon	50
Cheddar cheese	1 square	115
Cottage cheese	½ cup	100
Cream cheese	2 tablespoons	100
Parmesan cheese	2 teaspoons	110
Roquefort cheese	2 teaspoons	105
Swiss cheese	2 teaspoons	105

Meat, fish, poultry, eggs, nuts

Bacon, medium fat, cooked	3 strips	150
Beef, medium fat, hamburger cooked	¼ pound	225
Chicken, fried	¼ pound	275
Chicken, broiled	quarter chicken	332
Chicken liver	¼ pound	85
Corned beef, canned	4 ounces	240
Frankfurter	1	124
Ham, broiled	¼ pound	300
Ham, smoked, cooked	¼ pound	400
Ham, canned, spiced	¼ pound	290
Lamb, medium fat, leg roast, cooked	¼ pound	270
Lamb, rib chop, cooked	¼ pound	140

309

Appendix C

| ***TABLE C-1*** | Caloric Content of Food Groups (*Continued*) | |

Meat, fish, poultry, eggs, nuts

	Amount	*Calories*
Liver (beef)	1 slice	85
Pork, medium fat	¼ pound	365
Pork loin or chops, cooked	1 chop	265
Rib roast, cooked	2 slices (lean to fat)	200 to 400
Rump, cooked	2 slices	190
Sirloin, cooked	¼ pound (lean to fat)	200 to 300
Turkey, medium fat	¼ pound	270
Veal, medium fat, cutlet	¼ pound	220
Veal, medium fat, roast	¼ pound	360
Venison	¼ pound	140
Clams, long and round	¼ pound	80
Cod	1 piece	70
Crab, canned or cooked, meat only	½ cup	85
Flounder	¼ pound	200
Halibut	¼ pound	200
Lobsters	1 (¾ pound)	300
Oysters	5 to 8 medium	80
Salmon, Pacific, cooked	¼ pound	180
Salmon, canned	½ cup	190
Sardines, canned in oil	5 medium	180
Scallops, fried	5 to 6 medium	425
Shrimps, canned, drained	10 to 12 medium	45
Trout	¼ pound (brook/lake)	210 to 290
Tuna	3 ounces	247
Eggs, whole	1 medium	75
Egg white, raw	1 medium	15
Egg yolk, raw	1 medium	60
Almonds, salted	15	100
Brazil nuts	5	100
Cashews, roasted or cooked	10	200
Chestnuts	2 large	200
Peanuts, roasted	½ cup	440
Pecans	1 teaspoon	52
Walnuts	2 teaspoons	95

Soup

Bean soup	1 cup	260
Beef soup	1 cup	115
Beef soup with vegetables	1 cup	80
Chicken noodle soup	1 cup	68
Lentil soup	1 cup	600
Pea soup, creamed	1 cup	270
Tomato soup	1 cup	100
Vegetable soup	1 cup	90

TABLE C-1 Caloric Content of Food Groups (*Continued*)

Fruits, fruit juices, and vegetables

	Amount	*Calories*
Apples	1 sweet	60 to 90
Apple juice, fresh	1 cup	120
Apple sauce, sweetened	½ cup	80
Apricots	1 medium	18
Avocados, fresh	½	279
Bananas	1 (about 6 inches)	88
Blackberries, fresh	½ cup	40
Blackberries, canned, sweetened	½ cup	85
Blueberries, fresh	½ cup	45
Blueberries, canned, sweetened	½ cup	110
Cantaloupe, fresh	½	40
Cherries, canned, sweetened	½ cup	100
Cranberry sauce	2 teaspoons	60
Dates, dried	5 pitted	100
Fruit cocktail, canned	½ cup	80
Grapes, fresh	½ cup	65
Grape juice	½ cup	75
Grapefruit	½ (4¼-inch diameter)	75
Grapefruit juice, fresh	½ cup	45
Lemons, fresh	1 (2-inch diameter)	25
Limes, fresh	1	25
Olives, green	2 medium	15
Oranges, fresh	1 (3-inch diameter)	70
Orange juice, fresh	½ cup	55
Peaches, fresh	1 medium	45
Peaches, canned, sweetened	2 halves	85
Pears	1 (2½-inch diameter)	95
Pineapple, canned, sweetened	1 cup	200
Pineapple juice, canned	1 cup	120
Plums	1 (2-inch diameter)	30
Prunes, dried, uncooked	4 large	121
Raisins, dried	½ cup	190
Raspberries, fresh	½ cup	50
Raspberries, canned, sweetened	1 cup	100
Strawberries, fresh	10 large	35
Strawberries, frozen, sweetened	½ cup	125
Beans, kidney	½ cup	90
Beans, lima, fresh	½ cup	90
Beans, lima, canned	½ cup	95
Beans, snap, fresh	1 cup	35
Beans, wax, canned	½ cup	20

311

TABLE C-1 Caloric Content of Food Groups (*Continued*)

Fruits, fruit juices, and vegetables

	Amount	Calories
Beets (beetroots), peeled, fresh	½ cup	34
Broccoli, fresh	½ cup	22
Brussels sprouts, fresh	½ cup	30
Cabbage, fresh	Wedge	25
Carrots, canned	½ cup	30
Carrots, fresh	1 (6 inches)	20
Cauliflower, fresh	½ cup	30
Celery	2 stalks	17
Corn, fresh	1 ear with butter	90
Corn, canned	½ cup	70
Cucumbers	½ (7½ inches)	20
Eggplant, fresh	½ cup	25
Kale, fresh	1 cup	40
Lentils	½ cup	110
Lettuce, fresh	½ head	15
Mushrooms (field)	½ cup	20
Onions	1 (2½-inch diameter)	40
Peas, green, fresh	½ cup	60
Peas, canned	½ cup	70
Peppers, green, fresh	1 large	24
Potato chips	7 to 10	110
Potatoes, raw	1 medium	90
Potatoes, french fried	20 pieces	275
Radishes, fresh	4 small	4
Rhubarb, fresh	½ cup	10
Spinach, canned	½ cup	25
Sweet potatoes, fresh	1 small	150
Sweet potatoes, candied	1 medium	300
Sweet potatoes, canned	½ cup	120
Tomatoes, fresh	1 medium	30
Tomatoes, canned	½ cup	25
Tomato catsup	2 teaspoons	40
Tomato juice, canned	½ cup	25

Breads, flour, cereals

Brown bread, enriched	1 slice	100
Corn muffins, enriched	2	220
French bread	1 slice	70
Raisin bread, enriched	1 slice	65
Rye bread, American	1 slice	55
White bread, enriched	1 slice	63
Whole wheat bread	1 slice	55
Cornflakes	1 cup	100
Graham crackers	2	60
Saltine crackers	2	30

TABLE C-1 Caloric Content of Food Groups (*Continued*)

Breads, flour, cereals

	Amount	Calories
Soda crackers	10 small	40
Flour	1 cup	401
Macaroni, cooked	½ cup	70
Noodles, cooked	½ cup	54
Oatmeal, cooked	1 cup	75
Pancakes, wheat	2	150
Pie	1 slice	300 to 400
Popcorn, popped	1 cup	60
Pretzel sticks	15 small	15
Rice, cooked	½ cup	75
Spaghetti, cooked	1 cup	220
Sweet rolls	1	175
Tapioca, cooked	½ cup	130
Waffles, baked	1	225
Wheat germ	1 cup	365

Fats, sweets, alcohol

	Amount	Calories
Butter or margarine	1 tablespoon	100
Mayonnaise	1 tablespoon	100
Olive oil	1 tablespoon	125
Peanut butter	1 tablespoon	85
Salad dressing (French, thousand island)	1 tablespoon	60 to 100
Chocolate, sweetened	2½ ounces	335
Chocolate, milk	4 ounces	542
Chocolate, plain	4 ounces	471
Chocolate creams	2	110
Fudge	1 piece	120
Honey	1 tablespoon	65
Jams	1 tablespoon	55
Jellies	1 tablespoon	50
Jelly beans	10 pieces	70
Molasses	1 tablespoon	150
Sugar, maple	1 tablespoon	55
Sugar, cane or beet	1 tablespoon	50
Syrup (corn)	½ cup	427
Beer	1 cup	115
Brandy	1 ounce	70
Eggnog	½ cup	335
Highball	1 cup	165
Port, vermouth, muscatel	½ cup	155
Rum	1 jigger (1½ ounces)	140
Whiskey	1 jigger (1½ ounces)	130

TABLE C-1 Caloric Content of Food Groups (*Continued*)

Fats, sweets, alcohol

	Amount	*Calories*
Wine, white, rosé	½ cup	85 to 105
Carbonated soft drinks	1 cup	80
Chocolate milk	1 cup	250
Cocoa	1 cup	175
Coffee, black	1 cup	1
Coffee with cream and sugar (1 teaspoon each)	1 cup	45
Tea	1 cup	0

Big-calorie culprits

Chocolate milk	1 cup	250
Chocolate candy	3 ounces	453
Chocolate creams	2 ounces	220
Malted milk	1 cup	281
Nuts, cashews	2 ounces	328
Soda with ice cream	1 glass	325
Sundae, chocolate, with 2 teaspoons of syrup	½ cup	330
Whipping cream	1 teaspoon	50

Popular fast foods

Jack-in-the-Box		
Hamburger	1	263
Cheeseburger	1	310
French fries	1 serving	270
Onion rings	1 serving	351
French toast	1 serving	537
Pancakes	1 serving	626
Scrambled eggs	1 serving	719
Kentucky Fried Chicken		
Wing and thigh	1 dinner	661
Drumstick and thigh	1 dinner	643
Wing and thigh, extra crispy	1 dinner	812
Drumstick and thigh, extra crispy	1 dinner	765
McDonald's		
Hotcakes with butter and syrup	1 serving	500
Big Mac	1	563
Quarter pounder	1	424
Regular fries	1 serving	220
Chocolate shake	1	383
Taco Bell		
Beef burrito	1 serving	466

TABLE C-1 Caloric Content of Food Groups (*Continued*)

Popular fast foods

	Amount	*Calories*
Burrito supreme	1 serving	457
Enchirito	1 serving	454
Wendy's		
Single hamburger	1 serving	470
Double hamburger	1 serving	670
Triple hamburger	1 serving	850
Double hamburger with cheese	1 serving	800
French fries	1 serving	330
Frosty	1 serving	390

TABLE C-2 Energy Values for Common Snack Foods

	Amount or average serving	Energy (in Kcal)
"Just a little sandwich"		
Hamburger on bun	3-inch patty	330
Peanut butter sandwich	2 tablespoons peanut butter	330
Cheese sandwich	1 ounce cheese	280
Ham sandwich	1 ounce ham	320
TV snack		
Pizza (cheese)	⅛ of 14-inch diameter pie	185
Popcorn with oil and salt	1 cup	40
Pretzel, thin, twisted	1	25
Cheese fondue	½ cup	265
Dips (sour cream)	½ cup	248
Chippers	10	150
Beverages		
Carbonated drinks, soda, root beer, etc.	6 ounces	80
Cola beverages	12 ounces	150
Club soda	8 ounces	5
Chocolate malted milk	10 ounces	500
Ginger ale	6 ounces	60
Tea or coffee, straight	1 cup	0
Tea or coffee, with 2 tablespoons cream and 2 teaspoons sugar	1 cup	90
Alcoholic drinks		
Ale	8 ounces	155
Beer	8 ounces	110
Highball (with ginger ale)	8 ounces	185
Manhattan	Average	165
Martini	Average	140
Wine, muscatel, or port	2 ounces	95
Sherry	2 ounces	75
Scotch, bourbon, rye	1½-ounce jigger	130
Fruits		
Apple	1 (3-inch diameter)	75
Banana	1 (6 inches)	130
Grapes	30 medium	75
Orange	1 (2¾-inch diameter)	70
Pear	1	65
Salted nuts		
Almonds, filberts, hazelnuts	12 to 15	95
Cashews	6 to 8	90
Peanuts	15 to 17	85
Pecans, walnuts	10 to 15 halves	100

Source: From *Health and Physical Fitness* by William P. Marley. Copyright © 1982 by Saunders Publishing Co., a Division of Holt, Rhinehart & Winston, Inc. Reprinted by permission of the publisher.

TABLE C-2 Energy Values for Common Snack Foods (*Continued*)

	Amount or average serving	*Energy (in Kcal)*
Candies		
Chocolate bars		
Plain, sweet milk	1 bar (1 ounce)	155
With almonds	1 bar (1 ounce)	140
Chocolate-covered bar	1 bar	270
Chocolate cream, bonbon, fudge	1 piece, 1-inch square	90 to 120
Caramels, plain	2 medium	85
Hard candies, Lifesaver type	1 roll	95
Peanut brittle	1 piece (2½-inch square)	110
Desserts		
Pie		
Fruit—apple, etc.	1/6 pie, 1 average serving	410
Custard	1/6 pie, 1 average serving	265
Mince	1/6 pie, 1 average serving	400
Pumpkin pie with whipped cream	1/6 pie, 1 average serving	460
Cake		
Chocolate layer	3-inch section	350
Doughnut, sugared	1 average	150
Sweets		
Ice cream		
Plain vanilla	1/6 quart	200
Chocolate and other flavors	1/6 quart	260
Orange sherbet	½ cup	120
Sundaes, small chocolate nut with whipped cream	Average	400
Ice-cream sodas, chocolate	10 ounces	270
Midnight snacks for icebox raiders		
Cold potato	½ medium	65
Chicken leg (fried)	1 average	88
Milk	7 ounces	140
Mouthful of roast	½ inch X 2 inches X 3 inches	130
Piece of cheese	¼ inch X 2 inches X 3 inches	120
Leftover beans	½ cup	105
Brownie	¾ inch X 1¾ inches X 2¼ inches	140
Cream puff	4-inch diameter	450

TABLE C-3 Major Characteristics of Water-Soluble Vitamins

Vitamin	Human deficiency symptoms	Major functions	Food sources	RDA† established	Remarks
Vitamin C	Scurvy: loose teeth, bleeding gums, painful joints, bruising, skin hemorrhage.	Healing wounds, collagen formation, use of other nutrients, body metabolism.	Citrus fruits, strawberries, cantaloupes, kale, broccoli, sweet peppers, parsley, turnip greens, potatoes.	Yes	Undesirable effects from excess dose. Very unstable substance.
Vitamin B₁	Beriberi: fatigue, mental depression, poor appetite, polyneuritis, decreased muscle tone.	As coenzyme. Metabolism of carbohydrate, fat, and protein.	Pork, liver and other organ meats, grain (whole or enriched), nuts, legumes, milk, eggs.	Yes	Unstable in food processing.
Vitamin B₂	Cheilosis: cracked lips, scaly skin, burning/itching eyes. Glossitis: smooth, red, sore tongue, with atrophy.	As coenzyme. Metabolism of fat, carbohydrate, and protein.	Liver, milk, meat, eggs, enriched cereal products, green leafy vegetables.	Yes	Very susceptible to UV or visible rays of sunlight.
Vitamin B₆	In infants: convulsion, irritability. In adults: microcytic hypochromic anemia, irritability, skin lesions, and other nonspecific signs.	As coenzyme. Metabolism of protein.	Pork, beef, liver, bananas, ham, egg yolks.	Yes	Pharmacological dose occasionally relieves morning sickness.
Niacin	Pellagra (the 4 D's): dermatitis, diarrhea, dementia, death. Also sore mouth, delirium, darkened teeth and skin. Hyperpigmentation.	As a coenzyme in the metabolism of fat, carbohydrate, and protein.	Meat, fish, liver, poultry, dark green leafy vegetables, whole or enriched grain products.	Yes	May be synthesized from tryptophan in body.

318

TABLE C-3 Major Characteristics of Water-Soluble Vitamins (*Continued*)

Vitamin	Human deficiency symptoms	Major functions	Food sources	RDA† established	Remarks
Folic acid	Megaloblastic anemia.	Formation of nucleic acids (DNA, RNA). Metabolism of methyl (CH_3) groups. Rapid turnover of cells, e.g., red blood cells.	Pork, liver and other organ meats, peanuts, green leafy vegetables, yeast, orange juice.	Yes	Deficiency probably most prevalent in western societies.
Vitamin B_{12}	Megaloblastic anemia; neurodegeneration.	Same as above.	Animal products: meat, poultry, fish, eggs, etc. Not found in edible plant products.	Yes	Pernicious anemia infers a lack of the intrinsic factor (see text).
Pantothenic acid	Nonspecific symptoms; weight loss, irritability, intestinal disturbances, nervous disorders, burning sensation of feet.	As a coenzyme in the metabolism of fat, protein, and carbohydrate.	Widespread in nature. Meat, poultry, fish, grains, some fruits and vegetables.	No	Sensitive to dry heat.
Biotin	In infants: dermatitis. In adults: anorexia, nausea, muscle pain, depression, anemia, dermatitis, and other nonspecific symptoms.	As a coenzyme in metabolism of fat, carbohydrate, and protein.	Organ meats (liver, kidney), egg yolk, milk, cheese.	No	Antagonist, avidin, found in egg white.

+ RDA = Recommended Dietary Allowance established by the National Research Council of the National Academy of Sciences.

319

TABLE C-4 Major Characteristics of Fat-Soluble Vitamins

Vitamin	Human deficiency symptoms	Major functions	Food sources	RDA† established	Remarks
Vitamin A	Eye: night blindness, Bitot's spot, partial and total blindness. Skin: dryness, scaliness, hardening and epithelial changes (affecting body surface), mucosa along respiratory, gastrointestinal, and genitourinary tracts.	In the eye: synthesis of rhodopsin, visual pigment. In the epithelium: differentiation. In the bones and teeth: proper development.	Carotene: dark green and yellow leafy vegetables. Dark yellow fruits. Vitamin A: liver, butter, whole milk and other fortified dairy products.	Yes	Large doses may be toxic.
Vitamin D	Infancy and childhood: rickets. Adults: osteomalacia.	Calcium metabolism, especially its absorption from the intestine and mobilization from bones.	Fish, especially liver and oil; liver and fortified whole milk.	Yes	Large doses may be toxic.
Vitamin E	Uncommon in adults. Infants (especially premature): RBC susceptibility to hemolysis.	Not known. An antioxidant in food industry.	Wheat germ, vegetable oils, nuts, legumes, green leafy vegetables.	Yes	Therapeutic effects of large doses not substantiated.
Vitamin K	Prolonged blood-clotting time. Hemorrhage. Delayed wound healings.	Responsible for prothrombin synthesis in liver.	Dark green leafy vegetables; alfalfa.	No	Synthesized by intestinal bacteria.

†RDA = Recommended Dietary Allowance established by the National Research Council of the National Academy of Sciences.

TABLE C-5 Approximate Mineral Composition and Recommended Daily Mineral Intake, Adult Males

Mineral	Approximate amount of mineral in body (g)	Recommended daily dietary intake or suggested level of intake (mg/day)[†]
Macrominerals		
Calcium*	1400	800
Phosphorus	770	800
Potassium	245	1875–5625
Sulfur	175	?
Sodium*	105	1100–3300
Chlorine	105	1700–5100
Magnesium	35	350
Microminerals		
Iron*	2.8	10
Zinc	1.6	15
Trace Elements		
Copper	0.1	2–3
Iodine	0.003	0.15
Manganese	0.002	2.5–5
Chromium	<0.006	0.05–0.2
Cobalt	?	Provided in vitamin B-12
Newer Trace Elements		
Fluorine	?	1.5–4
Selenium	?	0.05–0.2
Tin	?	?
Silicon	?	?
Nickel	?	?
Vanadium	?	?
Molybdenum	?	0.15–0.5
Arsenic	?	?

*Minerals meriting the greatest consideration when making decisions on food selection.
†Recommended by the NAS-NRC.

D

Sexually Transmitted Diseases

Gonorrhea is caused by a bacteria and is so widespread, a new infection occurs every twelve seconds. If untreated, gonorrhea can cause sterility in men and pelvic inflammatory disease in women.

Symptoms: Men notice a discharge and painful urination within two to ten days after infection. Women may have no early symptoms but later may develop discharge, abdominal pain, and fever. A sore throat may result if contacted through oral sex.

Treatment: Gonorrhea can be quickly cured with antibiotics. Some strains, however, are resistant and may need more treatment.

Syphilis is caused by a corkscrew-shaped bacteria. Unless treated it can cause heart and brain damage and even death. Pregnant women can transmit the infection to unborn babies.

Symptoms: First symptoms occur up to twelve weeks after infection in the form of a painless sore (chancre) that appears on genitals, mouth, or rectal area. About six weeks later symptoms include fever, rash, and flu-like symptoms. These symptoms will disappear but if untreated, lead to serious complications later in life.

Treatment: Even if no symptoms appear, diagnosis can be made by blood test, but results may be negative for up to twelve weeks after initial exposure. Syphilis is treated with antibiotics. Early treatment is essential because symptoms may disappear but disease remains in the body.

Herpes is caused by two types of viruses. Over 20 million people have herpes. At present there is no cure. Many people have only one outbreak, others learn to control the infection.

Symptoms: Within ten days after infection, symptoms begin with one or more fluid blisters that open into sores. Sores may be painful and accompanied by swollen glands and flu-like symptoms.

Treatment: Herpes cannot be cured but can be controlled. Some drugs speed healing and prevent recurrence. Pregnant women should notify the doctor so that precautions can be taken and the baby is not infected.

Venereal warts are caused by a virus. Many warts are so small they are difficult to detect. Babies, whose mothers have venereal warts, can be born with warts. There is also a link between venereal warts and genital cancer. If the warts are caught early, they can be easily treated.

Symptom: Venereal warts can be flat or shaped like little cauliflowers. They usually appear within eight months of infection, causing local irritation and itching. They can grow on the penis, vagina, cervix, and in and around the rectum and throat.

Treatment: Immediate treatment is essential. They can be removed surgically or chemically.

Vaginitis is really a group of diseases. The three most common are trichomoniasis, yeast infection, and gardnerella. This disease is mainly a woman's disease but can be spread by men, who act as carriers.

Symptoms:

Trichomoniasis: Frothy, yellow discharge, itching and burning and unpleasant odor.

Yeast infection: Discharge like cottage cheese with intense itching.

Gardnerella: Grayish, white watery discharge with strong odor.

Treatment:

Trichomoniasis: Is treated with metronidazole.

Yeast infection: Is treated with nystatin vaginal suppositories or creams.

Gardnerella: Is treated with ampicillin or metronidazole.

Chlamydia is now more widespread than gonorrhea especially among young people fifteen to twenty-five. It is caused by a bacteria, which in many cases is symptomless and may not be tested for.

Symptoms: Early symptoms, if they occur, are often mild with odorless discharge and burning similar to gonorrhea. A complication in women is Pelvic Inflammatory Disease (PID). Both chlamydia and PID may cause sterility in women and tubal pregnancy. PID symptoms include fever, pain during sex, and abdominal pain.

Treatment: Chlamydia can be cured easily with antibiotics. Men diagnosed with chlamydia should notify their partners right away.

AIDS (acquired immune deficiency syndrome) is the deadliest STD; the virus destroys the body's immune system. Most people who have the virus do not have AIDS but they can pass it on. High-risk groups are gays, bisexual men, people who share IV needles, hemophiliacs, and sex partners of these groups. AIDS is spread through infected blood or semen, not casual contact. If an infected partner's blood or semen enters your body through a break in the lining of the rectum, vagina, or mouth or through a needle puncture, you can be infected with the virus.

Symptoms: Swollen lymph glands, fever, night sweats, severe fatigue and weight loss are early symptoms. Many symptoms are similar to other diseases, only they persist and get worse.

Treatment: See a doctor immediately if you experience AIDS symptoms. Currently AIDS has no cure, but treatments are being tested.

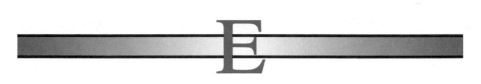

Fitnessgram: Fit for Life
Activity Log

The FITNESSGRAM "Fit for Life" program is designed to promote exercise as an important part of each day. It provides a means of monitoring physical activity over an 8- to 10-week period, and makes incentives available to individuals who record good exercise habits. Children, youth and adults are encouraged to exercise together. Here's what to do:

1 Try to get some kind of physical activity at least three or four days each week.

2 Consult the table below to determine how many points you have earned each day and record them on the activity log. Be proud of each point! Points may be earned from one or several activities. You should try to earn at least 2 points each day.

3 Earn as many points each week as you'd like. However, only the maximum number of points per week listed below will count toward successful completion.

4 Try to accumulate the total goal for your age group (see below) in an 8 week period. You may increase the time to 10 weeks if you are sick or injured.

Activity	Time	Points
Badminton	15 minutes	1
Basketball	20 minutes	2
Calisthenics	15 minutes	1
Cross Country Skiing	10 minutes	2
Cycling	15 minutes	1
Dance (Aerobics)	20 minutes	2
Dance (Tap, Ballet, Modern)	30 minutes	2
Field Hockey	20 minutes	2
Gymnastics	30 minutes	2
Ice Hockey/Field Hockey	20 minutes	2
Jogging/Running	10 minutes	2
Lacrosse	20 minutes	2
Martial Arts	20 minutes	1
Racquetball/Handball/Squash	20 minutes	2
Rope Jumping (Individual)	10 minutes	2
Skating (Ice/Roller)	15 minutes	1
Soccer	20 minutes	2
Swimming (Laps)	10 minutes	2
Tennis	15 minutes	1
Volleyball	30 minutes	2
Walking	15 minutes	2
Weight Training	15 minutes	1
Wrestling (Competitive)	20 minutes	2

Some activities will be more vigorous than others. Certain activities develop strength and flexibility, while others develop aerobic endurance. Point values are intended only for use in recording your activity.

Age	Total Points Needed	Maximum Points Per Week
13–17	160	20
17+	192	24

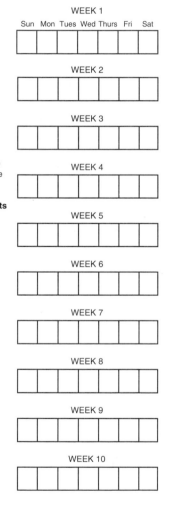

WEEK 1
Sun Mon Tues Wed Thurs Fri Sat

WEEK 2

WEEK 3

WEEK 4

WEEK 5

WEEK 6

WEEK 7

WEEK 8

WEEK 9

WEEK 10

Total Points Earned _____

Signature _____

Suggested Readings

Aerobics

Floyd, Patricia, and Janet Park. *Walk, Jog, Run for Wellness Everyone.* Winston-Salem, N.C.: Hunter Textbooks, 1994.

Kisselle, D., and K. Mazzou. *Aerobic Dance: A Way to Fitness.* Denver, Colo.: Morton, 1983.

Macceo, Karen, and Judy Kisselle. *Aerobic Dance: A Way to Fitness,* 2d ed. Denver, Colo.: Morton, 1987.

Penrod, James, and Janice Plastine. *The Dancer Prepares: Modern Dance for Beginners.* Palo Alto, Calif.: Mayfield, 1970.

Sheppard, Roy J. *Aerobic Fitness and Health.* Champagne, Ill.: Human Kinetics, 1994.

Sorensen, Jackie. *Aerobic Dancing.* New York: Rawson Wade, 1979.

Town, Glen, and Todd Kerney. *Swim, Bike and Run.* Champagne, Ill.: Human Kinetics, 1994.

Van Gelder, Naneene. Aerobic Dance-Exercise Instructor Manual, IDEA Foundation, Santiago, Calif., 1987.

Vincent, L. M. *The Dancer's Book of Health.* Kansas City, Kans.: Sheed Andrews & McMeel, 1978.

Age

Shepard, R. *Physical Activity and Aging.* Chicago: Year Book Medical Publishers, 1978.

Smith, E., and R. Serfass. *Exercise and Aging.* Hillside, N.J.: Enslow, 1981.

Spirruso, Waneen, and Helen Eckart. *Physical Activity and Aging.* Champagne, Ill.: Human Kinetics, 1989.

Tamaris, P. S. *Developmental Physiology and Aging.* New York: Macmillan, 1972.

Athletic Injuries

Anderson, J. L. *The Yearbook of Sports Medicine.* Chicago: Year Book Medical Publishers, 1981.

Mirkin, Gabe, and Marshall Hoffman. *Sports Medicine Book.* Boston: Little, Brown, 1978.

Olsen, O. C. *Prevention of Injuries, Protecting the Health of Student Athletes.* Philadelphia: Lea & Febiger, 1971.

Bicycling

Burke, Edmund. *The Science of Cycling.* Champagne, Ill.: Human Kinetics, 1986.

Delong, Fred. *Delong's Guide to Bicycles and Bicycling.* Radnor, Pa.: Chilton, 1974.

Kingbay, Keith. *Inside Bicycling.* Chicago: Contemporary Books, 1977.

Sloane, Eugene A. *The New Complete Book of Bicycling.* New York: Simon & Schuster, 1974.

Cross-Country Skiing

Caldwell, John. *New Cross-Country Ski Book.* 4th ed. Brattleboro, Vt.: Greene, 1973.

Gillette, Ned. *Cross-Country Skiing with John Dostal.* Seattle: The Mountaineers, 1979.

Thronton, Pat. *Contemporary Cross-Country Skiing.* Chicago: Chicago Books, 1978.

Heart Disease

American Heart Association Handbook. New York: E. P. Dulton, 1980.

Fisher, Arthur. *The Healthy Heart.* Chicago: Time-Life Books, 1981.

Friedman, Meyer, and Ray H. Rosenman. *Type A Behavior and Your Heart.* Greenwich, Conn.: Fawcett, 1974.

Halhuber, Canula, and Max Halhuber. *Speaking of Heart Attacks.* New York: Consolidated Book Publisher, 1978.

Pollock, Michael, and Donald Schmidt. *Heart Disease and Rehabilitation.* Boston: Houghton Mifflin, 1979.

Solomon, Henry A. *The Exercise Myth.* New York: Harcourt Brace Jovanovich, 1984.

Zohman, Lenore. *The Cardiologist's Guide to Fitness and Health through Excellence.* New York: Simon & Schuster, 1979.

Nutrition and Weight Control

Briggs, George M., and Doris H. Calloway. *Bogert's Nutrition and Physical Fitness.* Philadelphia: Saunders, 1979.

Brody, Jane. *Jane Brody's Nutrition Book.* New York: Norton, 1981.

Clark, Nancy. *Sports Nutrition Guidebook.* Champaign, Ill.: Leisure Press, 1990.

Clarkson, Priscilla, ed. *International Journal of Sport Nutrition.* Champagne, Ill.: Human Kinetics, 1994.

Coleman, Ellen. *Eating for Endurance.* Menlow Park, Calif.: Bull Pub., 1988.

Guthrie, Helen. *Introductory Nutrition.* St. Louis: C. V. Mosby, 1983.

Katch, Frank I., and William D. McArdle. *Nutrition, Weight Control and Exercise.* Boston: Houghton Mifflin, 1977.

Ornish, Dean. *Eat more, Weigh less.* New York: Harper Perennial, 1993.

Whitney, Eleanor N., and Corinne B. Cataldo. *Understanding Normal and Clinical Nutrition.* St. Paul: West, 1983.

Orienteering

Disley, John. *Orienteering.* Harrisburg, Pa.: Stackpole Books, 1969.

Kjellstrom, Bjorn. *Be Expert with Map and Compass, The Orienteering Handbook.* New York: Charles Scribner & Sons, 1976.

Physical Fitness and Health

The ACSM Fitness Book. Champagne, Ill.: Human Kinetics, 1994.

Allsen, Phillip E., Joyce M. Harrison, and Barbara Vance. *Fitness for Life.* 4th ed. Dubuque, Iowa: Wm. C. Brown Communications, Inc., 1989.

Cooper, Kenneth. *Aerobics.* New York: Evans, 1969.

Cooper, Kenneth. *Aerobics Program for Total Well Being.* New York: Evans, 1982.

Corbin, Charles, and Ruth Lindsey. *Concepts of Physical Fitness with Laboratory.* 5th ed. Dubuque, Iowa: Wm. C. Brown Communications, Inc., 1985.

Di Gennaro, Joseph. *The New Physical Fitness: Exercise for Every Body.* Englewood, Colo.: Morton, 1983.

Dintiman, George B., Stephan E. Stone, Jude C. Pennington, and Robert G. Davis. *Discovering Lifetime Fitness.* St. Paul: West, 1984.

Falls, Arnold B., Ann M. Baylor, and Rud K. Dishman. *Essentials of Fitness.* Philadelphia: Saunders, 1980.

Getchell, Bud. *Physical Fitness, A Way of Life.* 3d ed. New York: Wiley, 1983.

Marley, William. *Health and Physical Fitness.* Philadelphia: Saunders, 1982.

Pollock, Michael, Jack H. Wilmore, and Samuel M. Fox. *Exercise in Health and Disease.* Philadelphia: Saunders, 1984.

Rosensweig, S. *Sports Fitness for Women.* New York: Harper & Row, 1982.

Wilmore, Jack. *Sensible Fitness.* Champaign, Ill.: Leisure Press, 1986.

Physiology of Exercise

Brooks, George A., and Thomas D. Fahey. *Exercise Physiology.* New York: John Wiley & Sons, 1984.

Devries, Herbert A. *Physiology of Exercise for Physical Education and Athletics.* 3d ed. Philadelphia: Saunders, 1980.

Fox, E. L. *Sports Physiology.* Philadelphia: Saunders, 1979.

Lamb, David R. *Physiology of Exercise.* New York: Macmillan, 1984.

Shaver, Larry G. *Essentials of Exercise Physiology.* Minneapolis: Burgess, 1981.

Wells, C. L. *Women, Sport and Performance: A Physiological Perspective.* Champaign, Ill.: Human Kinetics, 1985.

Wilmore, Jack H. *Training for Sport and Activity, The Physiological Basis of Conditioning.* 2d ed. Boston: Allyn & Bacon, 1982.

Running

Anderson, Bob. *Stretching.* Bolinas, Calif.: Shelton, 1980.

Costill, David L. *A Scientific Approach to Distance Running.* Los Altos, Calif.: Track and Field News, 1979.

Daniels, Jack, Robert Fitts, and George Sheehan. *Conditioning for Distance Runners.* New York: Wiley, 1978.

Fix, James F. *The Complete Book of Running.* New York: Random House, 1977.

Fix, James F. *Second Book of Running.* New York: Random House, 1980.

Galloway, Jeff. *Galloway's Book on Running.* Bolinas, Calif.: Shelton, 1984.

Glasser, William. *Positive Addiction.* New York: Harper & Row, 1976.

Sheehan, George. *Running and Being.* New York: Simon & Schuster, 1978.

Sheehan, George. *Personal Best.* Emmaus, Pa.: Rodale Press, 1989.

Smith, Nathan J. *Food for Sport.* Palo Alto, Calif.: Bull, 1976.

Ullyot, Joan. *Running Free.* New York: G. P. Putman & Sons, 1982.

Strength and Muscle Development

Darden, Ellington. *The Nautilus Book.* Chicago: Contemporary Books, 1982.

Darden, Ellington. *The Nautilus Woman.* New York: Simon & Schuster, 1983.

Fox, E. L., and D. K. Mathews. *Interval Training, Conditioning for Sport and General Fitness.* Philadelphia: Saunders, 1974.

Jarrell, Steve. *Working Out with Weights.* New York: Anco, 1982.

Kirkley, George W. *Weight Lifting and Weight Training.* New York: Anco, 1981.

Leon, Edie. *Complete Woman Weight Training Guide.* Mountain View, Calif.: Anderson World, 1976.

Moran, Gary, and George McGlynn. *Dynamics of Strength Training.* Dubuque, Iowa.: Wm. C. Brown Communications, Inc., 1990.

O'Shea, J. P. *Scientific Principles and Methods of Strength Fitness.* Reading, Mass.: Addison-Wesley, 1979.

Pearl, Bill, and Gary Moran. *Getting Stronger.* Bolinas, Calif.: Shelter, 1986.

Sobey, Edwin. *Strength Training Book.* Mountain View, Calif.: Anderson World, 1981.

Westcott, Wayne. *Strength Fitness, Physiological Principles and Training Techniques.* Boston: Allyn & Bacon, 1982.

Swimming

Colwin, Cecil. *Swimming into the Twenty First Century.* Champagne, Ill.: Human Kinetics, 1992.

Counsilman, James E. *The Complete Book of Swimming.* New York: Atheneum, 1977.

Elder, Terry, and Kathy Campbell. *Aquatic Fitness Everyone.* Winston-Salem, N.C.: Hunter Textbooks, 1994.

Midtlyng, Joanna. *Swimming.* Philadelphia: Saunders, 1974.

Testing and Evaluation

Golding, Lawrence A., Clayton R. Meyers, and Wayne E. Sinning. *The Y's Way to Physical Fitness*. Rosemont, IL.: National Board of YMCA, 1982.

Guidelines for Exercise Testing and Prescription. 3d edition. The American College of Sports Medicine. Philadelphia, Pa.: Lea and Febiger, 1986.

Pollock, Michael, Jack Wilmore, and Samuel M. Fox. *Health and Fitness through Physical Activity*. Philadelphia, Pa.: Saunders, 1984.

Wilson, Phil, ed. *Adult Fitness and Cardiac Rehabilitation*. Baltimore: University Park Press, 1975.

Index

Heart
  cardiorespiratory endurance and, 99–101
  enlarged (hypertrophy), 116–18, *117,* 119
  increasing strength of, 9
  irregular heartbeats, 102, 119
  maximum oxygen uptake and, 44, 101, 119, 293
  preparing for demands of exercise, 80
  rapid beat during weight lifting, 157–58
  stroke volume, 101, 119
  structure and function of, *100,* 100–101
  training levels for, 284
  work capacity of, 3
  See also Coronary heart disease
Heart attack (MI; myocardial infarction), 26–27, 42
  exercise and, 40
  symptoms of, 25, 27, 114
Heart disease. *See* Coronary heart disease
Heart murmurs, 103
Heart rate, 103–8, 108t, 113
  age and, 284
  anaerobic threshold, 107
  checking, 23, 122
  elevated after exercise, 116
  maximum (HRmax), 104, 283, 293
  measuring, 103, *104*
  METS, 105, 106t
  perceived exertion and, 107–8, 108t
  resting, 104
    cardiorespiratory training and, 118, 118t
  in swimming program, 127
  ten-second rate, 105
Heart rate training effect, 103–5, 119
Heat stroke, 269
Hector, M., 17
Heel raise, *150*
Hemoglobin, 36
Hernia, weight lifting and, 157
Herpes, 323–24
High blood pressure (hypertension), 28, 31t, 32–33, 42
High-density lipoprotein (HDL), 33, 34t, 35, 42, 179
High-low arm stretch, *90*
Hip flexor, *86*
Hollow sprints, 291

Hormones, 161
  anabolic steroids and, 237, 239
  estrogen, 35, 39–40, 282
  growth (somatrophic), 161
  norepinephrine, 245
  testosterone, 161, 237
Hostility, 40
Hot reactors, 38–39
Hot weather, 269–72, 270t
HRmax (maximum heart rate), 104, 283, 293
Hyde, R. T., 3
Hydra-Fitness training equipment, 161
Hyperextension, 81, 91, 98
  of lumbar spine, 11
Hyperplasia, 210
Hypertension (high blood pressure), 28, 31t, 32–33, 42
Hypertrophy
  asymmetrical, 118
  cardiac, 116–18, *117,* 119
  of muscle, 137, 160–61, 283

Ice massage, 267
Individual differences, competitive sports and, 286–87
Injuries
  Achilles tendon problems, 267
  common, 264, 265t
  leg cramps, 266
  shinsplints, 267
  shoe selection and, 268
  sprains, 264–65
  strains, 265
  stress fractures, 267
  tennis elbow, 266
Insulin, 210
Intensity of exercise, 109, 119
  for older persons, 284–85
Intensity of training, 293
  for competition, 287
Interval training for advanced fitness, 289, 290t, 291, 292
Intrauterine device (IUD), 281
Intrinsic motivation, 17, 23
Iron
  female need for, 280–81
  in vegetarian diet, 192
Irregular heartbeats, 102, 119
Ischemia, 158

Pain
  associated with exercise, 2
  of sprains and strains, 264–65
Painter, P., 63
Participation in sports, increase in, 7–8
Pate, R. R., 63
Patience, 22
PC (phosphocreatine), 102, 119, 160
Peak cycle in periodization, 163
Pedersen, N. L., 210
Pelvic inflammatory disease (PID), 324
Perceived exertion, 107–8, 108t, 119
Perceptions
  motivation and, 16
  stress and, 253
Performance levels, age and, 283–84
Performance-related fitness, 8
Periodization, 162–63, 166
Peripheral blood flow, age and, 283
Personality type, 245, 252t, 252–53
Personal self-concept, 22–23
Phosphocreatine (PC), 102, 119, 160
Phospholipids, 174
Physical activity
  coronary heart disease and, 37–38, 39t
  effects of alcohol on, 234
  fat loss and, 216–17
Physical Activity Readiness Questionnaire
    (rPAR-Q), 112, 113t
Physical examinations, 113
Physical fitness
  advanced, 287–92
    interval training, 289, 290t, 291, 292
    long-distance running, 287–89
    other options for, 291–92
    over-distance training, 291, 292
  age and, 282–86
    benefits of exercise, 285
    nutrition, 285–86
    performance levels, 283–84
    types of exercise, 284–85
  components of, 43–44
  flexible programs for, 7
  misconceptions about, 8
  time in training and, 12–13
Physiological trainability, age and, 284
PID (pelvic inflammatory disease), 324
Pinault, S., 210
Plaque, 26, 26, 42
Plyometric loading, 140, 166

PNF (proprioceptive neuromuscular
    facilitation), 81
Polaris training equipment, 161
Pollock, M. L., 66, 68
Polysaccharides, 171
Polyunsaturated fat, 205
Polyunsaturated fats, 174–75
Powell, K. E., 3
Power, strength training and, 136–37
Preeclampsia, 170, 205
Preexercise screening, 111–14, 112t, 113t
  precautions, 113–14
Pregnancy
  exercise during, 279–80
  nutrition and, 170
  preeclampsia and toxemia in, 170, 205
Preparation phase of autogenic
    training, 260
President's Council on Physical Fitness and
    Sports, 8–9
Progressive overload principle, 23
Progressive relaxation exercise, 254,
    255–60, 261
  read-aloud directions for, 257–60
Progressive resistance, 137, 166
Proprioceptive neuromuscular facilitation
    (PNF), 81
Proteins, 177–78, 205
  toxic byproducts of, 183
  in vegetarian diet, 177, 192
Psychoactive drugs. See Drugs,
    psychoactive
PTFE-film fabric, 272
Pulldown, 144
Pull-ups, 130
Pulse
  monitoring, 215–16
  at radial artery, 104
Push-ups, 67, 68t, 69, 76t, 151
Pyramid method of advanced strength
    training, 156

Quadriceps stretch, 84

Race, risk of coronary heart
    disease and, 40
Racquetball sports, 95
Range of motion, 12
  flexibility and, 80–81
  in isometric exercise, 153